Arteriovenous Malformations in Functional Areas of the Brain

edited by

Shokei Yamada, MD, PhD, FACS

Note: The illustration on the cover is modified from Figure 7 in Chapter 1, drawn by Robert Harold Knabenbauer.

To my patients who endured the
hardships of AVM surgery.

To all personnel who maintained the high
standard patient care.

To my family - Rachel, Vivian, Cheryl, and Brian
for their encouragement and support.

Arteriovenous Malformations in Functional Areas of the Brain

edited by

Shokei Yamada, MD, PhD, FACS

Professor of Neurosurgery
Division of Neurosurgery
Loma Linda University School of Medicine
Loma Linda, California

FUTURA

Futura Publishing Company, Inc.
Armonk, NY

Library of Congress Cataloging-in-Publication Data

Arteriovenous malformations in functional areas of the brain / edited by Shokei Yamada.
p. cm.
Includes bibliographical references and index.
ISBN 0-87993-424-7 (alk. paper)
1. Cerebral arteriovenous malformations—Surgery. 2. Cerebral arteriovenous malformations—Pathophysiology. I. Yamada, Shokei.
[DNLM: 1. Cerebral Arteriovenous Malformations—surgery. 2. Cerebral Arteriovenous Malformations—complications. 3. Cerebral Arteriovenous Malformations—physiopathology. WL 355 A787 1999]
RD594.2.A78 1999
617.4′81—dc21
DNLM/DLC
for Library of Congress 98-37766
CIP

Published by
Futura Publishing Company, Inc.
135 Bedford Road
Armonk, NY 10504

LC #: 98-37766
ISBN #: 0-87993-424-7

Printed in the United States of America.
This book is printed on acid-free paper.

Contributors

Issam A. Awad, MD, MSc, FACS
The Nixdoff-German Professor of Neurosurgery
Director of Neurovascular Surgery Program
Department of Neurosurgery
Yale University School of Medicine
New Haven, Connecticut

Nikolay I. Baev, MD, PhD
Post Doctoral Associate in Vascular Biology
Neurovascular Surgery Program
Department of Neurosurgery
Yale University School of Medicine
New Haven, Connecticut

Floyd S. Brauer, MD, FACP
Diplomate of American Board of Anesthesiology
Professor and Former Chairman
Department of Anesthesiology
Loma Linda University School of Medicine
Loma Linda, California

Daniel J. Cole, MD
Professor, Department of Anesthesiology
Director of Neuroanesthesiology and
Director of Anesthesiology Research
Loma Linda University School of Medicine
Loma Linda, California

Lloyd Dayes, MD, PhD, FACS
Professor, Division of Neurosurgery
Loma Linda University School of Medicine
Loma Linda, California

Jacob I. Fabrikant, MD, PhD
Late Professor
University of California, Berkeley
Donner Pavilion and Donner Laboratory and
Lawrence Berkeley Laboratory
Berkeley, California;
Professor, Department of Radiology
University of California, San Francisco
San Francisco, California

John C. Flickinger, MD
Professor, Department of Radiation Oncology
University of Pittsburgh School of Medicine
Pittsburgh, Pennsylvania

Christopher Gallen, MD, PhD
Vice President, Premier Research Worldwide
Philadelphia, Pennsylvania

John P. Girvin, MD, PhD, FRCS(C)
Professor and Chairman
Department of Clinical Neurological Sciences
Western University
London, Ontario, Canada

Shwan Kim, MD
Resident, Department of Radiology
Montefiore Medical Center
Bronx, New York

David S. Knierim, MD, FACS
Associate Professor
Division of Neurosurgery
Director of Pediatric Neurosurgery
Loma Linda University School of Medicine
Loma Linda, California

Douglas Kondziolka, MD, MSc, FRCS(C)
Professor
Departments of Neurological Surgery
and Radiation Oncology
University of Pittsburgh Medical Center
Pittsburgh, Pennsylvania

Richard P. Levy, MD, PhD
Associate Professor
Department of Radiation Medicine
Loma Linda University School of Medicine
Loma Linda, California;
Department of Neurosurgery
School of Medicine
Stanford University
Stanford, California

Boleslaw Liwinicz MD, PhD
Professor, Department of Pathology
Chief, Section of Neuropathology
Loma Linda University School of Medicine
Loma Linda, California

Eng H. Lo, PhD
Associate Professor
Harvard Medical School
Head
Neuroprotection Research Laboratory
Department of Neurology and Radiology
Massachusetts General Hospital
Boston, Massachusetts

Russell R. Lonser, MD
Resident, Department of Neurosurgery
University of Utah Medical Center
Salt Lake City, Utah;
Fellow of Surgical Neurology Branch
National Institute of Neurological Diseases and Stroke
National Institute of Health
Bethesda, Maryland

L. Dade Lunsford, MD, FACS
Professor and Chairman
Department of Neurological Surgery
University of Pittsburgh Medical Center
Pittsburgh, Pennsylvania

George Mandybur, MD
Assistant Professor
Department of Neurological Surgery
University of Mississippi Medical Center
Jackson, Mississippi

Michael P. Marks, MD
Chief of Interventional Radiology
Director of Neuroradiology and Stanford Stroke Center;
Associate Professor
Department of Radiology
Stanford University School of Medicine
Stanford, California

Ajay Niranjan, MCh
Visiting Fellow
Center for Image Guided Neurosurgery
Department of Neurological Surgery
University of Pittsburgh
Pittsburgh, Pennsylvania;
Consultant Neurosurgeon
Indraprastha Apollo Hospital
New Delhi, India

Glenn Rouse, MD
Associate Professor
Department of Radiology
Director of Inpatient Ultrasonography
Loma Linda University School of Medicine
Loma Linda, California

James B. Slater, PhD
Assistant Professor
Department of Radiology
Director of Radiopharmaceutical Laboratory
Loma Linda University School of Medicine
Loma Linda, California

Jerry D. Slater, MD
Associate Professor
Department of Radiation Medicine
Loma Linda University School of Medicine
Loma Linda, California

Robert F. Spetzler, MD, FACS
Director, Barrow Neurological Institute
Professor, Neurological Surgery
University of Arizona
Phoenix, Arizona

Gary K. Steinberg, MD, PhD, FACS
Professor and Chairman
Department of Neurosurgery
Stanford University Medical Center
Stanford, California

Sigmund Teichman, MD
Associate Professor
Department of Medicine
Chief, Division of Nephrology
Loma Linda University School of Medicine
Loma Linda, California

Thomas M. Wascher, MD
The Neuroscience Group of Northeast Wisconsin
Appleton, Wisconsin

Daniel Won, MD
Assistant Professor
Division of Pediatric Neurosurgery
Loma Linda University School of Medicine
Loma Linda, California

John H. Wong, MD, MSc, FRCS(C)
Instructor of Neurosurgery
Fellow, Neurovascular Surgery Program
Department of Neurosurgery
Yale University School of Medicine
New Haven, Connecticut

Brian S. Yamada, BA
Senior Student
Wake Forest University School of Medicine
Winston-Salem, North Carolina

Shokei Yamada, MD, PhD, FACS
Professor of Neurosurgery
and Former Chairman
Division of Neurosurgery
Loma Linda University School of Medicine
Loma Linda, California

Shoko M. Yamada, MD, PhD
Attending Staff
Department of Neurosurgery
Nippon Medical School
Tokyo, Japan

Foreword

The surgery of arteriovenous malformations remains one of the most challenging aspects of neurosurgery. The modern era of the surgery of arteriovenous malformations may be said to have begun with the monograph by Olivecrona, which gathered many observations about their structure and natural history into an easily accessible source. Since that time, a number of neurosurgeons have made notable contributions to understanding the pathophysiology of arteriovenous malformations and have described classification systems to be used for planning treatment and have developed surgical techniques for their removal. Therefore, this is an opportune time to again gather together these observations. Dr. Yamada is uniquely qualified to bring this material together into a new monograph because of his extensive surgical experience with complex arteriovenous malformations which led him to develop a meticulous analysis of the vascular anatomy of arteriovenous malformations and of the surgical steps that are necessary to expose that anatomy for a successful excision of the malformation. A careful study of his methods will be repaid by improved surgical outcomes.

In addition to the detailed exposition of the microsurgical techniques of removal of arteriovenous malformations, this monograph presents the work of an outstanding group of experts who join Dr. Yamada in presenting up-to-date methods of neuroanesthesia, of perioperative care, of techniques for resection of malformations in eloquent areas, and of the use of embolization and radiosurgery as adjunctive methods of treatment. This monograph will be an important reference for all physicians who care for patients with cerebral arteriovenous malformations.

Robert G. Grossman, MD, FACS
Professor and Chairman
Department of Neurological Surgery
Baylor University College of Medicine
Houston, Texas

Foreword

President George Bush declared the 1990s as the "Decade of the Brain." The book, *Arteriovenous Malformations in Functional Areas of the Brain,* is a timely contribution toward the fulfillment of this proclamation. It is a difficult task to make introductory remarks on a book that speaks for itself. Certainly, the scope of the subject and the history of surgical intervention makes one realize the value of this book. Dr. Yamada's years of meticulous research and clinical experience have culminated in the perfection of his AVM surgery. Throughout the book, his originality, accuracy, and persistence are evident. Unquestionably, Dr. Yamada is one of three neurosurgeons who have attained the highest level of AVM surgery.

Despite the successful treatment of AVMs in silent areas, those in functional areas were barely within the scope of neurosurgical treatment. For the first time, this book addresses the challenges of this extremely difficult problem and then delineates the specific treatments with their acceptable risks. Dr. Yamada has skillfully structured the book to present the three modes of treatment (microsurgery, intravascular intervention, and radiosurgery) individually or in conjunction with each other.

The expertise of each contributing author brings current concepts and methods to forefront. Radiosurgery treatment is convincingly appropriate for elimination of small lesions in the basal ganglia, internal capsule, and thalamus; however, the combined approach of either two or three modes can be an alternative for large AVMs in or near functional areas. Surgical treatment of cavernous hemangiomas is now practical as described with extreme precision. The basic science in hemodynamics theory, the amazing advances in the field of medical technology, and angiogenesis of AVMs are components not only of current treatment, but also for future management of AVMs in functional areas.

The innovative surgical procedure that Dr. Yamada devised is the main focus of the microsurgical treatment. It is based on the understanding of the hemodynamics of AVMs, as well as the meticulous planning and careful execution of the surgical procedure. The patients and their quality of life are evidence of the success and effectiveness of his surgery. The vital element in using his technique lies in the experience, knowledge, and skill of the neurosurgeon. This book will become a standard for those who will study and apply the specific guidelines for the surgery for AVMs in the functional areas of the brain.

George M. Austin, MD, FACS
Director,
Brain Aneurysm Research Institute
Attending Neurosurgeon at
Cottage Hospital and St. Francis Hospital
Santa Barbara, California

Preface

This book is the culmination of my desire to promote the multidisciplinary treatment of arteriovenous malformations (AVMs) of the brain. When Professor Olivecrona published his monogram in 1957, the en bloc resection technique for this vascular disorder was established. However, the nature of AVMs and the brain precluded his surgical technique from being used for direct intervention to AVMs located in functional areas.

My interest was keenly engaged by the plight of 70% of the patients during my early practice who suffered neurological deficits or focal seizures closely related to an AVM in the functional areas. I directed my research toward developing systematic changes in the surgical technique for these AVMs while decreasing the patient mortality and morbidity to significantly less than that found in the natural history of this disorder. Each chapter in this book is dedicated to the treatment of these AVMs and the related anatomy and physiology, along with the complexity of the problems associated with the treatment of this condition.

Introduced in this book is the surgical technique that I developed for AVMs in the functional areas. It is based on the hemodynamic anatomy of AVMs relative to the brain, as well as a thorough comprehension of specific anesthesia techniques.

Each contributing author has individual expertise in the treatment of functional area AVMs and related pathophysiology. I am most grateful for the considerable effort made by each author.

I am particularly indebted to three outstanding neurosurgeons for their inspiration and advice during my training and early neurosurgical practice: Professor E. Harry Botterell (University of Toronto), who introduced hypothermia and hypotension for safe surgery of aneurysms and AVMs; Professor Sean F. Mullan (University of Chicago), who developed ingenious surgical techniques and wire embolization of aneurysms and AVMs; and Professor George M. Austin (University of Oregon Medical School and Loma Linda University School of Medicine), who developed an intravenous method of ^{133}xenon regional blood flow studies, correlated regional cerebral blood flow in patients with transient ischemic attacks, and extracranial-intracranial anastomosis.

I acknowledge the contributions of many neurosurgeons, neuroradiologists, radiosurgeons, neuroanesthesiologists, and neuropathologists who have influenced the various aspects in the field of AVM surgery. The following pioneers are recognized: Professors Charles Drake, Ladislau Steiner, Leonard Malis, Charles Wilson, Bennett Stein, Thoralf Sundt, Gazi Yaşarigil, Bernard Pertuiset, Lindsay Symon, Mario Brock, Jacques Moret, P. Lasjaunius, Grant Hieshima, Fernando Veñuela, Jacob Fabrikant, Roberto Heros, Robert Spetzler, and John Tew. To the numerous colleagues who assisted me in my research, I give my heartfelt gratitude: especially to Dr. Floyd Brauer for his exceptionally skillful anesthesia administrated to my patients, based on his thorough understanding of my surgical technique and controlled hypotension, and Dr. Myron Rosenthal for his continuous involvement in my research and his advice of the highest scientific quality. I wish to recognize the guidance of the late Joseph P. Evans (University of Chicago) whose instruction in the study and management of increased intracranial pressure was crucial, and Professor William Longheed for demonstrating innovative clinical and research work in cerebrovascular disorders.

I am thankful to Professor Robert Grossman for promoting my principle of AVM surgery in functional areas, and to Professors John Girvin, Steven Giannotta, Neil Martin, Phanor Perot, Julian Youmans, Duke Samson, L. N. Hopkins, Grant Gauger, Terry Joyner, Christopher Ogilvy, Issam Awad, Ronald Tasker, Fred Gentili, Charles Neblett, Laligam Sekhar, Magid Samii, Werner Usbeck, Helmut Pothe, Alice Felten, Keiji Sano, Norio Nakamura, Akira Hakuba, Hitoshi Fukui, Hiroshi Abe, Takanori Fukushima, and Kenichiro Sugita for their understanding and support.

I am appreciative of the cooperation and assistance of the staff of Loma Linda University School of Medicine and Medical Center, among whom the following were particularly helpful: Professors Lyn Behrens, David Hinshaw, Bruce Branson, Leonard Bailey, and Brian Bull (Administration); Professors Robert Knighton, David Knierim, Lloyd Dayes (Department of Neurosurgery); Drs. Delmar Sanders, David Zinke, William Hill, Stephen Ritland, Ronald Jutzy, Donald Soloniuk, Thomas Purtzer, Maged Abu-Assal (former neurosurgery residents); David Hinshaw Jr., Joseph Thompson, Anton Hasso (Department of Neuroradiology); Betty Behrends, Marie Hand, Patty Caldwell, Elaine Soloniuk, Thelma Chaffe, Betty Van Lant (operating room nurses); Paula Fedun (ward nurse coordinator); and William Hayward, Gary Haugen, and Hao Nguyen (laboratory associates).

I wish to thank Mr. Steven Korn, Chairman of the Board of Futura Publishing Company, for encouraging me by continually emphasizing the value of this book, and Ms. Linda Shaw for the editing of this manuscript. I acknowledge the guidance of Ms. Joanne Needham, AANS Publication Office, as editorial consultant, Mrs. Ellen Trammell for editing research papers, and Mr. Robert Knabenbauer for his fine art work for the illustrations. And finally, I thank my family for their patience and support in every phase of this endeavor, and my brother, Shotetsu Yamada, MD, and Mr. and Mrs. Earl Childers for encouragement and financial support in promoting my research.

Shokei Yamada, MD, PhD, FACS

Introduction

An arteriovenous malformation (AVM) is defined as a cluster of entangled anomalous vessels in which arteries are directly connected to veins, without intervening capillaries. In the brain, the circulation through an AVM is extremely complex, as will be explained in the chapters that follow. Nevertheless, the basic hemodynamic theory is that afferent vessels (arterial branches) provide arterial blood supply to the anomalous AVM core, from which efferent vessels (draining veins) direct blood flow to the venous system of the brain.

In treating AVMs, a major source of concern is preservation of the functional areas of the brain. These areas are the cerebral regions whose own specific functions cannot be replaced (compensated for) by any other region of the brain (Penfield). These regions include the motor and sensory cortices, the speech (Wernicke's and Broca's) areas, the visual area, and the dominant posterior parietal (visual cognitive function) area. Also to be considered as part of the functional areas to be preserved are the neuronal processes originating from these areas.

In this book, the phrase "eloquent areas" is not used as a synonym for the functional areas, because the frontal lobes, temporal lobes, posterior parietal lobe, and limbic lobes, which perform delicate and subtle functions (e.g., emotional control or various cognitive functions), can be compensated for, at least partially, by areas on the opposite brain hemisphere or by other parts of the brain. These areas are termed "silent areas."

Surgery for AVMs in functional areas of the brain requires techniques, understandings, and commitments that may be beyond those associated with general microneurosurgery. There is much to learn, even for neurosurgeons experienced in general AVM surgery, because successful surgical procedures for AVMs in functional areas differ significantly from those procedures used for AVMs in silent areas. A further complexity of AVM surgery in functional areas is that the techniques required are location-specific.

At first glance, one might believe that describing AVM surgery in functional areas is a straightforward task. Certainly, the basic principles of AVM surgery are similar to those for other neurosurgical procedures. It is intuitively obvious, for example, that surgeons should seek to avoid removal of essential brain tissue and to preserve microcirculation, especially in functional brain areas. Nevertheless, the authors are often asked such basic questions as:

1) Must the feeding arteries be obliterated while removing AVMs in functional areas?

2) Is it safe to approach an AVM through the sulcus, passing the draining vein?

3) Why is a staged operation necessary?

4) Does a venous approach result in a large excavation after AVM resection, similar to en bloc resection?

5) Is the hemodynamic structure of AVMs too complex to apply simplified principles of surgical techniques?

The goals of this book are to answer such questions and to explain certain basic concepts, principles, and procedures that are necessary to accomplish surgical extirpation of AVMs in functional areas without unacceptable morbidity and/or mortality. A clear and correct description of concepts, principles, and procedures of AVM surgery will motivate and enable neurosurgeons to achieve the level of competence required for AVM surgery in functional areas.

There are important issues that must be considered when decisions are made regarding which among the three modes of treatment of AVMs is to be selected. These treatment modes are: (1) surgical intervention; (2) embolization; and (3) radiosurgery. Each of these treatments is described, together with guidelines for considering its advantages and disadvantages. This book includes other aspects of AVM treatment considered essential by the editor, including anesthesia, cerebral blood flow, and basic science related to the surgery. Surgical approaches to cavernous hemangiomas, now accessible in the brain stem, are highlighted separately in this book. It is this author's hope that neurosurgeons will be stimulated *to understand why different approaches to AVMs in functional areas are necessary. This understanding is especially important in cases where surgery is required in subcortical locations, which is the most common situation.*

Shokei Yamada, MD, PhD, FACS

Contents

Chapter 1

Surgical Approach to Arteriovenous Malformations in Functional Areas of the Brain

Shokei Yamada, MD, PhD

Introduction

The fascinating history of recognizing arteriovenous malformations (AVMs) as a pathological entity dates back several centuries.[18,78,130] This chapter focuses on the key issues of surgical management of AVMs in functional areas: (1) how to delineate signs and symptoms, and diagnostic studies, (2) how to determine prognosis, (3) the indications for various modes of treatment, and (4) surgical treatment mode and results.

In recent years, vascular microneurosurgical techniques have become markedly improved.[24,35,56,65,100–102,104,115,119] As a result, there is now a potentially favorable risk:benefit ratio for surgery in patients with neurological symptoms associated with AVMs in functional areas. This group of patients includes those presenting not only with significant intracerebral hemorrhage (ICH), but also those with headaches, seizures, transient neurological deficits (similar to transient ischemic attacks [TIAs], and subtle symptomatology. Because of patients' awareness of the previous extreme risk for surgical resection, the surgeon must be confident in presenting the surgical options now available, along with the improved risk: benefit factor.

The fact that AVM surgery has become safer, even when performed in functional areas, is a major step forward in neurological surgery. Successful AVM surgery has relieved the suffering of many patients who have experienced the signs and symptoms associated with strokes or transient neurological deficits, seizures, severe paroxysmal throbbing headaches, mental deterioration, and psychiatric behavior. Symptomatology in patients with AVMs in functional areas is usually more serious and more frequent than that noted with AVMs in patients in silent areas. AVM surgery in functional areas has relieved the fear associated with the awareness of possible AVM ruptures, or the inexplicable fear associated with other symptoms, particularly with paroxysmal pulsatile headaches.

AVM Hemodynamics

There are two types of AVMs: compact and diffuse (dispersed).[119,130] Compact AVMs consist primarily of entangled anomalous venous loops that form a core or nidus. The AVM vessels are tightly packed with only microscopic islands of nonfunctional brain tissue found sparsely between the loops (Figures 1A and B). The venous loops of these AVMs are connected to shunting arterioles, which are approximately 50–250 μm in diameter, as well as to communicating venules of similar size. These loops are also connected to one or more draining veins. The shunting arterioles are terminal branches of feeding arteries and can only be identified individually under the microscope. Feeding arteries are much larger (0.5–2.5 mm) than the shunting arterioles and are angiographically demonstrable. They send many branches to the AVM, as well as to the normal cerebrovascular bed; therefore, clipping these arteries can result in transient or permanent ischemia. Furthermore, since the feeding arteries are usually located beneath the cortex, their exposure requires brain tis-

From Yamada S (ed): *Arteriovenous Malformations in Functional Areas of the Brain.* © Futura Publishing Co, Inc, Armonk, NY, 1999.

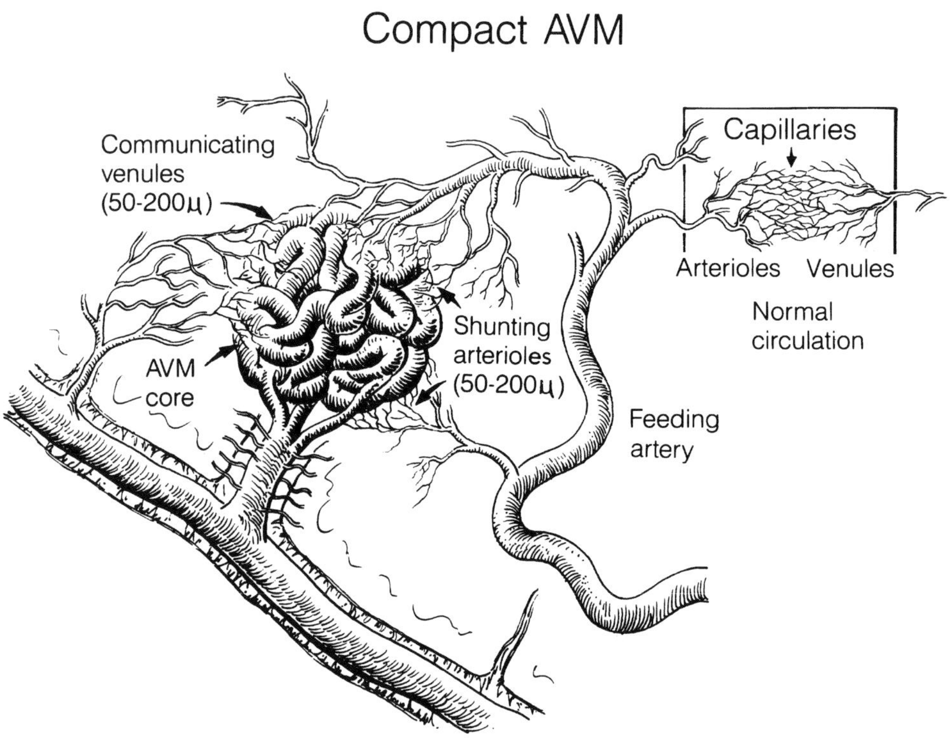

Figure 1A. A schematic drawing of a one-compartment AVM, representing the core, shunting arterioles, communicating venules, and a draining vein connected to a dilated cortical vein. The branches of the feeding artery terminate to the shunting arterioles as well as to the cerebral capillaries. *Continued*

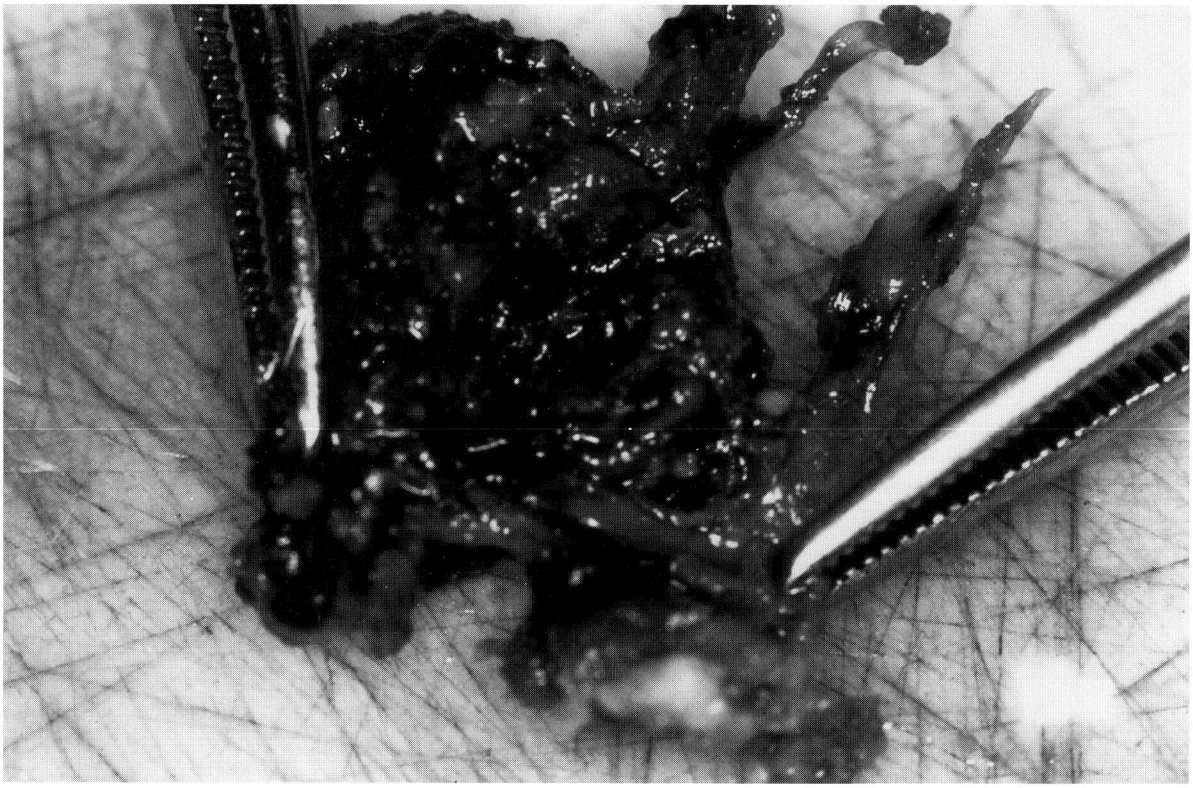

Figure 1B. A specimen of a compact AVM removed by the author's technique. No brain tissue is seen grossly on the surface of the core loops. Only microscopic islands of glial tissue were found between the loops by histological studies.

sue removal; however, the authors advocate that this type of AVM can be resected with few or no neurological deficits by using their special technique.

In diffuse AVMs, anomalous vessels are dispersed between normal brain tissue[119,130] (Figures 2A and B). These AVMs are frequently found in the basal ganglia and thalamus, and cannot be totally removed without disturbing brain function.

Hemodynamic Anatomy

An AVM is a cluster of entangled vessels in which arteries are directly connected to veins, without interposing capillaries. After circulating through the venous loops of the AVM core, arterial blood flows into collecting veins and then into the major draining vein. A compact AVM consists of four parts: (1) core, (2) arterial feeders (afferent system), (3) draining vein (efferent system), and (4) communicating venous system.[115,119] An AVM smaller than 3 cm in diameter usually has one compartment, with one or two feeding arteries and one or two draining veins. The following is a description of the one-compartment AVM.

AVM Core

The core of the AVM consists of dilated anomalous veins[115,119] (occasional transitional vessels, veins resembling arteries)[3,18,19,66,67] that are 0.5–3.0 mm in diameter (0.25 mm in some AVMs, particularly in children) during ordinary pulsation.[115,119] Blood flow in the venous loops is complex: slow flow before joining faster flow through longer loops that have numerous feeders, and extremely fast flow from the type 1 final feeding artery into one of the venous loops that are located near the junction to a draining vein. Core vessels dilate passively, secondary to increases in arterial core pressure and blood flow (due to lack of autoregulation) or to the relative congestion of venous flow. Venous loops are interconnected by small venules (<50 μm), and are identifiable only by endoscopic magnification. Blood flow through these vessels is extremely complex.

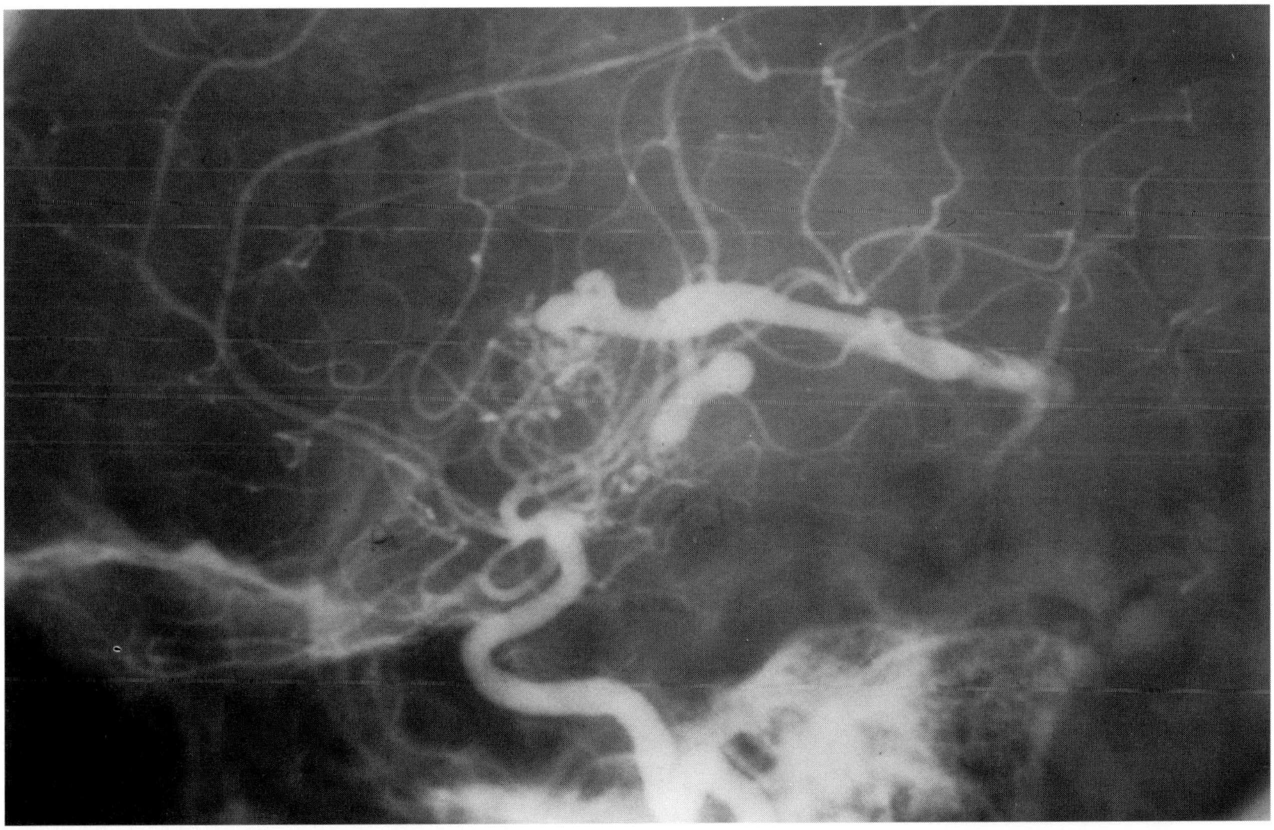

Figure 2A. A lateral angiogram **(A)** and an AP angiogram **(B)** of a diffuse AVM located in the capsulocaudatothalamic area showing brain tissue between abnormal arteriovenous loops. The AVM vessels were approached stereotactically, cauterized, and subtotally eliminated. Postoperatively, the patient was free from the transient neurological deficits experienced frequently before surgery. *Continued*

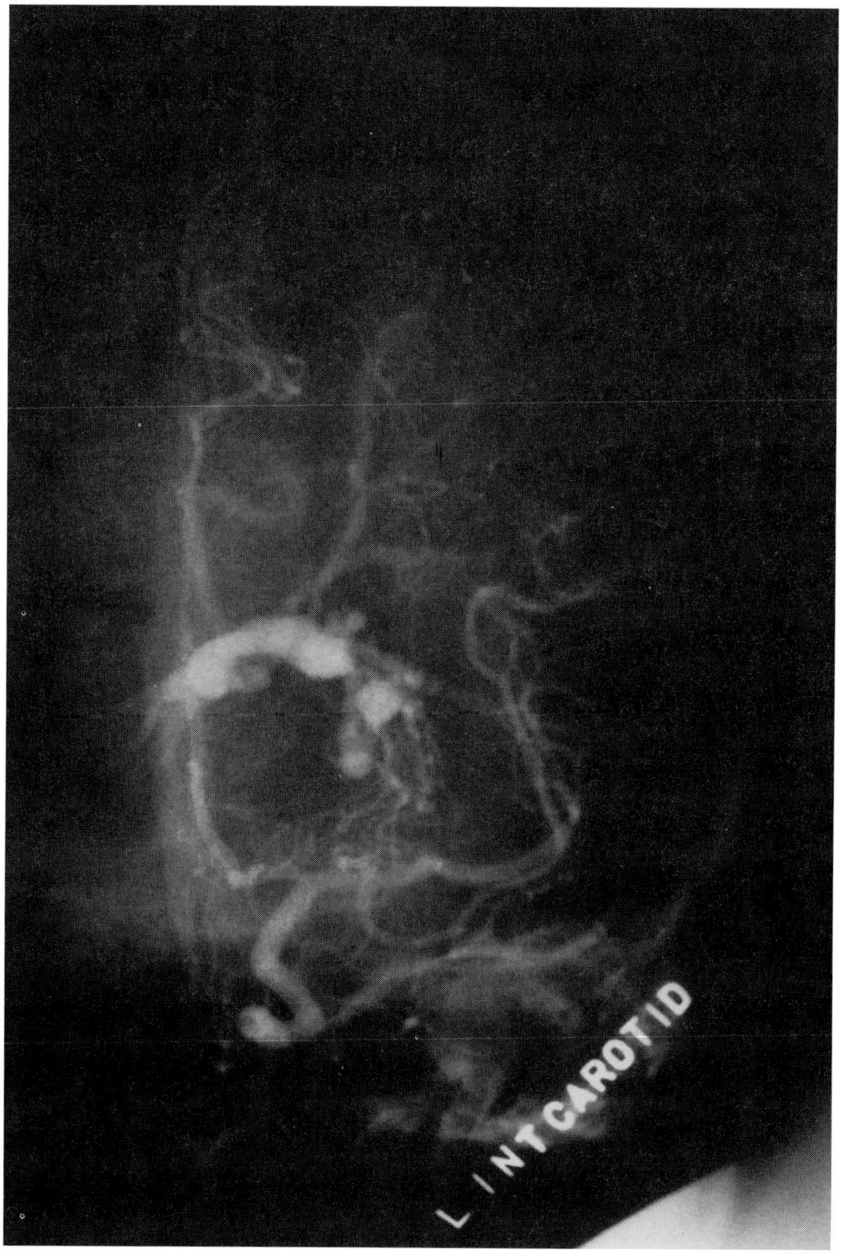

Figure 2B. AP view of a diffuse AVM located in the capsulocaudatothalamic area showing brain tissue between abnormal arteriovenous loops.

Arterial Feeders

The blood supply to the AVM core occurs mainly through multiple arterioles 50–200 μm in diameter, sometimes as large as 250 μm in diameter. These shunting arterioles are directly connected to venous loops of the core as terminal branches of the feeding arteries.[115,119] Angiographically demonstrable arteries that transfer arterial blood into the AVM core are customarily called "feeding arteries." There are three types of feeding arteries: (1) circumferential[119] (transitional),[130] (2) final[78,119] (terminal),[130] and (3) penetrating.[119,130]

Circumferential Feeding Artery: The circumferential (transitional) feeding artery surrounds the AVM core. It branches to small arteries and arterioles, many of which are connected to the AVM core venous loops and others which are connected to the capillaries of the brain (Figure 3).

A significant amount of arterial blood is diverted to the AVM from the feeding arteries; for example, regional cerebral blood flow in the area adjacent to the AVM is about 81% of normal in active AVM patients.[128] The cerebrovascular circulation must be autoregulated because blood flow into an AVM of 4–5 cm in diameter is about 800 mL per minute, or equal to the blood flow into the entire brain in the normal individual.[128]

Shunting arterioles have muscular layers capable of constriction. Therefore, shunting arterioles constrict and reduce blood flow to the AVM core when blood pressure is lowered below 60 mm Hg.[85,89,115,119]

Final Feeding Arteries: The final (terminal) feeding arteries have no branches for a certain distance, as described below, before they join the venous loops. These feeding arteries can be grouped into two types. Type 1 final feeding arteries are 0.5–2.0 cm long and 1.0–2.5 mm in diameter. They connect directly to one of the AVM loops, without tapering peripherally. Naturally, no shunting arterioles arise from a type 1 final feeding artery (Figures 4A and B). The wall of this artery is always hypotrophic, with a thin muscular layer, contrary to the angiographic appearance of

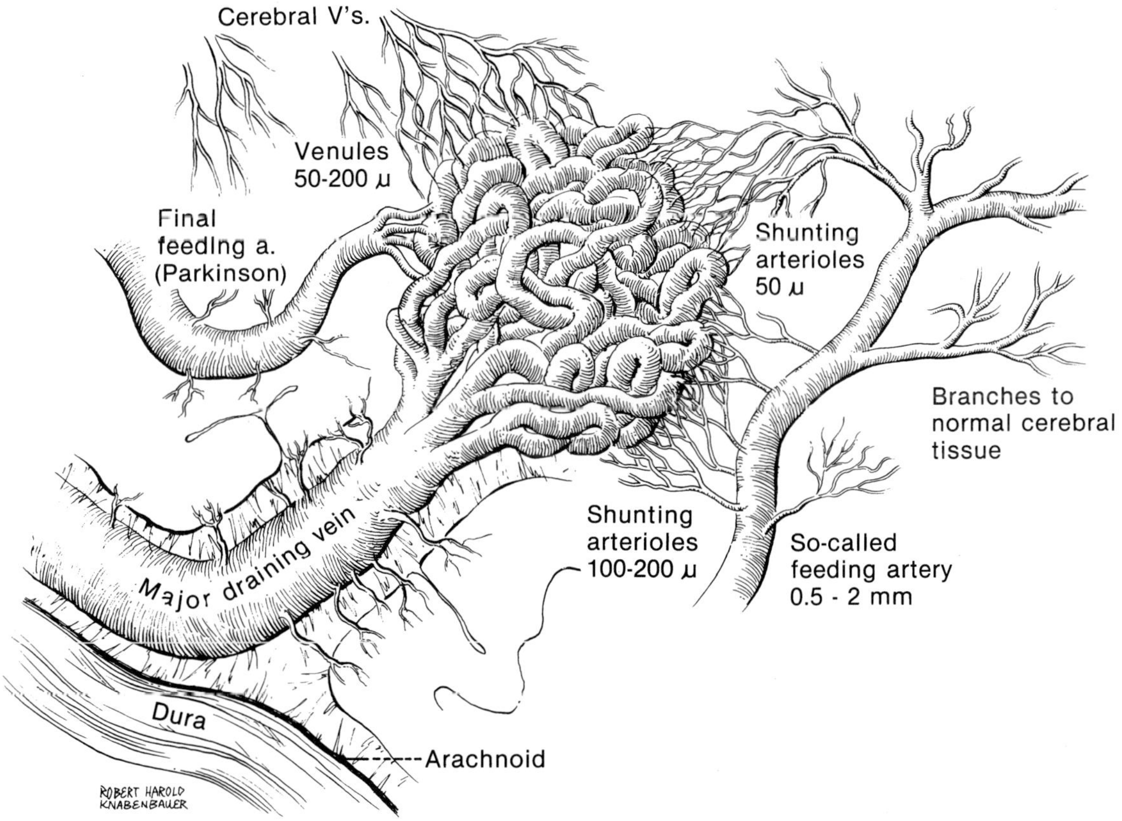

Figure 3. A compact AVM with a circumferential feeding artery and a type 2 final feeding artery that has no branches for a short distance before connecting to the core. Both feeding arteries send shunting arterioles that connect directly to the AVM loops. Venules of 50–200 μm connect the core vessels to the surrounding cerebral veins. Figure used with permission of the Journal of Neurosurgery.[119]

a seemingly hypertrophic artery. Type 2 final feeding arteries are smaller (200–300 μm) and shorter (1–3 mm) than type 1 arteries. Type 2 arteries often branch to shunting arterioles (Figure 3).

Descriptions of arteriovenous fistulae[6,7,37,73,130] are not well defined. Basically, angiographically demonstrable connections between an artery and the core vessels are called fistulae. These can represent either type 1 or type 2 final feeding arteries. However, what appears to be a type 1 final feeding artery is often found to further branch to type 2 final feeding arteries or shunting arterioles (Figure 5).

Type 2 feeding arteries were described by Parkinson[78] before the development of microneurosurgery. These final feeding arteries are difficult to recognize individually at their junctions to the core vessels on angiography because these (approximately 400 μm-sized) vessels in and around the AVM core are superimposed by the core vessels.

It is possible for the naked human eye to perceive cortical vessels as small as 50 μm in diameter with adequate illumination. In order to cauterize 50–200 μm-sized vessels, however, the surgeon must hold the vessel with two tips of the bipolar coagulator, separately touching the opposite sides of the vessel (see the section on surgical techniques). Without microscopic magnification, the tips of the forceps tend to touch each other, causing a short circuit. This short circuit makes coagulation ineffective or causes the vessel to rupture before coagulation occurs. Recently, the authors found, using the scanning electron microscope, numerous 20–25 μm (diameter) communicating venules connected to and between the core vessels.[57]

Penetrating Feeding Artery: The penetrating feeding artery[119,130] passes through the middle of the AVM, sending branches (shunting arterioles) to the

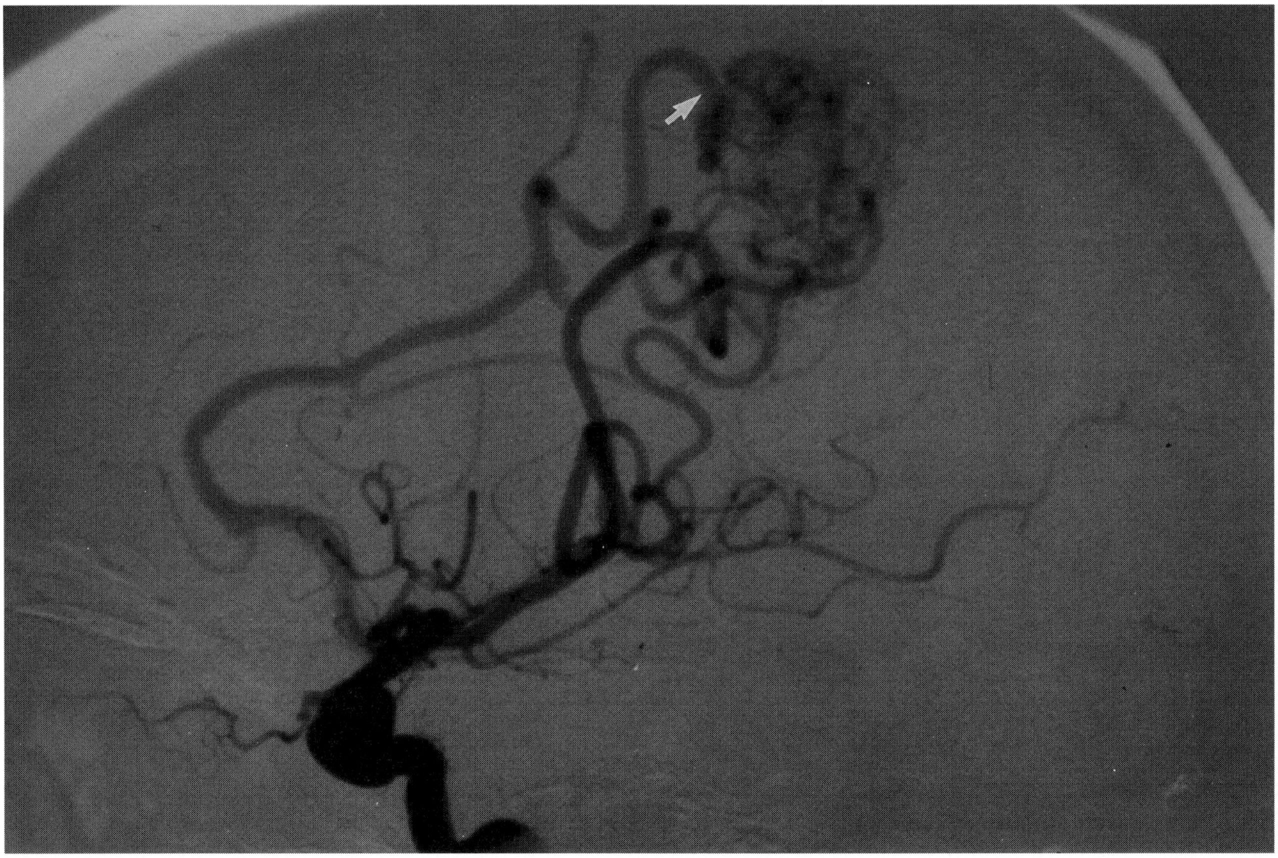

Figure 4A. A type 1 final feeding artery 1.5 mm in diameter originates from one of two large branches of the anterior cerebral artery, as indicated by the arrow (see illustrative case 2). The arrow indicates no branches to the brain peripheral to this point. Other feeding arteries with large diameters were found to be circumferential feeding arteries and terminated as shunting arterioles or type 2 final feeding arteries. The terminal segment (0.5 cm) of type 1 feeding artery (distal to the arrow) was removed and was proved histologically hypotrophic (see illustrative case 2). Figure used with permission of Neurological Research. *Continued*

AVM core. An AVM with this type of artery can be found in any part of the brain; however, it is readily recognizable in the territory of the posterior cerebral artery and its branches (Figures 6A and B). Because the AVM core is formed around this feeding artery (360_0 circumferential to the artery), embolization is usually effective, although homonymous hemianopia must be anticipated as a complication.[22] Embolization can result in motor or sensory dysfunction if the penetrating artery is located in the sensorimotor area.

Draining Venous System

After circulating through the AVM core, arterial blood flows into several collecting veins. These veins are greater in diameter than the core venous loops (see Figure 3). Most often, the collecting veins run parallel to each other, until they converge to connect to the major draining vein. Shunting arterioles and communicating venules are connected to each of the collecting veins. The major draining veins always travel in the sulcus and are surrounded by the sulcal cortex.[115,119] Many venules of 200–300 μm in diameter connect the draining vein and surrounding cortical veins. The external end of the major draining vein is connected to large cortical veins of the hemispheric surface, either on the convexity, lateral, or superior aspect. Arterial blood in these veins eventually pours into venous sinuses. Occasionally, the draining vein may be directly connected to the sinus.

Communicating Venous System

Communicating Venules: Communicating venules connect AVM venous loops or collecting veins with surrounding cerebral veins and venules (see Figure 3).[119] The venules of 50–200 μm in diameter can be perceived under the microscope. However, venules as small as 20 μm have been identified by using the endoscope,[124] as well as the scanning electron microscope.[57] These communicating venules are usually

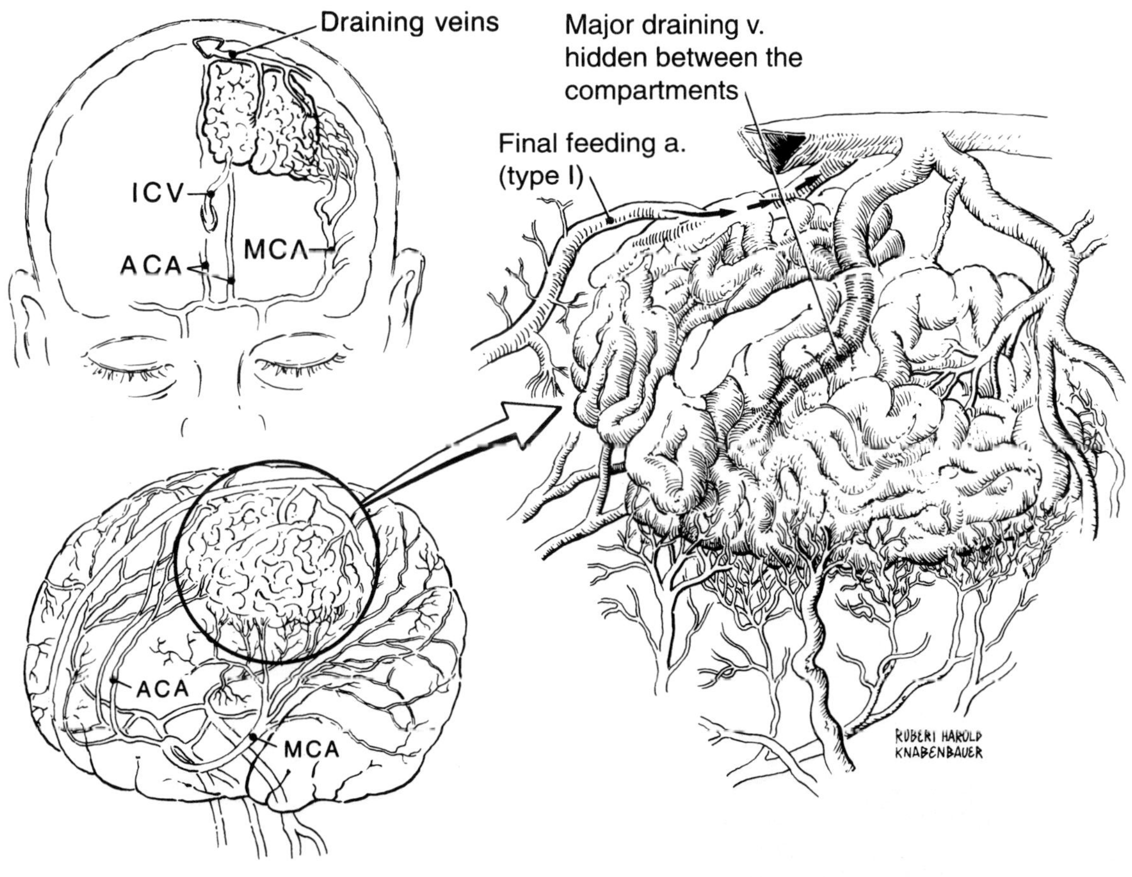

Figure 4B. A three-compartment AVM (posterior compartment omitted). Type 1 and type 2 final feeding arteries correspond to those seen in the angiogram in **A.** Major draining veins were first seen originating from the lateral compartment, second from the lateral aspect of the medial compartment (refer to text), and third from the medial aspect of the medial compartment. The draining vein from the lateral compartment was connected to the vein of Trolard and several other cortical veins.

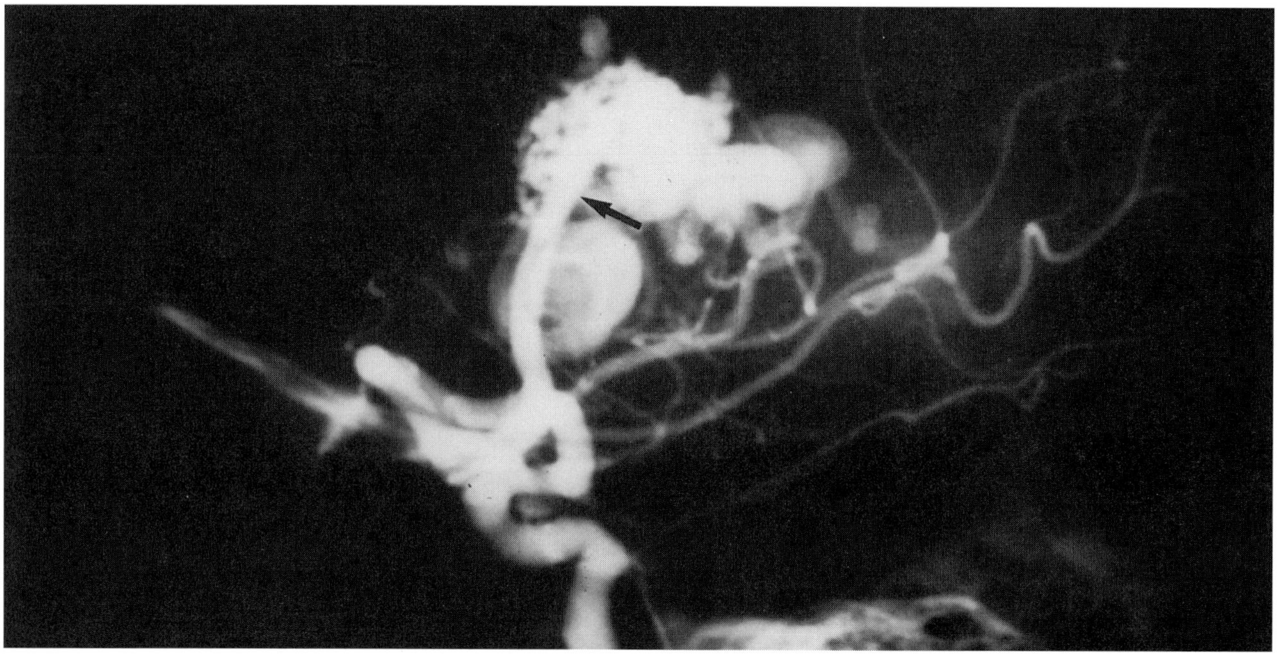

Figure 5. A sensorimotor area AVM angiogram. A feeding artery with a large diameter had several small branches that terminated to arterioles. This large artery (arrow) is sometimes called a fistula, which is a misnomer. An aneurysmal dilation of an AVM loop is superimposed on the artery in the lateral view and should not be mistaken for an arterial aneurysm.

equal to or greater in number than the shunting arterioles. The communicating venules are the free communication system of the AVM core. They likely function as a buffer to counteract (reduce or normalize) excessive blood flow and blood pressure in the AVM core.

Juxtanidal Veins: Juxtanidal veins,[119] which originate from the AVM core and detour around it, are connected to other parts of the core or to smaller cortical veins or venules (Figure 7). The juxtanidal veins (approximately 300 μm in diameter) are slightly smaller than the venous loops of the AVM core. The juxtanidal veins are often spiral shaped[41] and have been described as corkscrew-shaped feeding arteries;[24] however, from the author's experience, spiral vessels are usually found to be veins.

Compartments of AVMs

The concept of AVM compartments originated from segmental embolization of the AVM.[22,24,46,114] In 1987, Yasargil[130] drew schematic models of AVM compartments according to combinations of feeding arteries and draining veins. Yamada[115,119] and associates clearly demonstrated AVM compartments by angiography, which divided the AVM by feeding artery distribution (1990), and then additionally by draining vein pattern.[118]

AVMs are not compartmentalized in an anatomical manner, such as are the lobes of a lung. Rather, AVM compartments are hemodynamic in nature. Identification of AVM compartments provides advantages to any mode of treatment. Microsurgical elimination, embolization, or radiosurgical obliteration of each compartment can then be done effectively in steps until the entire AVM is eliminated.

Each compartment has its own feeding arteries and draining veins.[79,89,119,130] Venous loops of each compartment are also connected to their individual shunting arterioles and communicating venules. Large AVMs in the sensorimotor area are usually supplied by the middle cerebral artery branches for the lateral compartment, by the anterior cerebral artery branches for the medial compartment, and by the posterior cerebral arteries for the posterior compartment.

Feeding arteries to AVMs are not limited to those branching from these large cerebral arteries. In fact, the lenticulostriate, Heubner's, and the anterior and posterior choroidal arteries may be feeding arteries. Compartments supplied by those small arteries are small, and often considered to be satellite AVMs.

The number of AVM compartments usually increases with AVM size. Most often, AVMs of less than

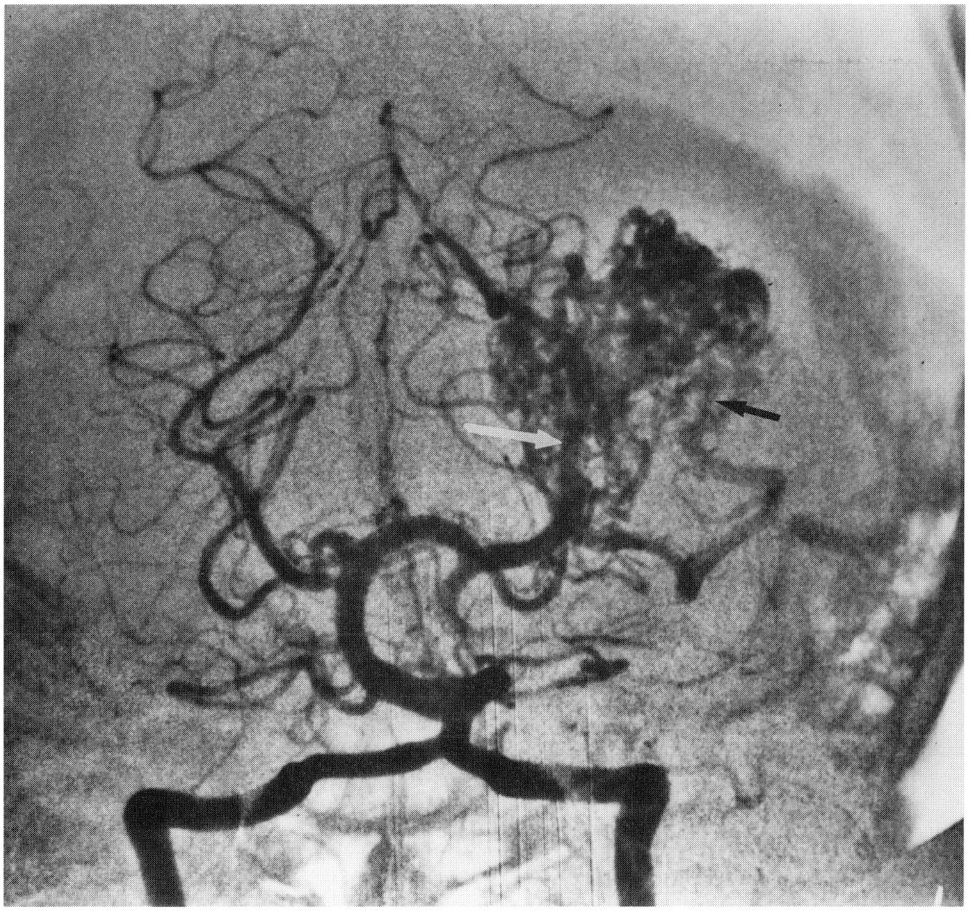

Figure 6. A penetrating feeding artery is surrounded circumferentially by the AVM as shown schematically in **A** and angiographically in **B**. The posterior cerebral artery or its branches frequently penetrate the AVM core (arrows). The middle or anterior cerebral arteries or their branches penetrate the AVM less frequently. Figures 6A and B used with permission of the Journal of Neurosurgery.[119] *Continued*

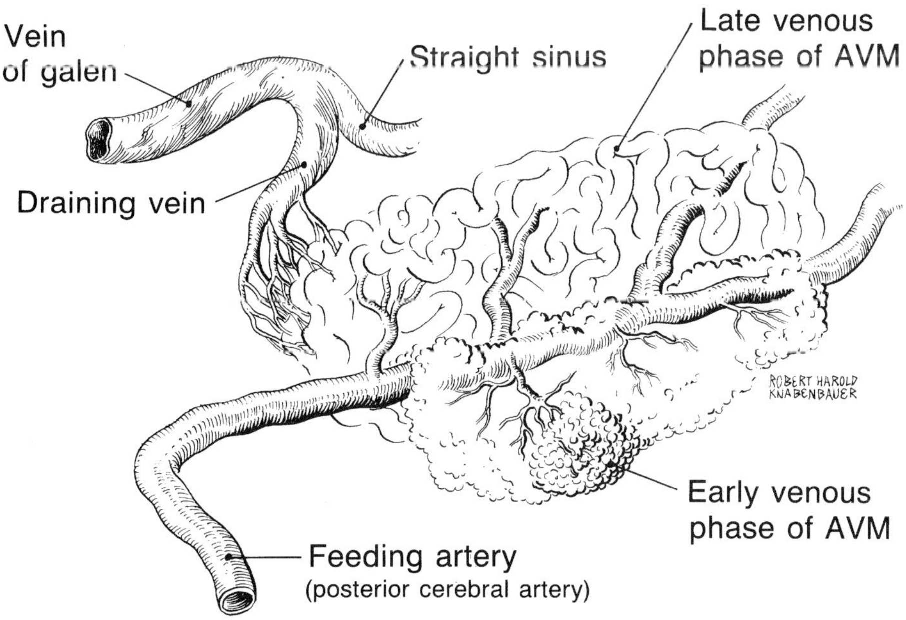

Figure 6B. A schematic drawing showing a penetrating feeding artery surrounded by an AVM.

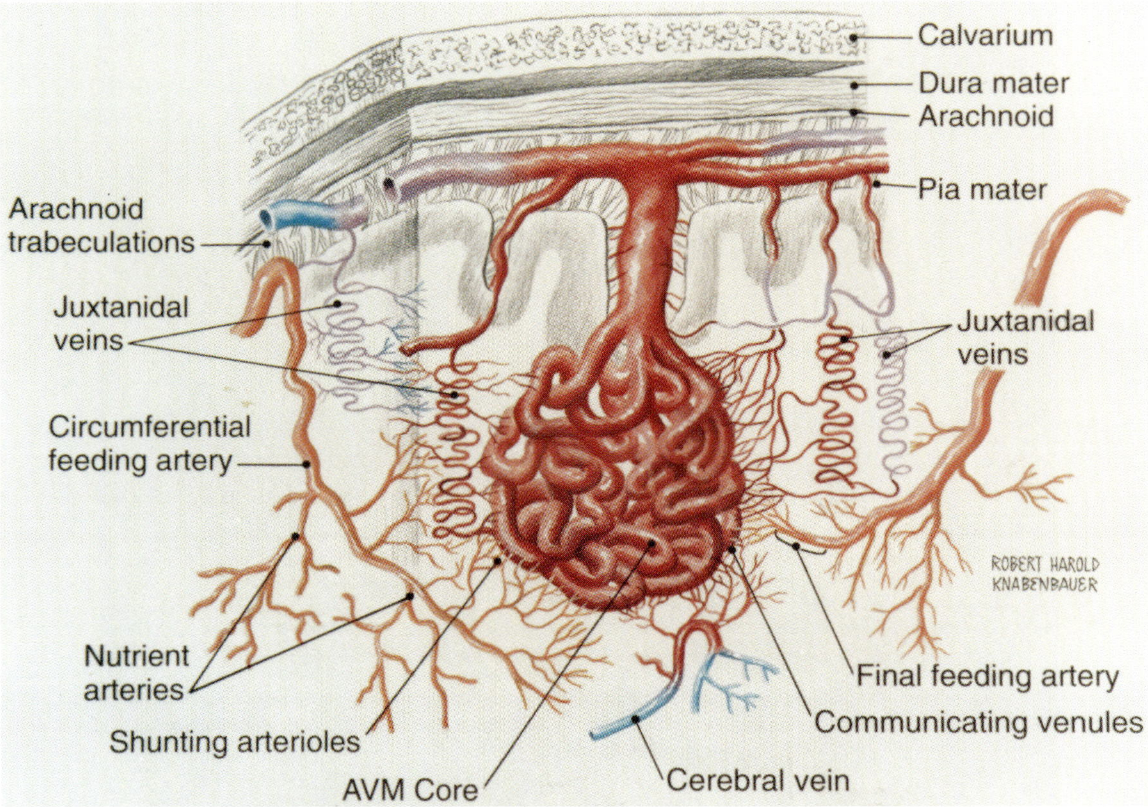

Figure 7. Juxtanidal vessels and their connections to the AVM core and to the cortical veins are dilated with arterial blood but are not a part of the AVM core. These cortical veins and the cortex in functional areas must be preserved. Also shown are a circumferential feeding artery, a type 2 final feeding artery, shunting arterioles, and communicating venules.

3 cm in diameter (14.2 cm^3 in volume) have one compartment. In larger AVMs, measuring 3–4 cm (33.5 cm^3 in volume), there are usually two compartments. In AVMs that measure greater than 4 cm in diameter, there are usually three compartments. In the author's experience, all AVMs of greater than 5 cm have been composed of three or more compartments.

Blood flow through AVMs increases proportionately to the increased number of compartments and AVM volume. For example, an AVM of 2 cm has a blood flow of 285 mL/min, and an AVM of 4–5 cm a flow of 800–1000 mL/min.[128]

Figures 8A-F show three hemodynamic compartments in a large AVM (5 cm in diameter), which were identified by angiography. The medial and lateral compartments are both demonstrated by left carotid angiography. In this example, right carotid angiography demonstrates a medial compartment through the anterior communicating artery and left anterior cerebral artery. Contrast material injected into the right carotid artery is too diluted in the left middle cerebral artery to fill in the lateral compartment. Furthermore, blood flow from the left carotid artery likely washes the contrast material from the left carotid bifurcation into the anterior cerebral artery.

A posterior compartment is identified by vertebral angiography. This compartment receives blood flow through the posterior cerebral artery, and is located immediately posterior to the medial compartment and partly medial to the lateral compartment. In the AVM shown in this example, surgery required isolating each compartment, as described later, and then resecting the entire AVM.

The compartment concept is not universally shared by neuropathologists. For example,[76] Okazaki demonstrated blood supply to an entire large AVM by injecting resin dye or x-ray contrast into one of the feeding arteries. This AVM filling can be explained by probable communications between different compartments by venules or small veins, as recently demonstrated by endoscopy (see Section 4, Chapter 10 on endoscopy-assisted microsurgery). On the other hand, this transcompartmental flow of contrast material is seldom demonstrated by angiography.

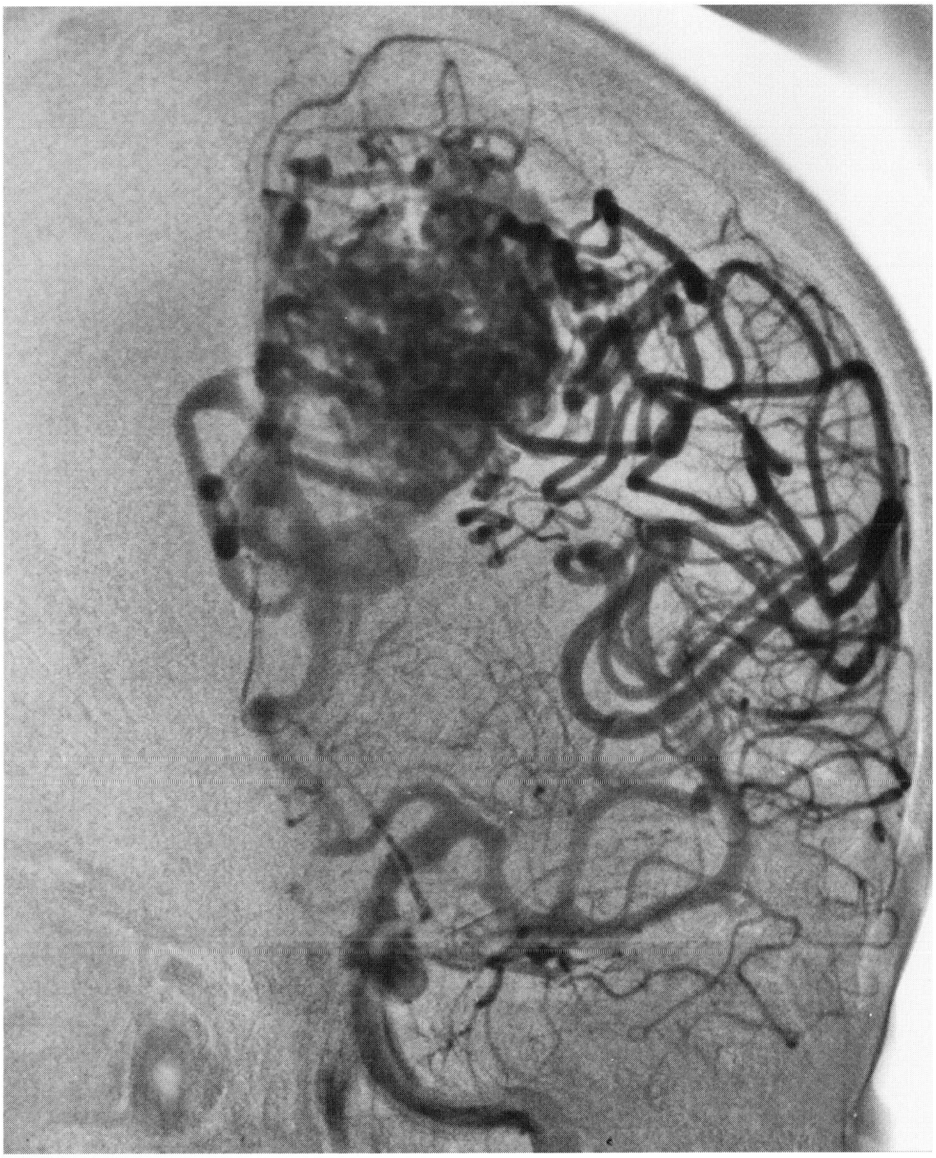

Figure 8. Angiograms clearly delineating three compartments: lateral, medial, and posterior (refer to text) **A.** AP view of left carotid injection. *Continued*

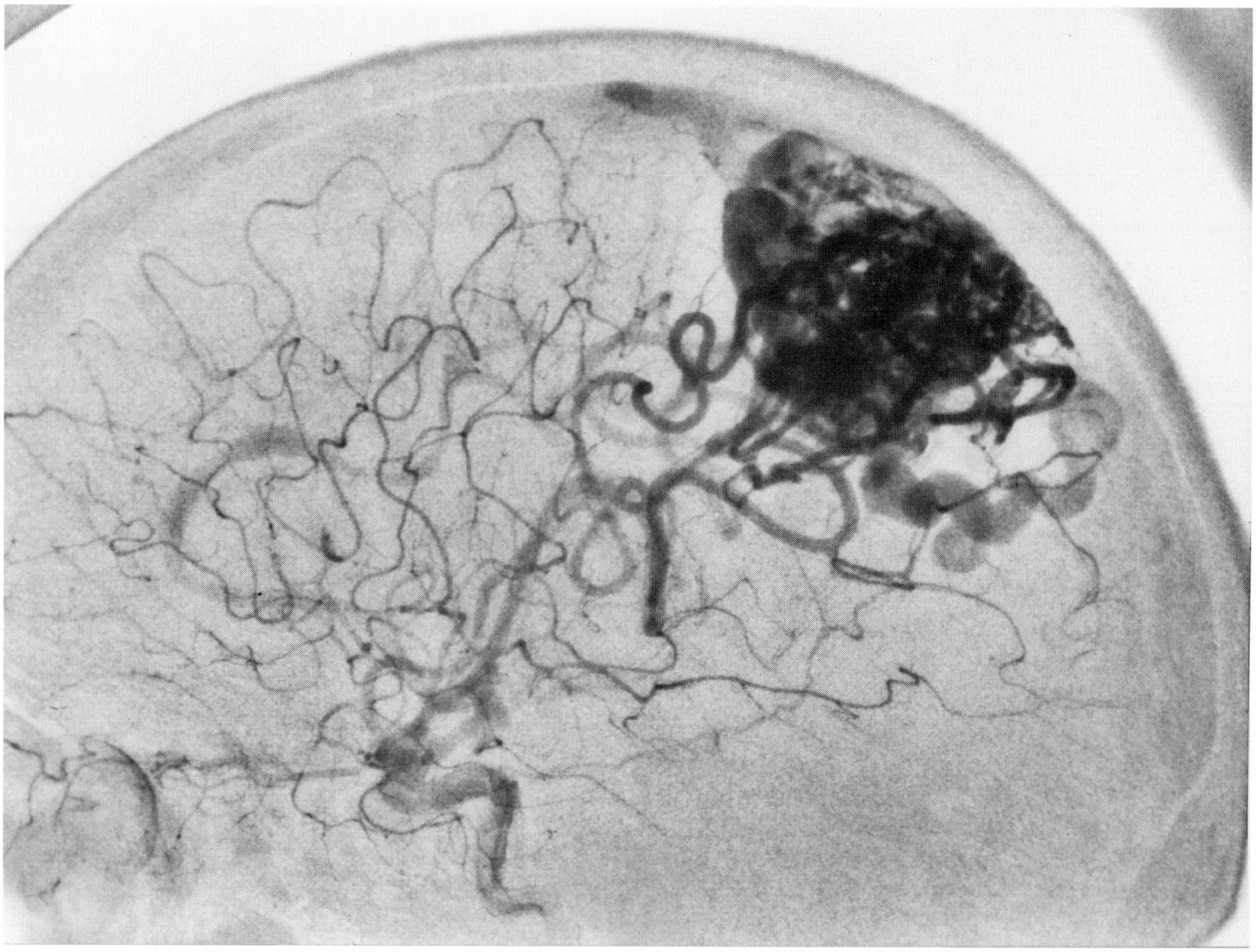

Figure 8B. Lateral view of left carotid injection. *Continued*

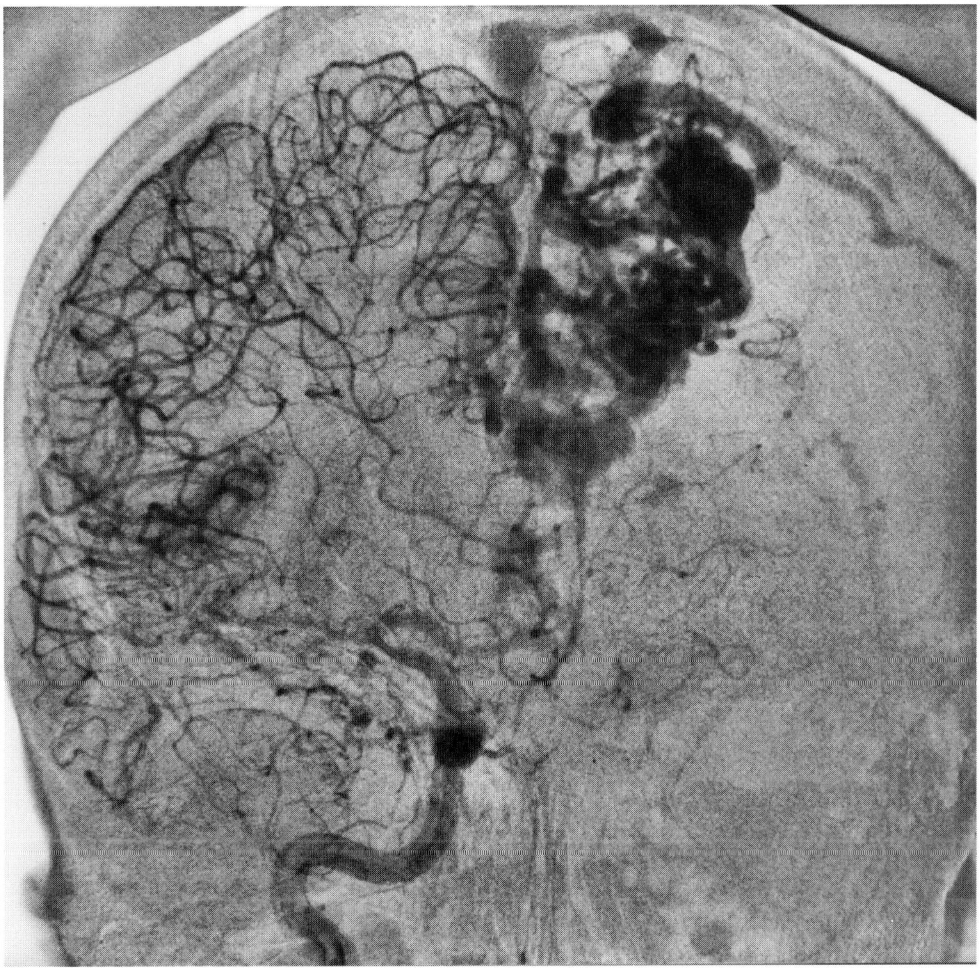

Figure 8C. AP view of right carotid injection. *Continued*

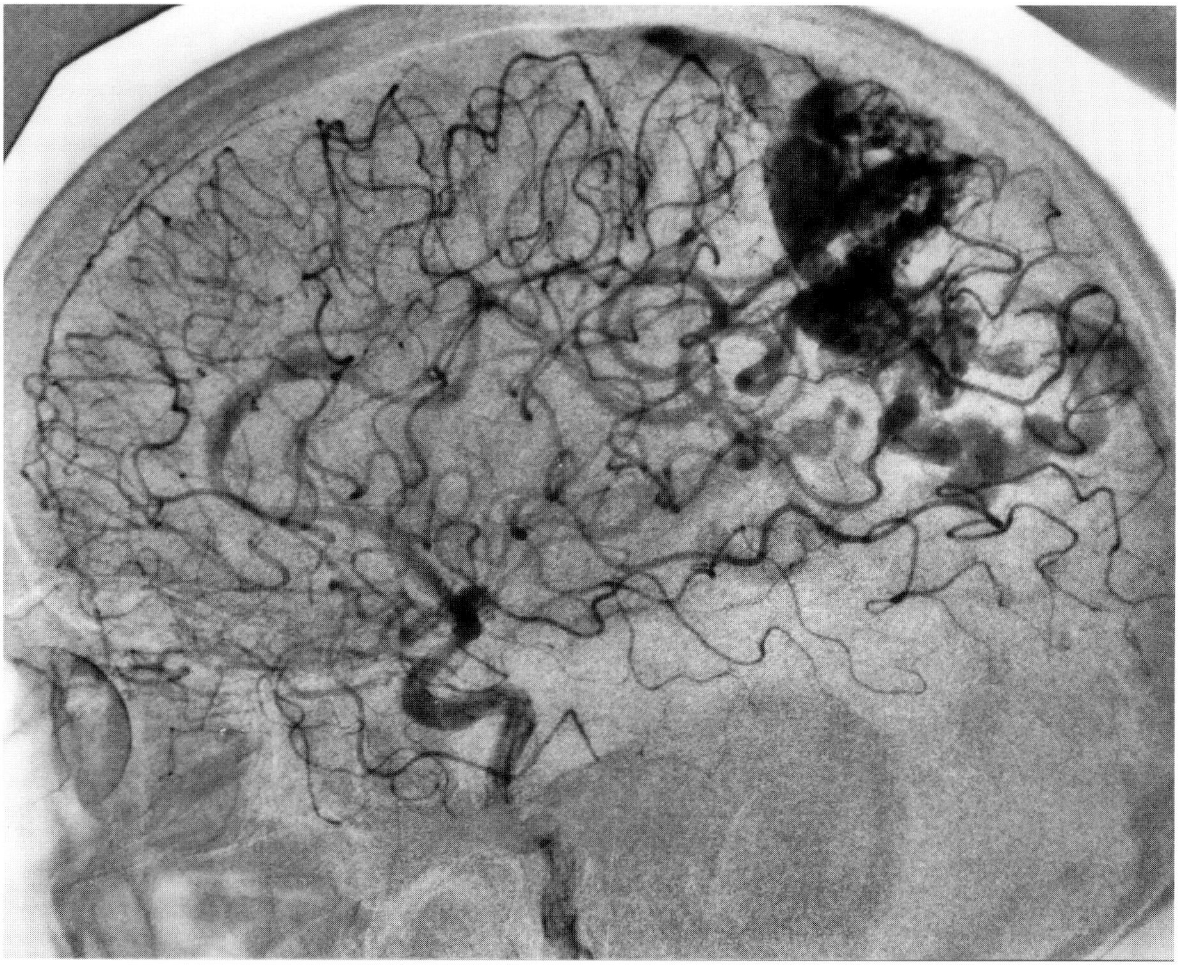

Figure 8D. Lateral view of right carotid injection. *Continued*

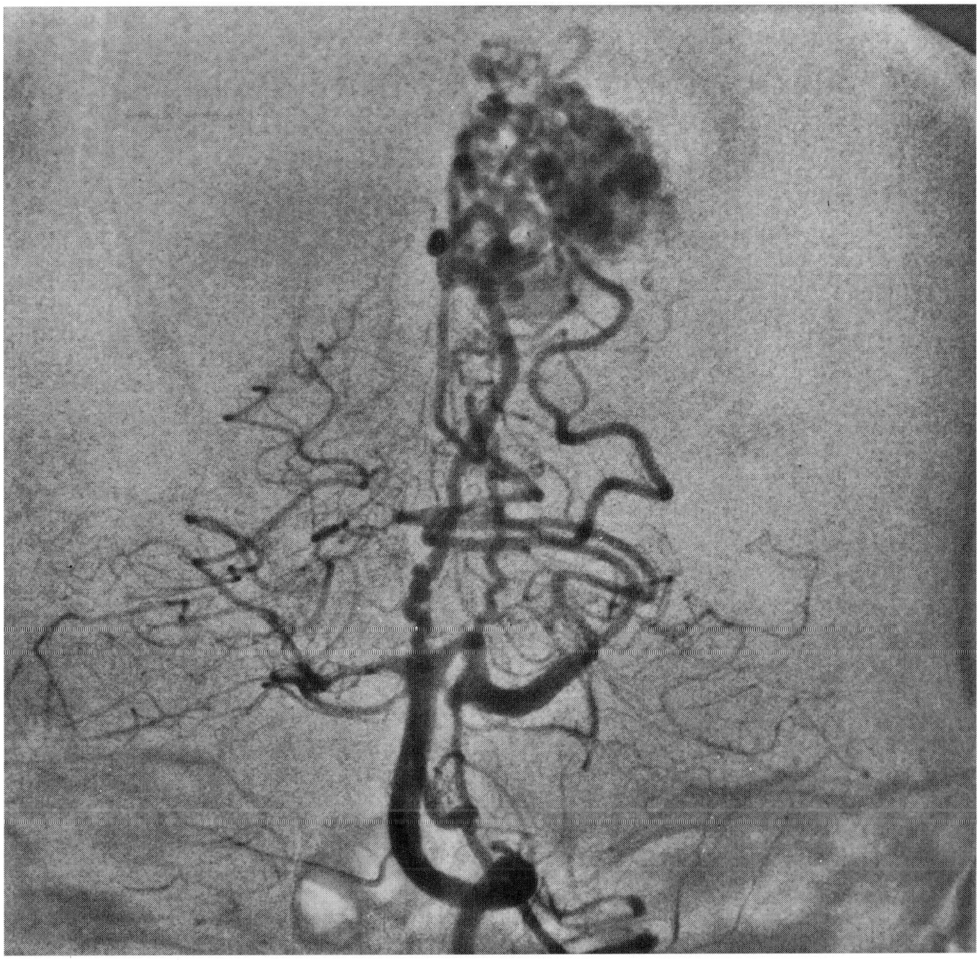

Figure 8E. AP view of vertebral artery injection. *Continued*

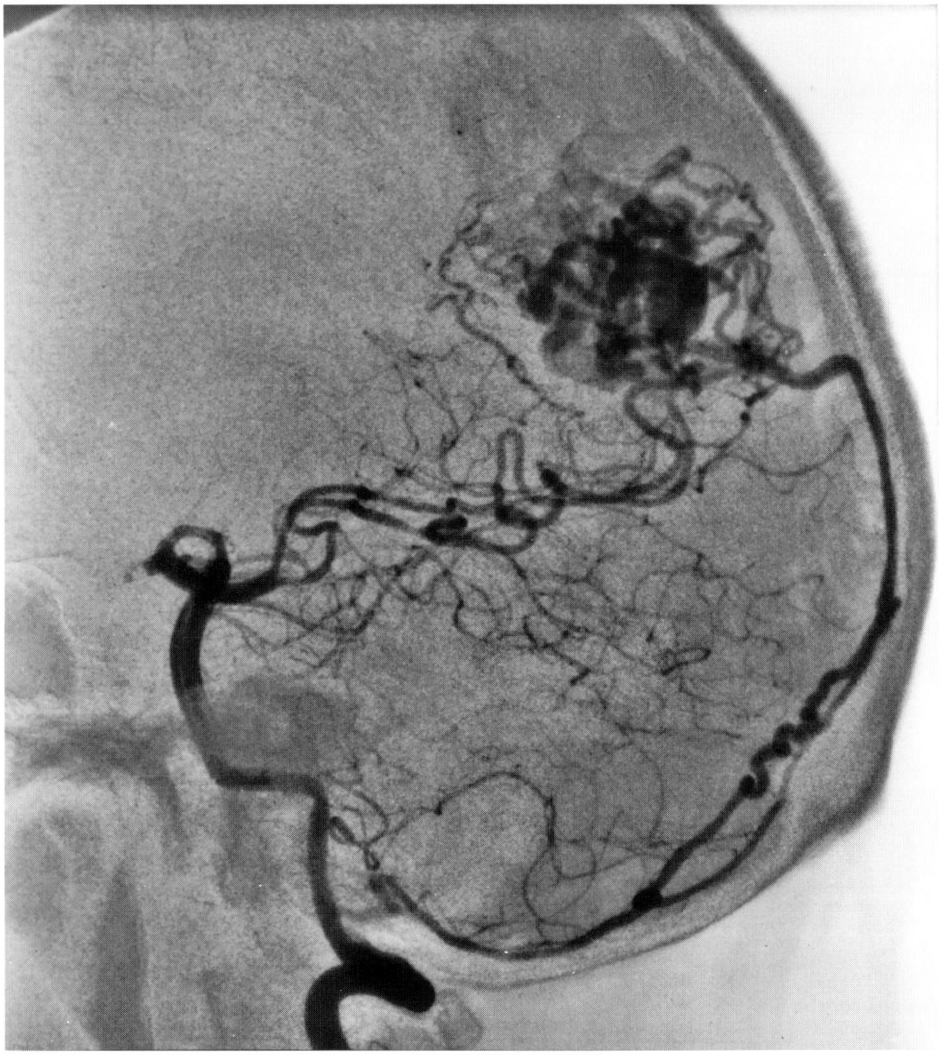

Figure 8F. Lateral view of vertebral artery injection. Figures 8A–F used with permission of the Journal of Neurosurgery.[119]
Continued

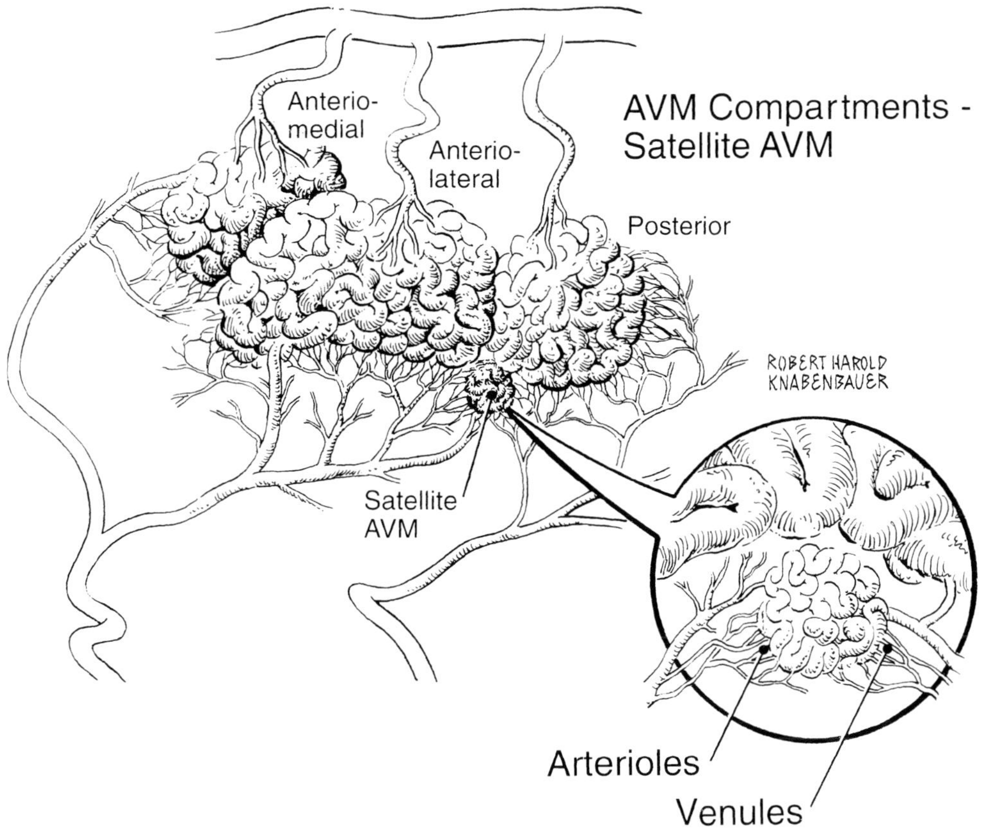

Figure 8G. Satellite AVMs are usually seen immediately outside the area where two compartments meet and have their own small feeding arteries and a draining vein, as shown schematically.

Consideration of the compartment concept provides a basis for understanding many aspects of treatment. For example, there is a much higher success rate of gamma knife irradiation for AVMs that are less than 2.5 cm in diameter than for larger AVMs.[105] The authors postulate that smaller AVMs are almost always composed of one compartment, and larger AVMs with two or more compartments usually have more complex arterial inflow and venous communication between the compartments. Therefore, larger AVMs are more resistant to radiational obliteration. Similarly, single-compartment AVMs can be surgically resected or obliterated by embolization more easily than multicompartment AVMs in the silent area. This rule may not always apply for AVMs in functional areas; therefore, the degree of radiation necrosis and embolization ischemia of arteries supplying these areas must be evaluated when planning treatment.

Draining veins have variable patterns of communication with cortical veins and sinuses. For example, veins draining the lateral compartment are connected to the veins of Trolard and/or Labbé, eventually draining into the superior sagittal sinus and/or the transverse sinus, respectively. The medial compartment draining veins are connected to cortical veins on the surface of the mesial hemisphere, and sometimes to the internal cerebral, thalamostriate, and choroid veins, and usually drain into the superior or inferior sagittal sinus and the vein of Galen. The posterior compartment draining vein usually flows into the sagittal sinuses or the vein of Galen through cortical veins. The major draining vein of the medial compartment may arise from its lateral aspect. Therefore, it is usually hidden between the medial and lateral compartments and cannot be visualized from either the medial or the lateral side of the AVM (Figure 4B). Inadvertent occlusion of this vein may result in catastrophic expansion of the medial compartment and its rupture, or localizing neurological deficit by subsequent obliteration of cortical veins.

Cortical veins connected to the major draining veins are more dilated than those seen in a one-compartment AVM. In addition, small cortical veins and venules are dilated passively with arterial blood by communicating with the AVM core through juxtanidal veins.[119] These dilated red veins spread out over a large area of the cortical surface, which is at least as wide as the diameter of the AVM core. These veins may provide a false impression that they are a part of the AVM core. During surgery in the functional area, these veins and the cortical tissue must be preserved (see the sections on operative techniques later in this chapter).

In a multicompartment AVM, a satellite AVM or nidus (Figure 8G) is frequently found.[118,119] This satellite AVM is commonly located near the multicompartment AVM in a notch formed by the edges of any two compartments.[119] The satellite AVM usually has its own small feeding artery and draining vein. These vessels are often imperceptible on preoperative angiography, but are sometimes demonstrated only after all compartments of the multicompartment AVM have been removed or obliterated. According to Mullan (personal communication, 1997) the draining vein of the satellite AVMs usually connects to a core draining vein and if the core is occluded, the satellite AVM usually disappears.

AVMs in the Spinal Cord

The term "AVM nidus" was coined by Doppman[23] to describe an AVM in the spinal cord. This type of AVM was described angiographically as a cluster of entangled vessels that is connected to an enlarged branch of the radicular artery as an arterial feeder. Blood flows through the entangled vessels into a draining vein (Figure 9A).

In the senior author's experience, a spinal cord AVM (particularly those of the dorsal type) consists of entangled anomalous veins (nidus) and usually has two sources of arterial blood supply. One source is a feeding artery that originated from one of the radicular arteries, and the other source is multiple shunting arterioles derived from the spinal cord circulation (Figure 9B).

Since the blood flows directly from the spinal cord vessels (shunting arterioles), clipping the feeding artery does not eliminate vigorous nidus pulsation unless all shunting arterioles are first interrupted at their junctions to the nidus. Recently, Spetzler (personal communication, 1998) and Malis (personal communication, 1998) measured the intravascular pressure in the spinal cord nidus with no difference found before and after clipping of the feeding artery. This finding supports our observation of the nidus pulsation in dorsal spinal cord AVMs. The authors' conclusion is that the large feeding artery connected directly to the dorsal spinal cord AVM corresponds to the type 1 final feeding artery of cerebral AVMs, and since shunting arterioles do not have an angiographically demonstrated main trunk (feeding artery) from which they originate, the concept of the nidus of spinal AVMs does not seem to be synonymous to the cerebral AVM core. Therefore, the authors use the term "AVM core" when describing cerebral AVMs and "nidus" for spinal cord AVMs. Spinal cord AVMs can be categorized as a variant of AVMs.

AVMs in the Superior Temporal Gyrus

AVMs in the superior temporal gyrus are unique for their anatomical relationship to functionally important areas. This relationship poses both serious technical and neurologically related challenges.

AVMs in this region extend into such areas as the frontal, temporal, and parietal opercula, lower sensorimotor area, Broca's area, basal ganglia, internal capsule, optic radiation, and Wernicke's area. Bleeding into these areas will result in temporary or permanent neurological deficits, including deficits in higher cortical functions and in seizures. The symptoms related to the secondary sensory area can be sensory seizures. AVMs in the superior temporal gyrus often surround the middle cerebral artery and may receive blood supply from several of its branches (Figure 10A). In larger AVMs, there are several draining veins that are connected to the superficial middle cerebral (sylvian) vein, cortical veins in the lateral and inferior temporal lobe, deep middle cerebral vein, basilar vein of Rosenthal, vein of Galen, or the internal cerebral vein. The sylvian vein shares the circulation of arterial blood with the vein of Trolard, the lateral temporal vein, and the vein of Labbé, or the inferior temporal vein, deep middle cerebral vein (Figures 10B and C), and rarely with the cavernous sinus. Many small feeding arteries originating from the sylvian group (the middle cerebral artery branches) and draining veins, both 0.5–1 mm or smaller, travel at a right angle to the sylvian vein. These arteries and veins take a parallel course, connecting to the AVM core and sylvian vein, respectively. This arterial and venous arrangement is unique to AVMs in the superior temporal gyrus. Technically, a bundle of the small feeding arteries and draining veins must be cauterized and sectioned together at one time because it is often difficult to separate each vessel without causing the rupture of neighboring vessels.

Another important role of the middle cerebral artery is that this artery sometimes sends branches to the AVM as it passes through the middle of the AVM core as a penetrating artery. It is mandatory to save not only the main trunk of the artery but also

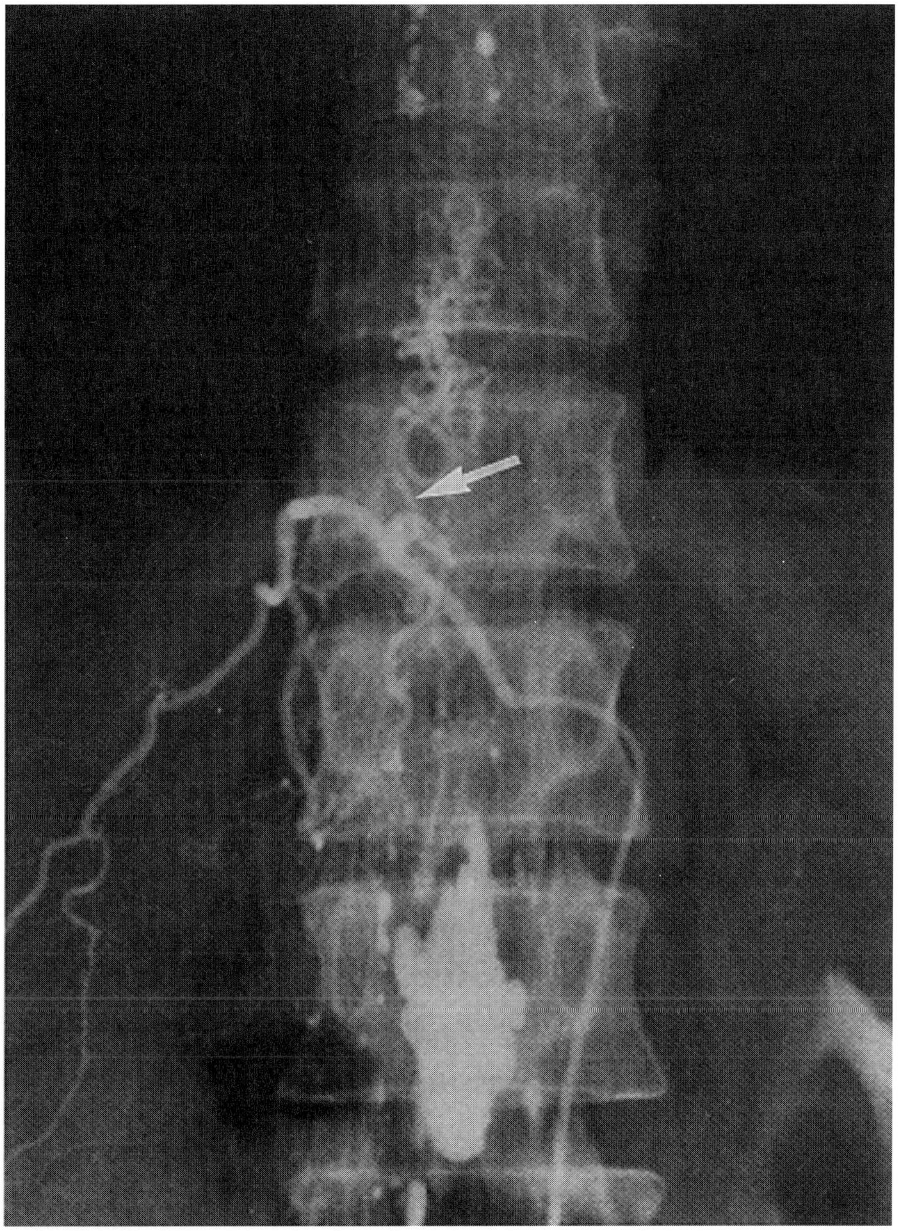

Figure 9A. Angiograms show the feeding artery (arrow) connected to the nidus of dorsal spinal cord AVM. *Continued*

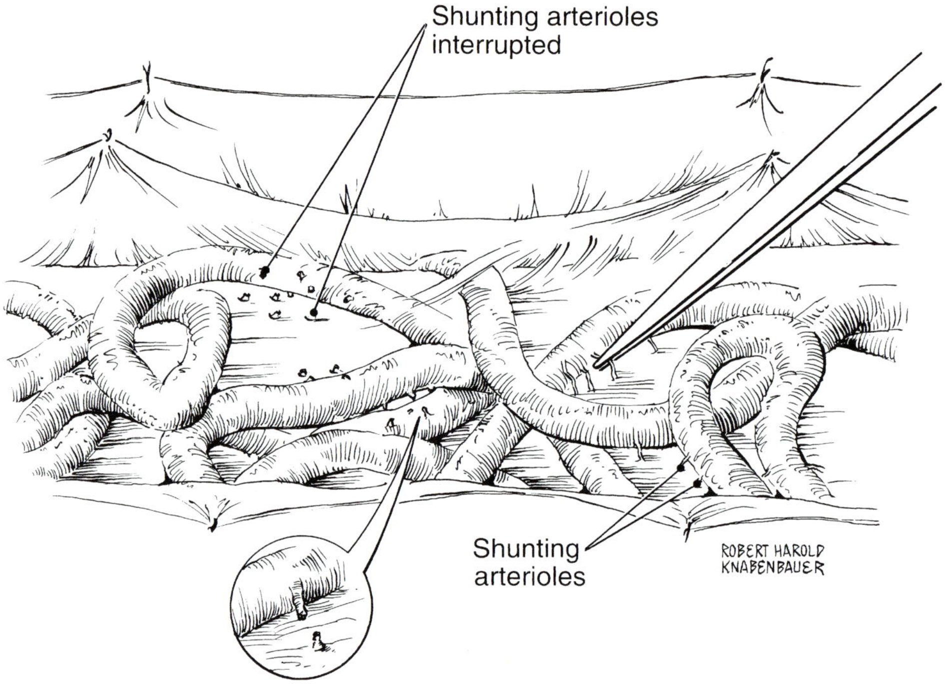

Figure 9B. A dorsal type spinal cord AVM always has shunting arterioles as terminal branches (50–100 μm) originating from arteries within the spinal cord. The inset depicts a magnified shunting arteriole already sectioned. What is called a feeding artery is not a single feeder to the AVM.

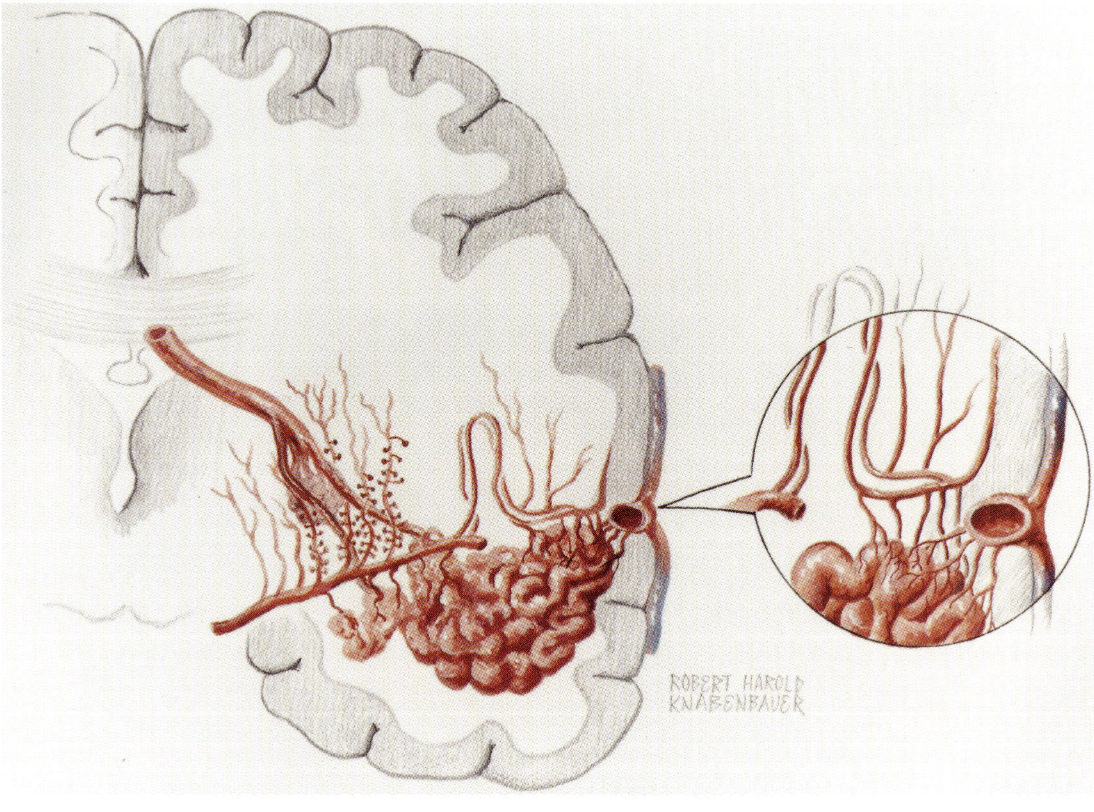

Figure 10A. An AVM in the superior temporal gyrus surrounds the middle cerebral artery branches, the lenticulostriate artery, and extends into the functionally important areas (refer to text). Small feeding arteries and small veins are densely packed around the sylvian vein (inset). *Continued*

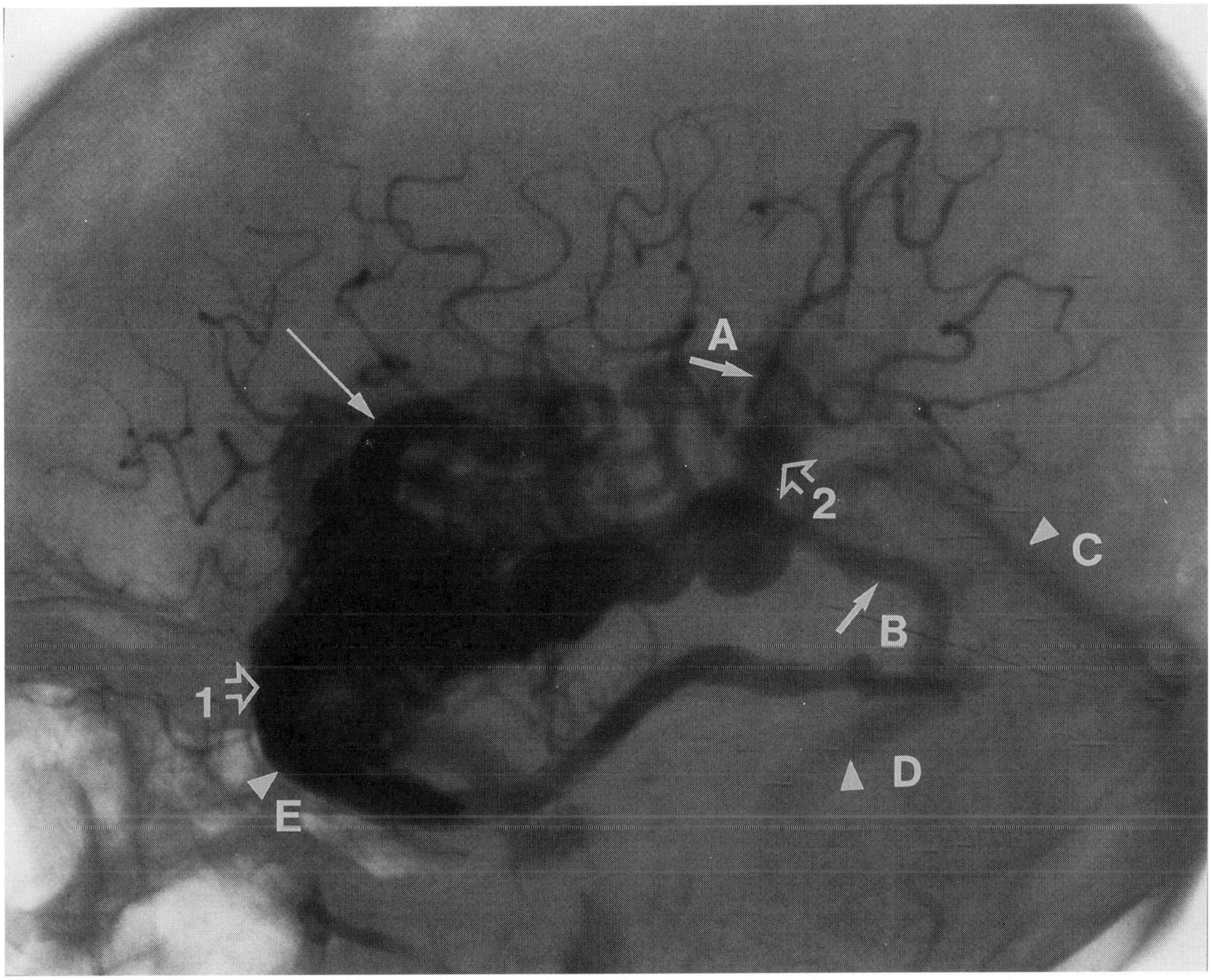

Figure 10B. The lateral view of the angiogram showing a feeding artery (narrow arrow), a draining vein (open arrow 1) that connects to the sphenoparietal sinus (E), and another draining vein (open arrow 2) that connects to the vein of Galen (arrow A) and then to the straight sinus (arrowhead C), and to the vein of Labbé (arrow B) that connects to the core vessel. *Continued*

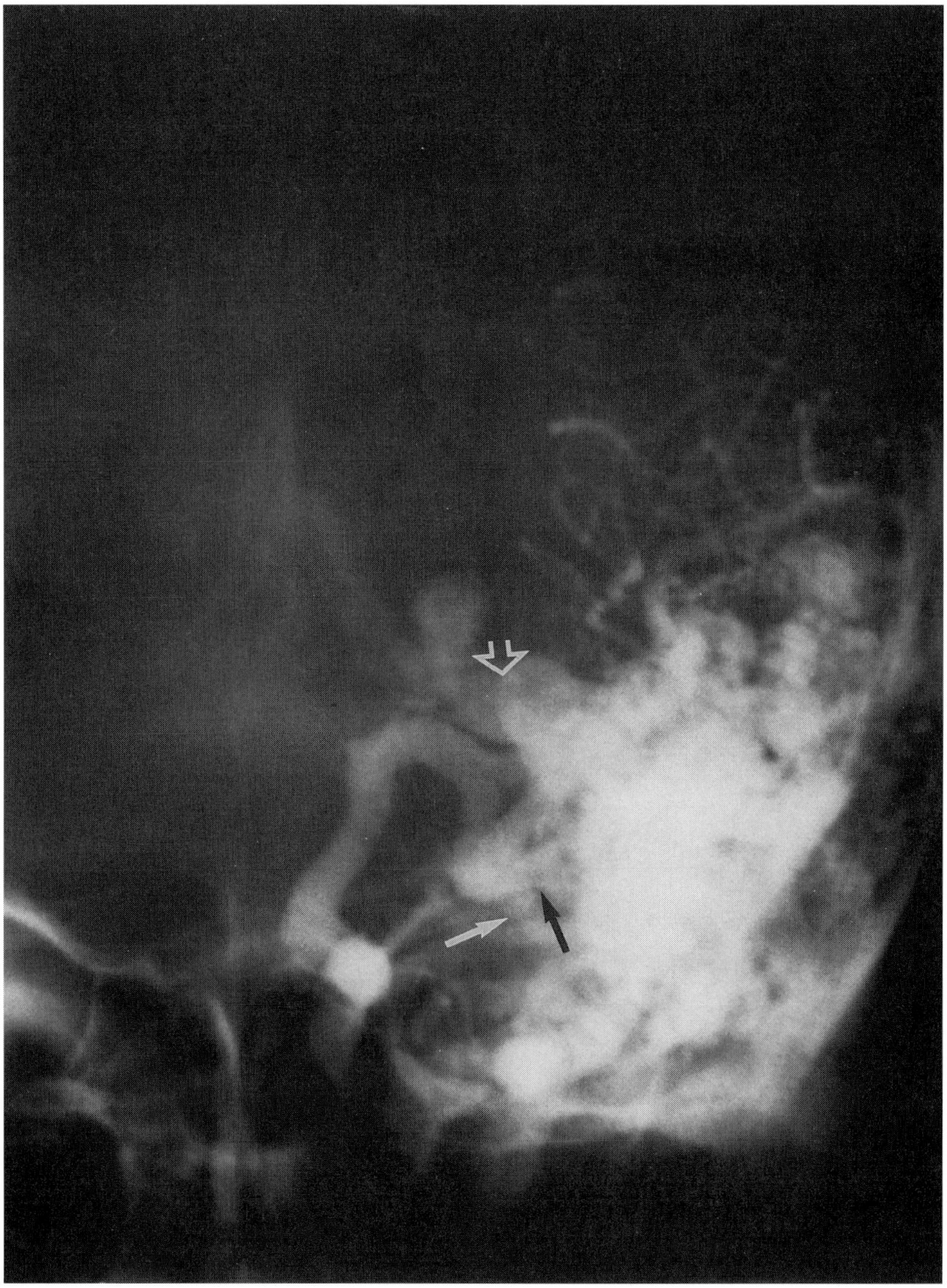

Figure 10C. The AP view, showing two feeding arteries and a major draining vein connected to the basilar vein and then to the vein of Galen. The draining veins are difficult to identify because they are superimposed by core vessels and cortical veins.

its branches that supply circulation to functionally important areas, as discussed previously.

AVMs in the Occipital Visual Area

The distance from the occipital convexity to the inferior medially located AVM is much greater than that from the sensorimotor cortex to the subcortically located AVM (Figure 11). The approach from the mesioinferior occipital surface to the AVM is extremely difficult to perform without damaging the striate cortex. Because the AVM is usually located subcortically, the access to the AVM (without removing brain tissue) must be done by following a draining vein from the occipital convexity. The angle of the operator's vision when following another draining vein on the mesioinferior surface is not favorable to safe isolation of this vessel.

Symptomatology of AVM Patients

AVMs in Functional Areas

Signs and symptoms manifested by patients with AVMs in all locations include: (1) intracerebral, subarachnoid, or intraventricular hemorrhage, (2) seizures, (3) progressive neurological deficits, (4) headaches, (5) transient neurological deficits, (6) mental deterioration, and (7) psychiatric manifestations.[111] The most common forms of presentation are ICH and seizures. These two manifestations occurred with equal frequency according to some published reports;[84,104] cerebral hemorrhage was reported by others[35] to be the initial event in 70% of the cases. The incidence rates for the other signs and symptoms are less than 5%.

In the authors' series of 135 patients with AVMs in functional areas, the primary signs and symptoms were hemorrhagic ictus in 79 patients (58.5%), seizures in 48 (35.6%), progressive neurological deficits in 4 (3%) (1 infant with mental deterioration associated with increasing head size and marked bruit in the head), and transient neurological deficits (similar to TIAs) in 1 (0.7%), and paroxysmal severe throbbing headaches that were incapacitating in occupational activities in 3 (2.2%).

A total of 66 patients (48.9%) had seizures, including 42 patients with seizures as the only symptom. This percentage corresponds to that reported by others,[35,84,104] who included AVMs in all locations (with focal or generalized seizures) whereas all but one of our cases presented with focal seizures. Among the remaining seizure patients, hemorrhagic ictus was found in 18, progressive neurological deficits in 2, transient deficits in 2, and transient as well as progressive deficit in 3. A total of 78 patients with hemorrhagic ictus was divided into five groups as shown below.

Patients with Hemorrhagic Ictus

Ictus only	59
With seizures	17
With progressive deficit	1
With transient deficit	1
With seizures and progressive deficits	1

Patients with Seizures

Seizures only	42
With progressive deficits	2
With TIA	2
With progressive deficits and TIA	2

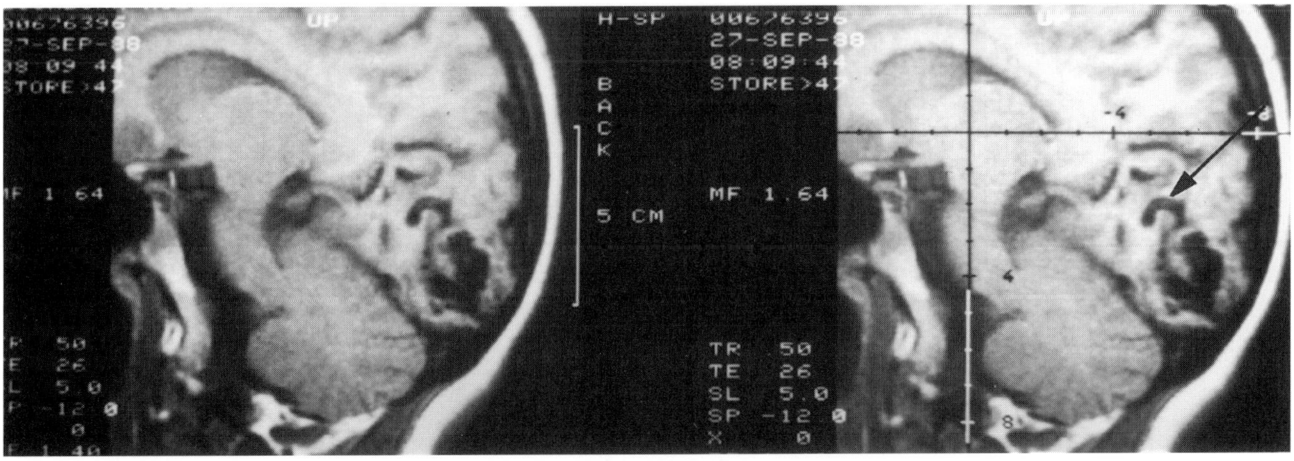

Figure 11. A large medial occipital AVM located partly in the striate cortex was approached by following the draining vein (arrow) from the convexity surface. The length of the tortuous draining vein was greater than the usual length of the draining veins connected to an AVM in the sensorimotor area (refer to illustrative case 8).

All of the patients had evidence of hemorrhage at operation: either frank intracerebral, subarachnoid, or intraventricular hemorrhage; hemosiderin-laden brain tissue adjacent to the AVM core, associated with or without a small area of liquefied blood; or marked arachnoid adhesion directly in contact with an AVM. The high rate of hemorrhage detection in this series is due partly to the surgical technique, which delineates the venous loops of the AVM core at its margin (where they make direct contact to surrounding brain tissue), and partly because there was no destruction of brain tissue or AVM loops while using the suction apparatus.

The highest incidence of hemorrhage from AVMs was previously reported to be in the second decade of the patient's life;[84] however, the patient's first visit to the physician for AVM detection was during the third decade.[84] Other reports indicate that the average onset of seizures was noted to be 25 years of age, as contrasted to the onset of hemorrhagic events, which was 30 years of age.[35] In the authors' series of 135 patients with AVMs in functional areas, the highest incidence of ictus onset, as well as seizure onset, was found to be in the fourth decade of life (Figure 12) (Figures 13A and B).

AVMs in the Superior Temporal Gyrus

The symptomatology of 22 patients in the authors' series of 135 patients who were treated surgically for AVMs in the superior temporal gyrus included:

1. Fourteen patients who presented with a history of hemorrhagic ictus, 6 of whom had both motor and speech deficits, 3 had sensorimotor deficits (1 of which was transient), 2 had speech difficulties, and 3 had signs of increased intracranial pressure.
2. Another 6 patients manifested with focal seizures only: 5 with temporal lobe seizures and 1 with sensorimotor seizures.
3. Seven patients presented with both ictus and seizures, 2 had temporal lobe seizures, and 5 had motor seizures or speech arrest.
4. Transient neurological deficit was manifested in 1 patient and progressive neurological deficit in 1 patient.

Preoperatively, 10 patients were neurologically intact, 11 patients had mild neurological deficits, and severe deficits were present in 1 patient with capsulocaudatothalamic involvement.

AVMs in the Occipital Visual Area

Patients with AVMs in the visual cortex area present with either visual seizures or a visual defect with sudden onset of headache, nausea, and vomiting.[65] Seizure patients see intermittent blinking lights in the homonymous field opposite to the AVM lesion. On clinical presentation some patients show visual field defect, alexia, or visual agnosia.

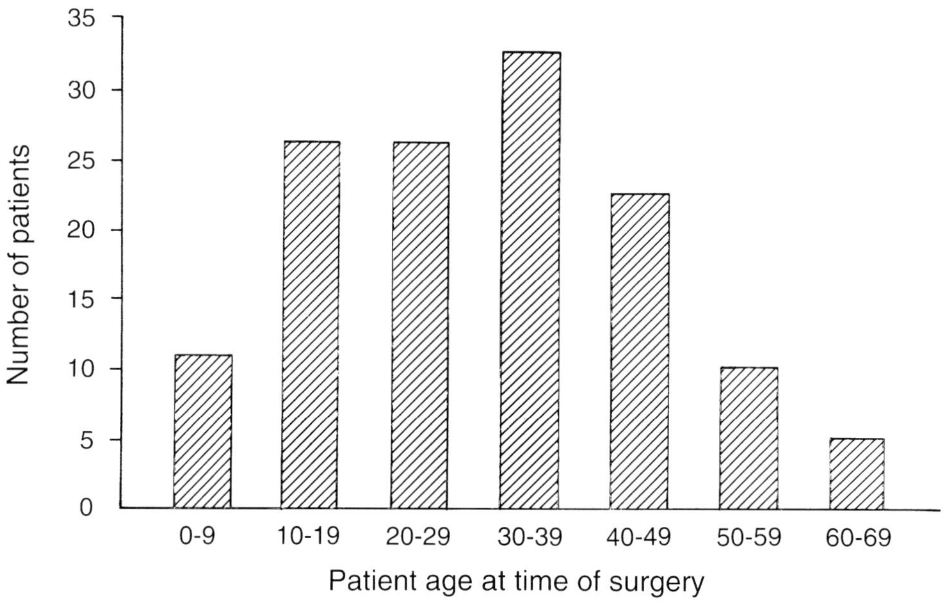

Figure 12. The bar graph from a study of 135 cases with AVMs in functional areas indicates the highest incidence of surgery in the 4th decade of life, followed by a high incidence in the 2nd, 3rd, and 5th decades, respectively.

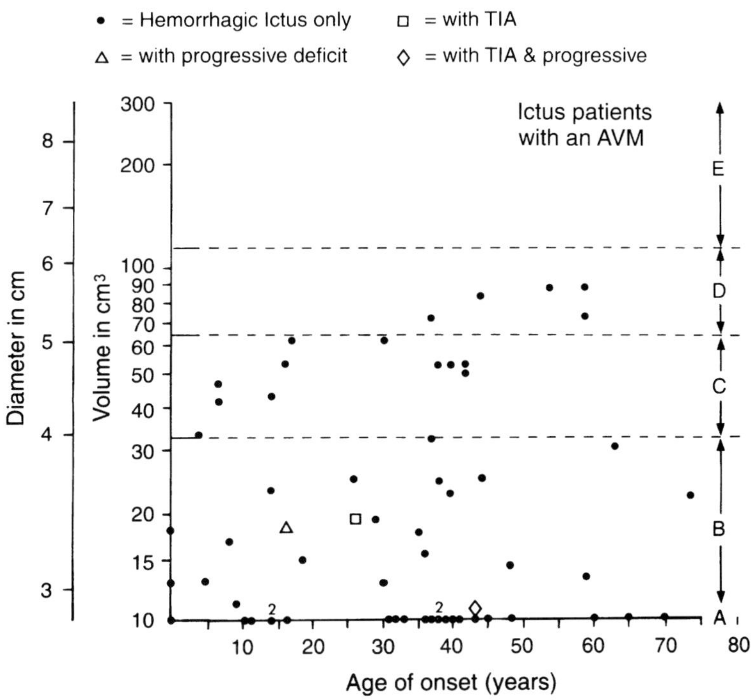

Figure 13. Graphic depiction of the relationship between the size of the AVM and the patient ages at the onset of hemorrhagic ictus (**A**), and at the onset of seizures (see **B**). **A.** The incidence for first hemorrhagic ictus is relatively high in patients with an AVM to ≤25.2 cm³, 4 cm sphere (indicated by dots). *Continued*

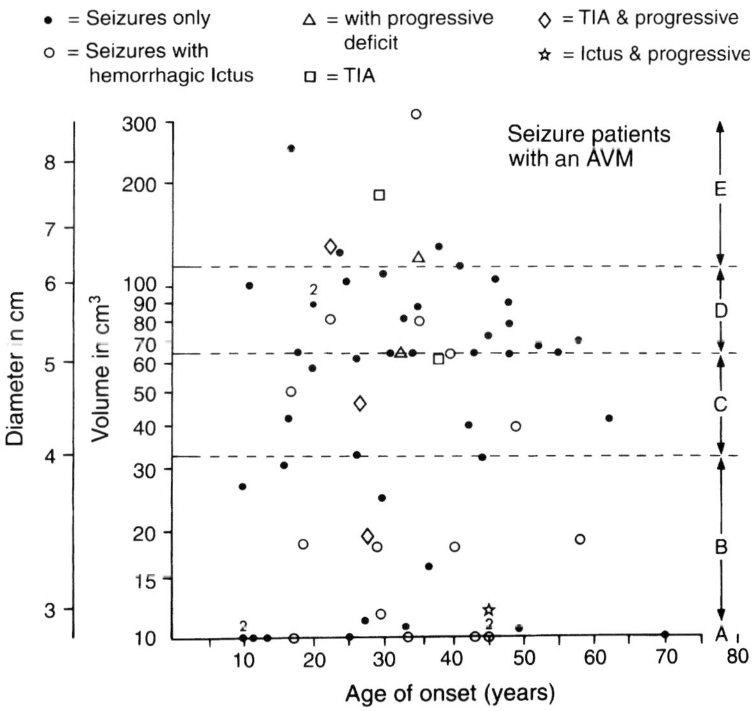

Figure 13B. The incidence of the first episode of seizures in 135 cases is relatively high in patients with AVMs ≥ 65.4 cm³, 5 cm diameter sphere (indicated by dots). The incidence of seizures and ictus is relatively high in patients with AVMs <25.2 cm³ (indicated by circles). The highest incidence of hemorrhagic ictus was noted in the 4th decade of life, followed by the 1st, 2nd, and 5th decades (see Figure 13A). The highest incidence of seizures was noted in the 5th decade, and no patient of the 1st decade presented with a seizure history.

AVMs in the Posterior Parietal Area

The posterior parietal area controls body images and orientation in space, and dysfunction of this area is manifested by anosognosia and autotopagnosia on the side opposite to the lesion (or bilateral with dominant hemisphere lesions). The area is surrounded by the sensory cortex, occipital cortex (area 9), Wernicke's area, visual cognitive area (including left and right orientation, finger discrimination, and calculation), and the optokinetic nystagmus center. Hemorrhages in this area are often associated with hemiparesis and hemianopia, dysphasia, agnosia, Guerstman syndrome, sensory or visual extinction, and optokinetic impairment loss of fast phase movement toward the side opposite to the lesion. These signs and symptoms are often subtle and unrecognized when they are transient.

AVMs in the Capsulocaudatothalamic Area

Symptoms and signs of AVMs in the basal ganglia, internal capsule, and thalamus are usually caused by hemorrhage and include hemiplegia, hemianesthesia, dysphasia, and hemianopia. Impaired short-term memory and cognition are also reported.[56] Hydrocephalus can result from hemorrhage that extends into a ventricle.

Other vascular malformations are often difficult to distinguish from AVMs because small AVMs (histologically proven) may not have distinct angiographically demonstrable feeding arteries and draining veins. Cavernous hemangiomas are often intermingled with venous malformations as confirmed by pathological studies. It is imperative to identify diffuse AVMs in this area because they are favored by radiosurgery or irradiation treatment, whereas a compact AVM in this area can be surgically removed safely[56,100,101] as seen in one of the illustrative cases.

AVMs in the Brain Stem

AVMs in the brain stem are frequently associated with extension into the cerebellum. Presenting symptoms are diplopia, facial weakness or pain, incoordination gait difficulties, numbness and paresthesia, weakness of extremities, and difficulty speaking and swallowing. Signs include oculomotor palsy, internuclear ophthalmoplegia, nystagmus, nuclear facial palsy, facial hypesthesia, hemisensory deficit, hemiparesis, and cerebellar ataxia. Compact AVMs located near the brain stem surface are candidates for surgical resection while deep-seated and diffuse AVMs in the brain stem are favored by radiosurgery.[25,56]

Preoperative and Intraoperative Diagnostic Studies

Computed tomography (CT), magnetic resonance imaging (MRI), magnetic resonance angiography (MRA), four-vessel cerebral angiography, and intraoperative color Doppler ultrasonography have each provided insights into the presence of AVMs, their location, size, arterial feeders, and draining system. Three-dimensional studies have helped surgeons understand the AVM hemodynamic arrangement. These images have provided a beneficial means to stereoscopically separate feeding arteries, draining veins, and various parts (compartments) of the AVM core. Further, angiographic holograms localize these vascular structures in true three dimensions. Magnetic source imaging (MSI) or functional MRI are of great value in localizing sensory and motor areas, which allows surgical planning accuracy in these areas.

Cerebral Angiography

Conventional cerebral angiography[47,73,109] is the most informative technique for demonstrating arterial feeders, the AVM core, and the draining veins in continuity and different phases of contrast filling in various portions of the AVM core (Figures 14A-D). Stereoscopic angiograms identify the course of each feeding artery and draining vein; however, it is extremely difficult to identify the connecting point of each shunting arteriole, or type 2 final feeding artery, to a venous loop of the AVM core (Figure 14C). Likewise, it is difficult to find the exact connection of the type 1 final feeding artery to the corresponding venous loop in a large AVM. CT angiography (Figure 14E) is informative in demonstrating the full size of the AVM core simultaneously with feeding arteries, the major draining veins, and venous sinuses, as well as other normal venous structures only passively dilated with arterial blood, such as cortical veins, the internal cerebral vein, and the vein of Galen. The core vessels are so densely packed that it is extremely difficult to determine the exact point of the junction between shunting arterioles or final feeding arteries and venous loops of the AVM. Superselective angiography of multiple feeding arteries may distinguish final feeding arteries individually (Figures 15A-C).

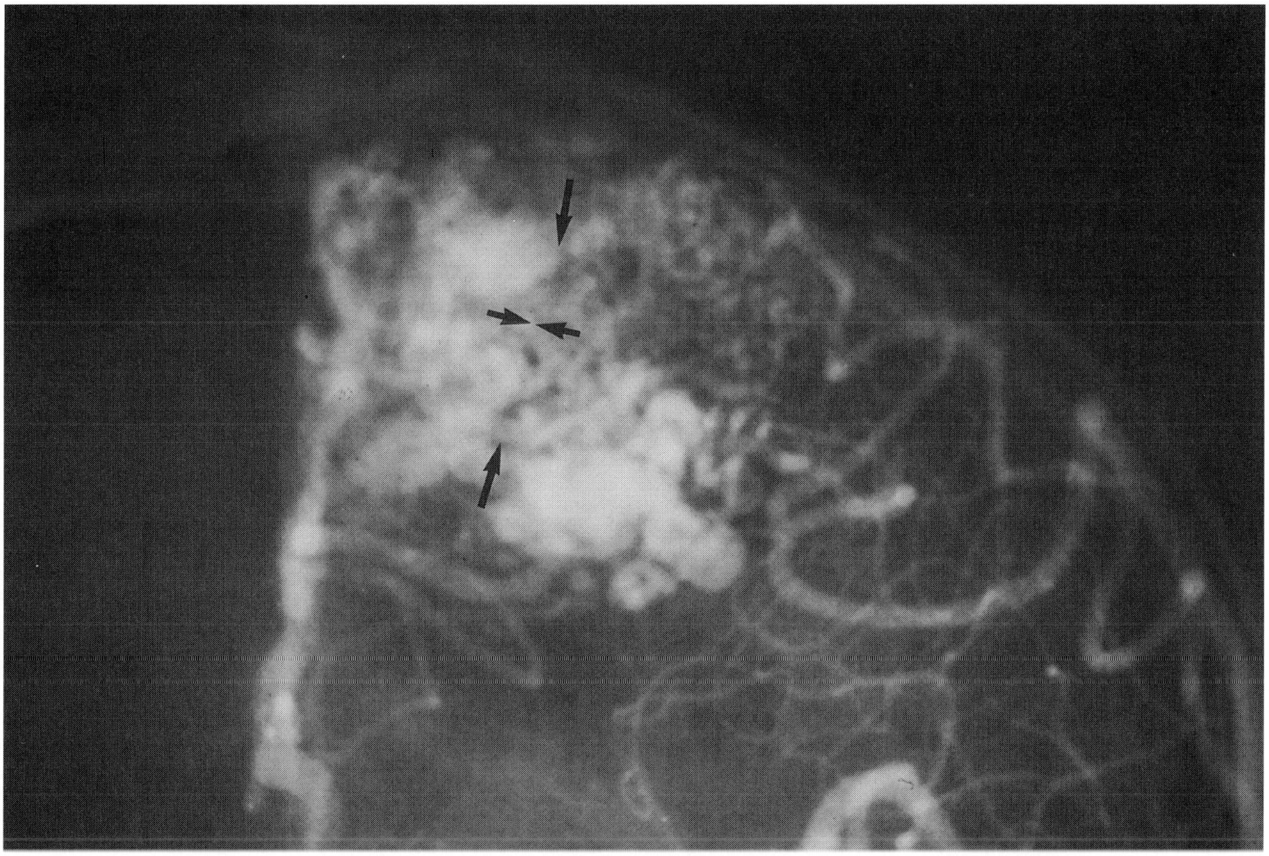

Figure 14. Angiograms of a sensorimotor area AVM showing that the size of the AVM appears different depending on the phase of contrast filling. **A.** AP view depicts both medial and lateral compartments of an AVM, with the medial compartment slightly more extensively filled than the lateral compartment, presumably due to the greater diameter of the feeding arteries of the former compartment. Arrows indicate the border between the medial and lateral compartments (see illustrative case 2). *Continued*

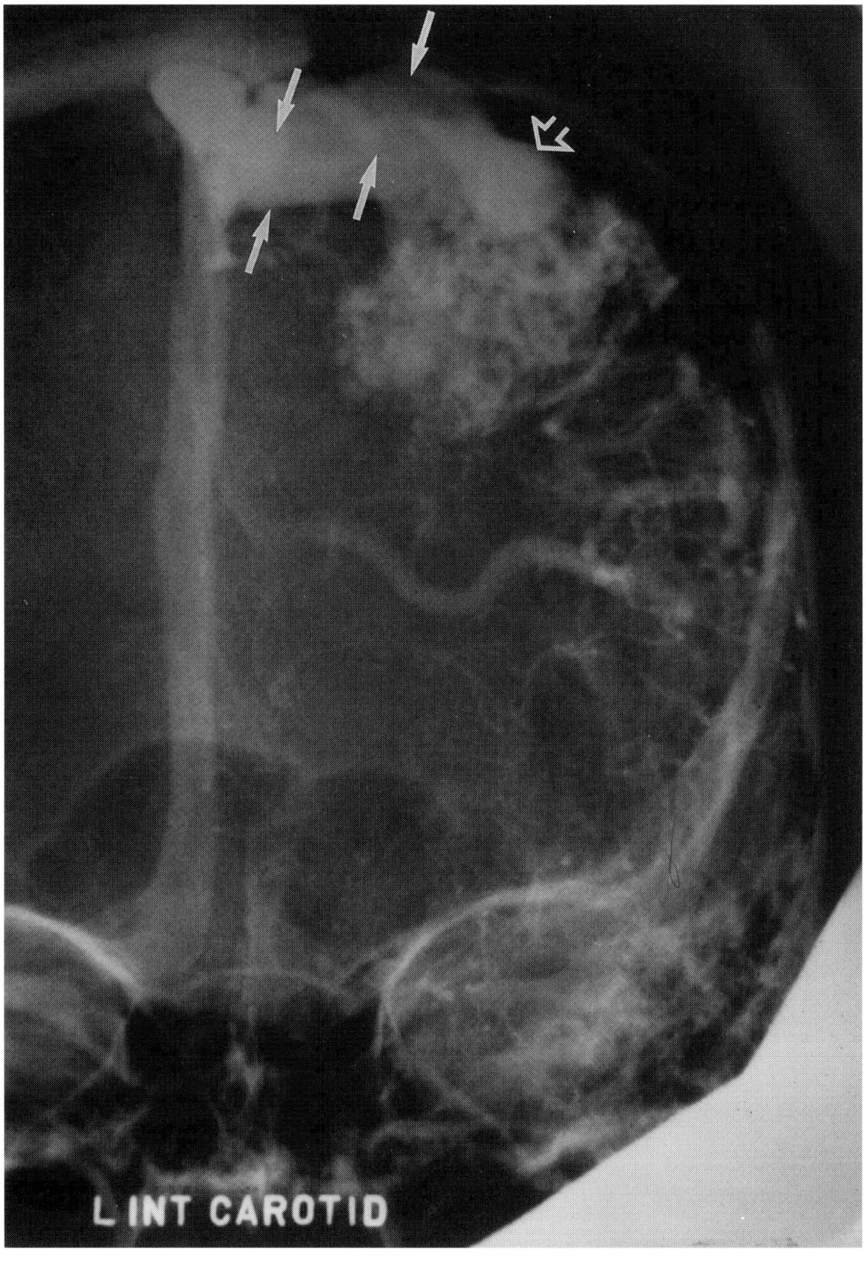

Figure 14B. The AP angiogram of a sensorimotor area AVM showing a large draining vein (open arrow) originating from the lateral compartment connected to two equally dilated cortical veins (arrows). Blood flow through the medial compartment was much faster than through the lateral compartment. Figure used with permission of Neurological Research. *Continued*

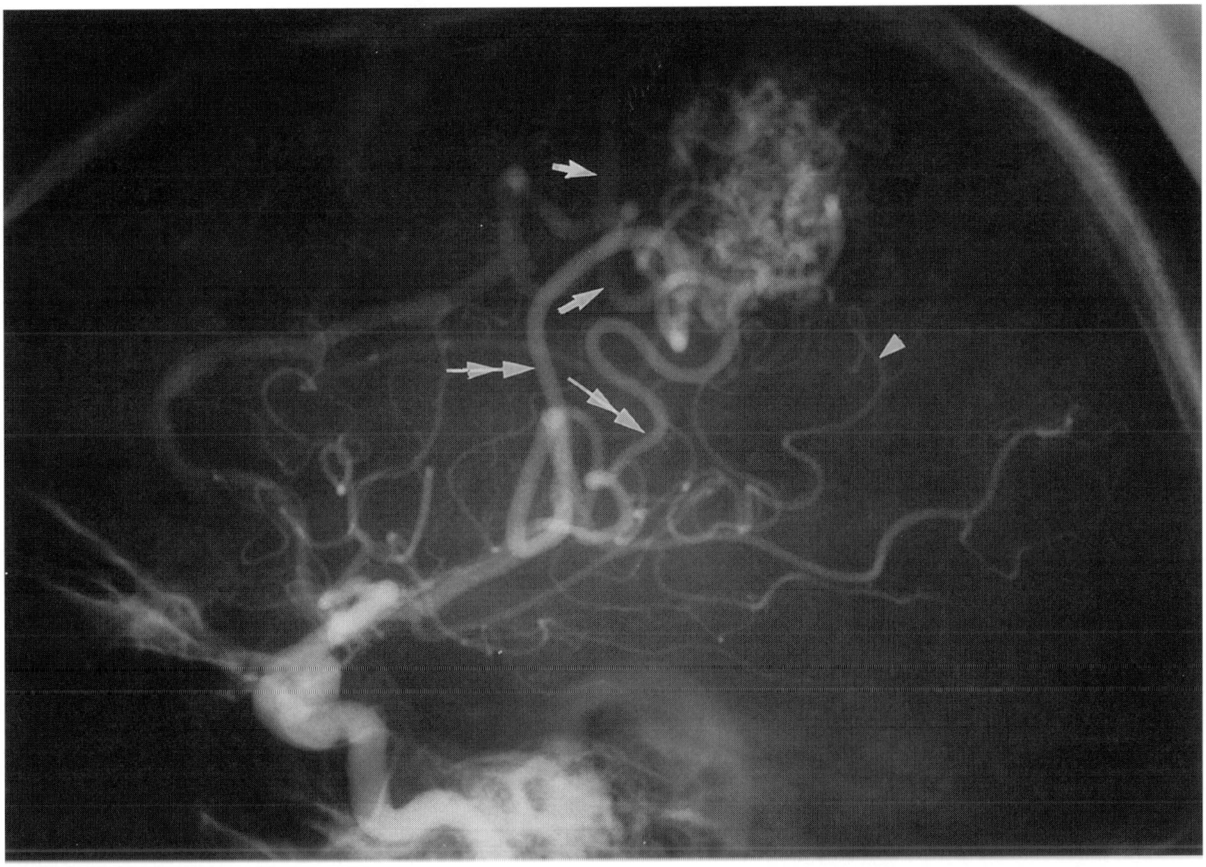

Figure 14C. Different AVM loops are depicted in different lateral films as filling of the AVM vessels progressed. A lateral view of the early angiographic phase shows several feeding arteries (branches of the middle cerebral artery) connected to the lateral compartment with two of them enlarged, as indicated by double arrows; single arrows indicate two enlarged feeding arteries (branches of the anterior cerebral artery), one of which was a type 1 final feeding artery connecting to the medial compartment. The diameter of the former two enlarged arteries reduced to normal size within several weeks after total AVM resection and that of the latter two arteries reduced to normal within several months. A small feeding artery (arrowhead) supplies the posterior compartment. *Continued*

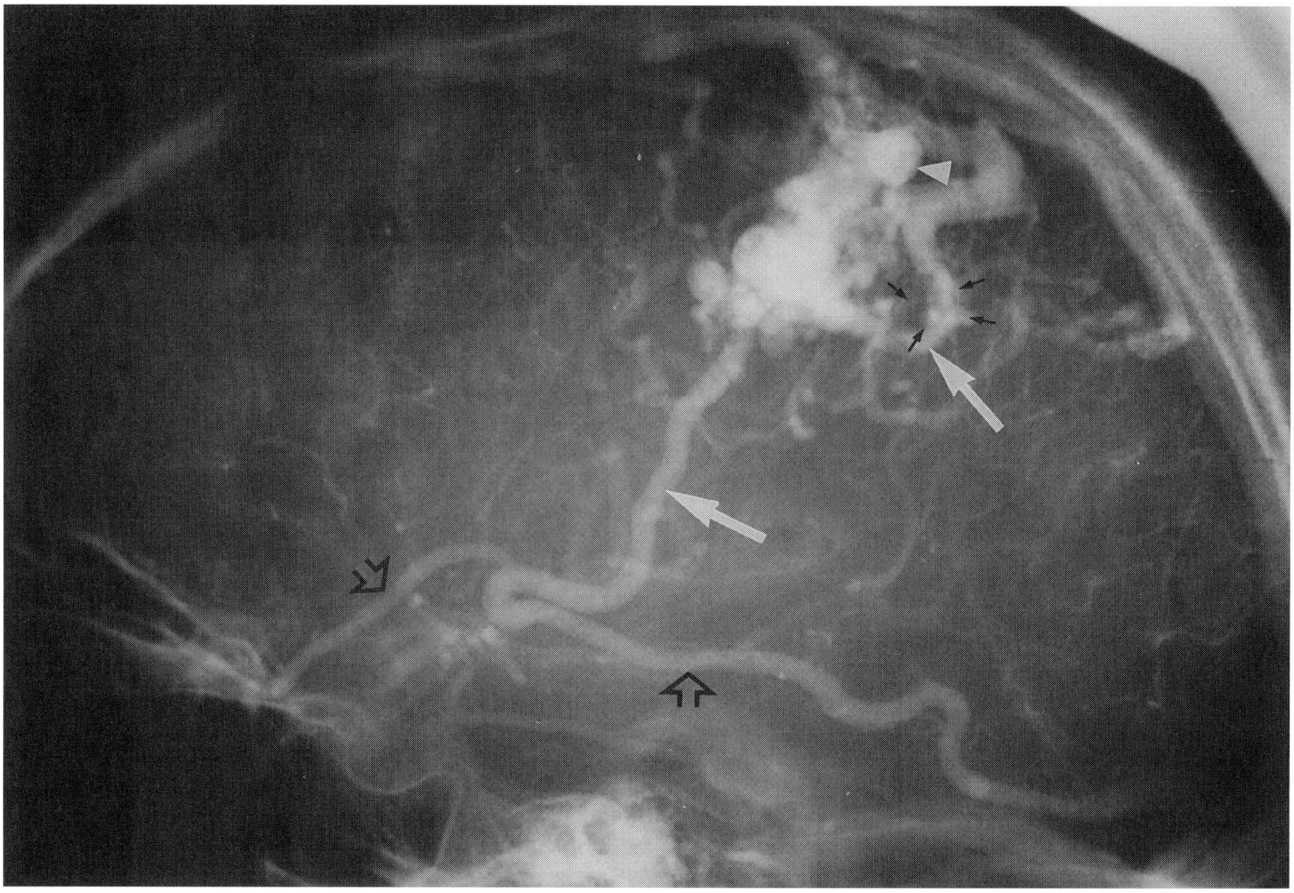

Figure 14D. A lateral view of the late angiographic phase. The smaller posterior compartment (small arrow) is shown inferior to the external end of the major draining vein (arrowhead). This vein is connected to the tortuous vein of Trolard (large arrows), which is continuous to the vein of Labbé (posterior open arrow) and to the sylvian vein (anterior open arrow) (see illustrative case 2). Figure used by permission of Neurological Research. *Continued*

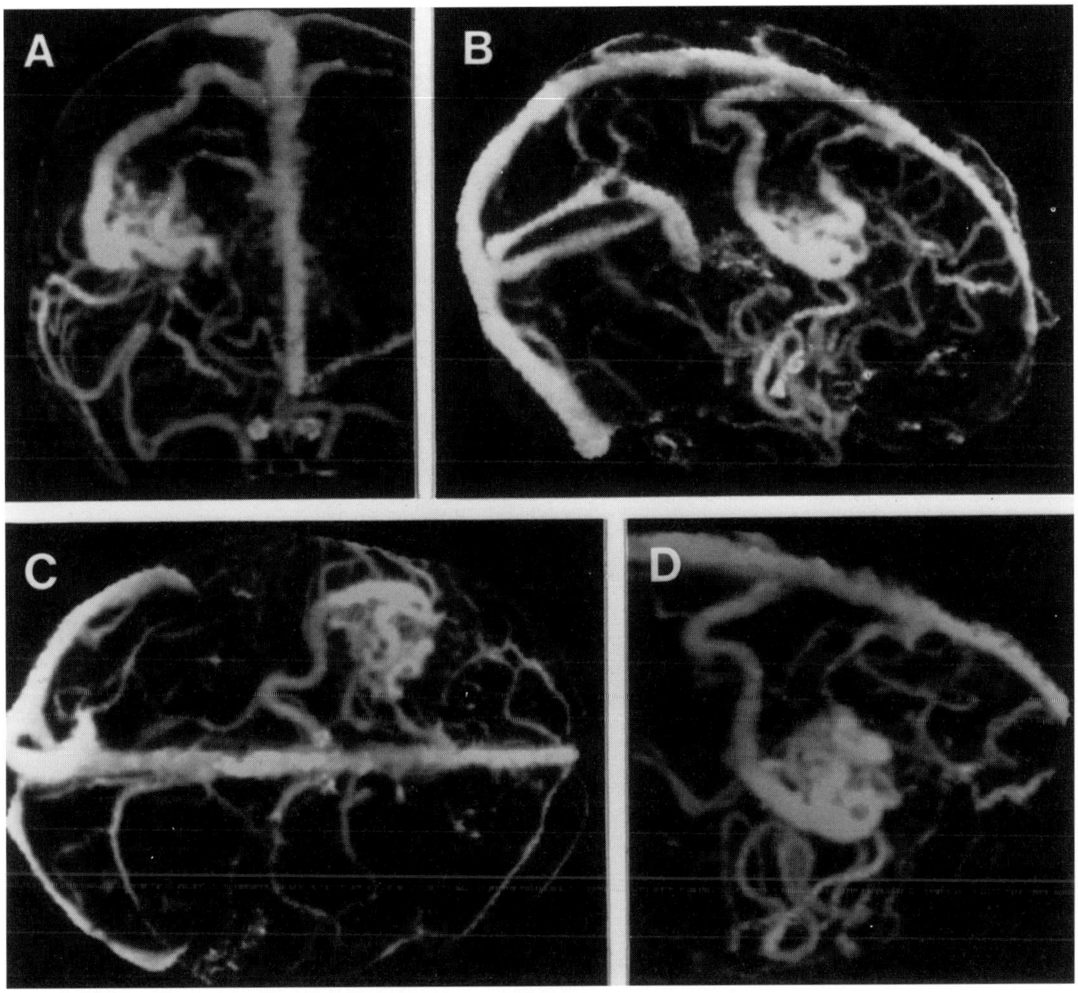

Figure 14E. Four films of a 3-D CT angiogram are shown, depicting different views of the AVM and surrounding vessels. When the films are demonstrated successively in order on the monitor, the observer can form a three-dimensional reconstruction of the vasculature in rotational image.

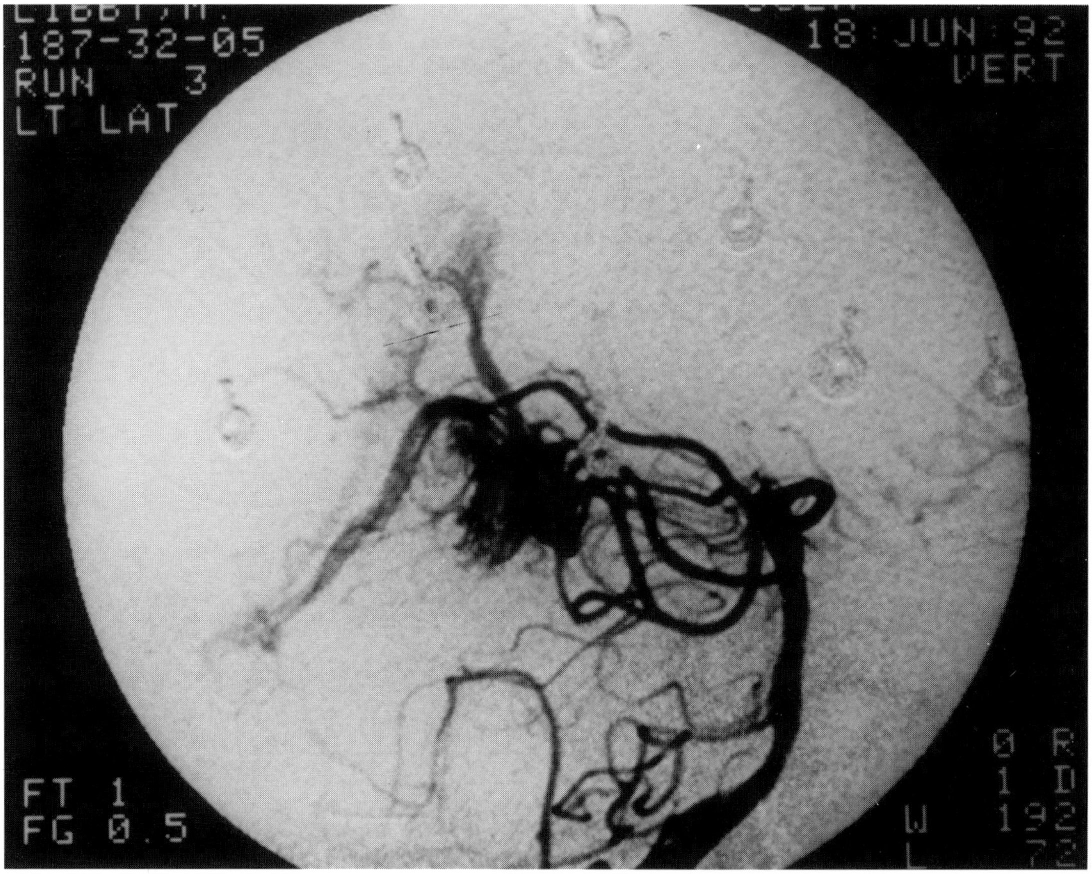

Figure 15A. Vertebral arteriogram demonstrating a cerebellar AVM. *Continued*

Magnetic Resonance Imaging

MRI is the most beneficial diagnostic tool for identifying the anatomical relationships between the AVM core and the feeding arteries, the draining veins, and surrounding vasculature (passively dilated cortical veins). Moreover, MRI is valuable for demonstrating the borders between different compartments (Figure 16A). MRI has the ability to anatomically relate brain structures on the images, such as important gyri and other areas of deep gray and white matter (such as the basal ganglia, thalamus, and internal capsule) with AVM structures. Furthermore, MRI localizes the projection fibers for sensorimotor function (such as in the corona radiata) or optic radiation, and commissural fibers (such as the corpus callosum or anterior commissure) in relation to the AVM. Identification of these fibers will alert surgeons to the proper dissection of the AVM in the future surgery.

Magnetic Resonance Angiography

MRA is especially helpful in defining the small venous loops of the AVM core that are not clearly demonstrated by conventional angiography (Figure 16B). On MRA, these venous loops are seen as small diffuse vascularities extending beyond the angiographically demonstrated AVM core. These vessels may contain juxtanidal vessels and satellite AVMs.

Magnetic Source Imaging

MSI[4,34,123] can demonstrate each small segment of a human body on the precise location of each segmental cortical representation (Figure 17). MSI localizes each segment of the sensory and motor areas in relation to bodily presentations, within an error of 1 mm. This technology detects an electromagnetic field of 50–150 femtotesla (fT, fT $= 10^{-15}$ tesla), generated around the dendrites of pyramidal fibers with the aid of a superconducting quantum interference device (SQUID). The magnetic field is activated by sensory stimulation of different parts of the body (by inflating a small airbag placed on the skin) for somatosensory localization and movement of different portions of the extremities or face for motor localization. Representation of the bodily images in the sulci can be best

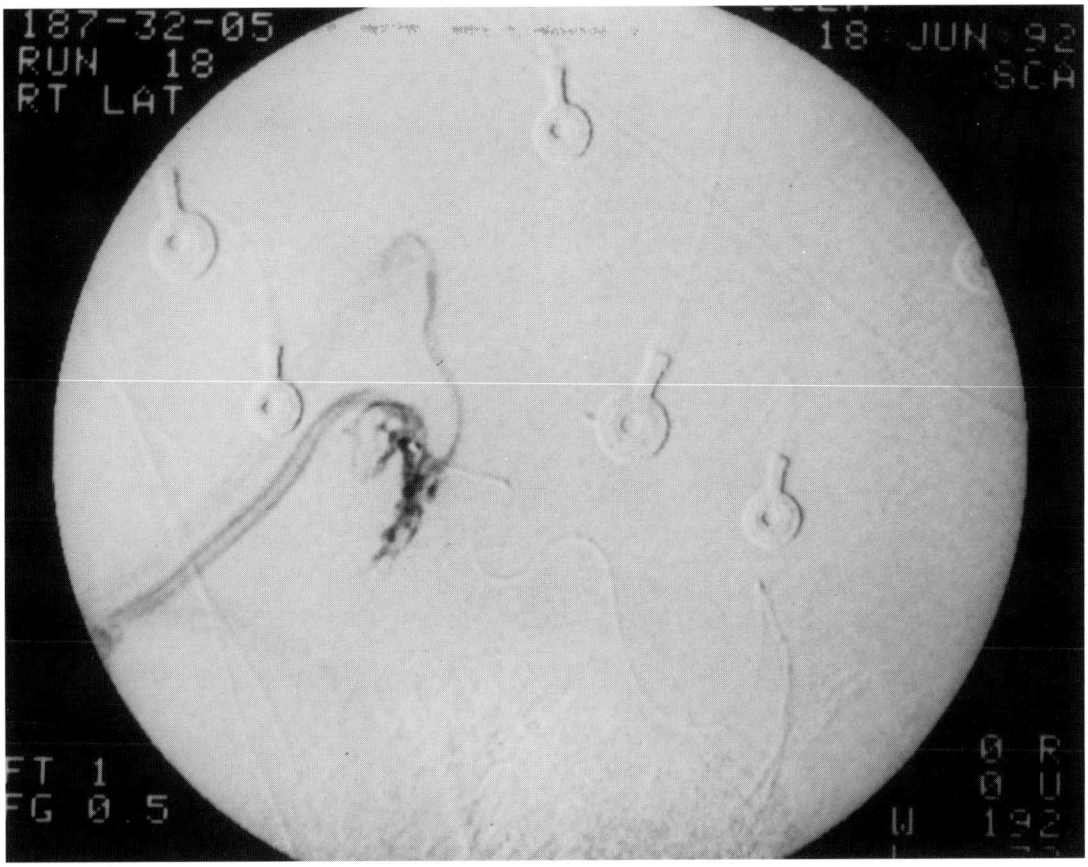

Figure 15B. Superselective angiogram during embolization procedure showing rapid obliteration of the AVM. *Continued*

identified by MSI whereas somatosensory evoked potential (SSEP) recordings, cortical stimulation, and functional MRI determine the localization of the bodily images in the superficial cortex.

MSI is effective in pinpointing the AVM's location beneath the sensorimotor area, as well as AVMs that partially intrude into this area. It electromagnetically determines the precise point of seizure foci, either with sharp waves or slow waves (Figure 18).

Preoperative MSI localization of sensory and motor areas provides a means to determine surgical indications (many neurosurgeons refrain from operating in the sensorimotor area) and plans for a surgical approach. The technique provides a basis for determining the area in the hemispheric surface to enter, where to start, how to extend dissection, and how to avoid damage to the sensorimotor cortex. Intraoperative SSEP recordings also confirm the accuracy of the MSI findings.

Color Doppler Ultrasonography

Intraoperative color Doppler ultrasonography[10,127] provides distinction of vascular structures as colored images: red for blood inflow directed toward the probe, and blue for flow away from it (Figure 19). It provides a practical means to localize AVMs and the course of feeding arteries and draining veins that share arterial blood with the core. It also offers a means to anatomically relate the AVM core to the craniotomy and dural opening, i.e., the depth from the exposed gyri to fissures, sulcal cortex, ventricles, basal ganglia, and thalamus. A three-dimensional (3-D) ultrasonographic imaging can distinguish a feeding artery from a draining vein, and separate the course of the feeding artery as it approaches the crowded AVM core vessels and surrounding cerebral vessels. Color Doppler ultrasonography detects arteries that approach a vascular malformation (venous malformation or cavernous hemangiomas) as the feeder from which shunting arterioles originate and connect to the malformation.

Holography

Holograms of CT angiography provide true 3-D images of the parent data. This technology is an advancement beyond so-called 3-D CT, 3-D MRI, or

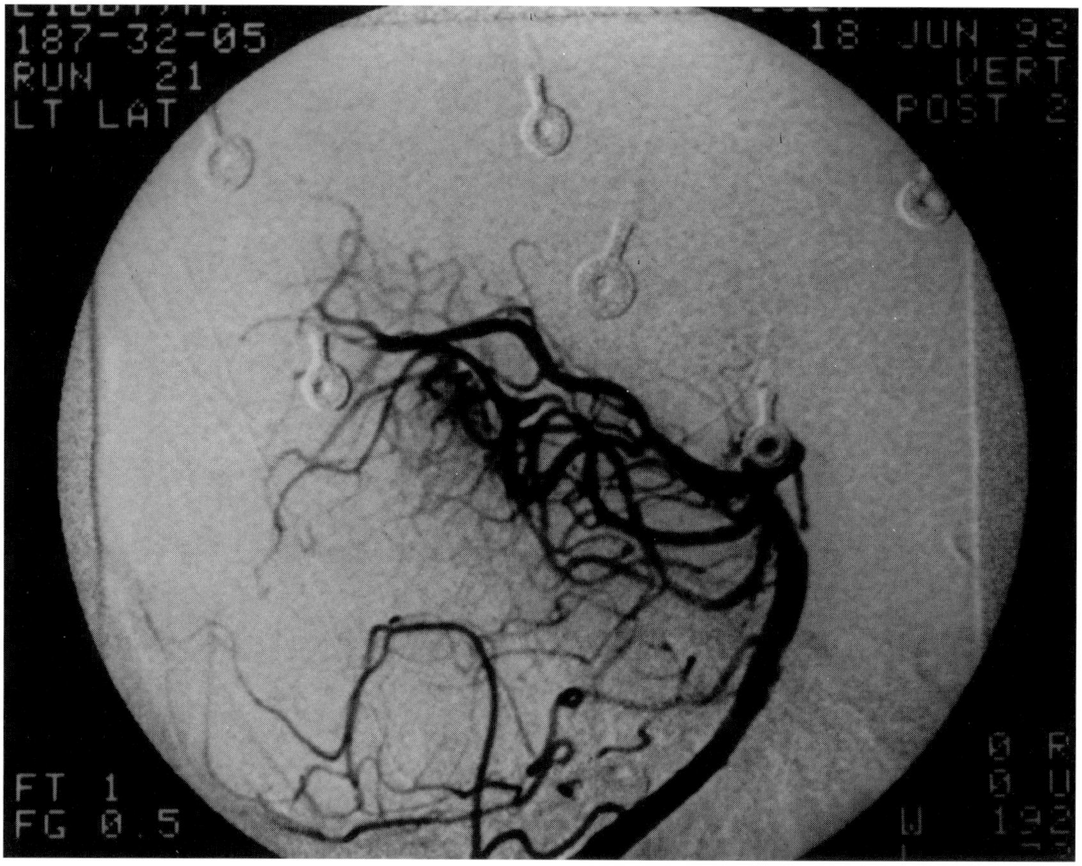

Figure 15C. Vertebral angiogram after embolization showing elimination of the AVM. Photographs courtesy of F. Viñuela, MD.

3-D MRA, where shaded surface renderings, volume renderings, or rotating maximum-intensity projection have been used to attempt depiction of the third dimension on flat display media.

In contrast, holograms are constructed from any number of cross-sectional images (slices) from CT or MRI. Using the Voxbox® equipped with proprietary componentry, the data are projected into space as tangible 3-D images.

Angiographic holograms, or Voxgrams® made from CT data, allow visualization of an AVM in the space inside the skull and demonstrate exact anatomical relationships. The anatomical structures in the rear of the volume are not obscured by those in front. Small vessels and the venous anatomy of AVMs can be clearly visualized, i.e., small draining veins are distinguishable from feeding arteries. Voxgram images permit clinical interaction with the data. Each of the feeding arteries and major draining veins can be traced with a instrument or pointer as it approaches the AVM core. The junction of the major draining vein to the cortical veins can be clearly visualized. This image demonstration facilitates identifying the junction of the external end of the major draining vein as it connects to the cortical vein. The crowded area between feeding arteries and AVM core indicates the presence of the connecting shunting arterioles. Careful observation of the 3-D images enables the surgeon to examine every characteristic of the pathology from an extensive range of angles and facilitates effective presurgical planning.[5,49]

Principles of AVM Treatment

It is generally accepted that treatment of AVMs is essential to prevent hemorrhage. A key to such treatment is defining what protocol best fits a patient's situation. Modern technology has made three modes of treatment practical for AVMs: (1) direct microsurgical intervention, (2) intravascular intervention, e.g., embolization, balloon insertion, or wire coiling,[28,36,39,45,51,59,98] and (3) radiosurgery.[15,26,31,52,60,105] Of these treatment modes, surgical resection will likely continue to be the primary treatment procedure, with embolization as an adjunct to the surgical treatment. Radiosurgery is indicated for treatment of AVMs that are less than 2.5–3.0 cm in diameter.[97,105] A combination of two or three

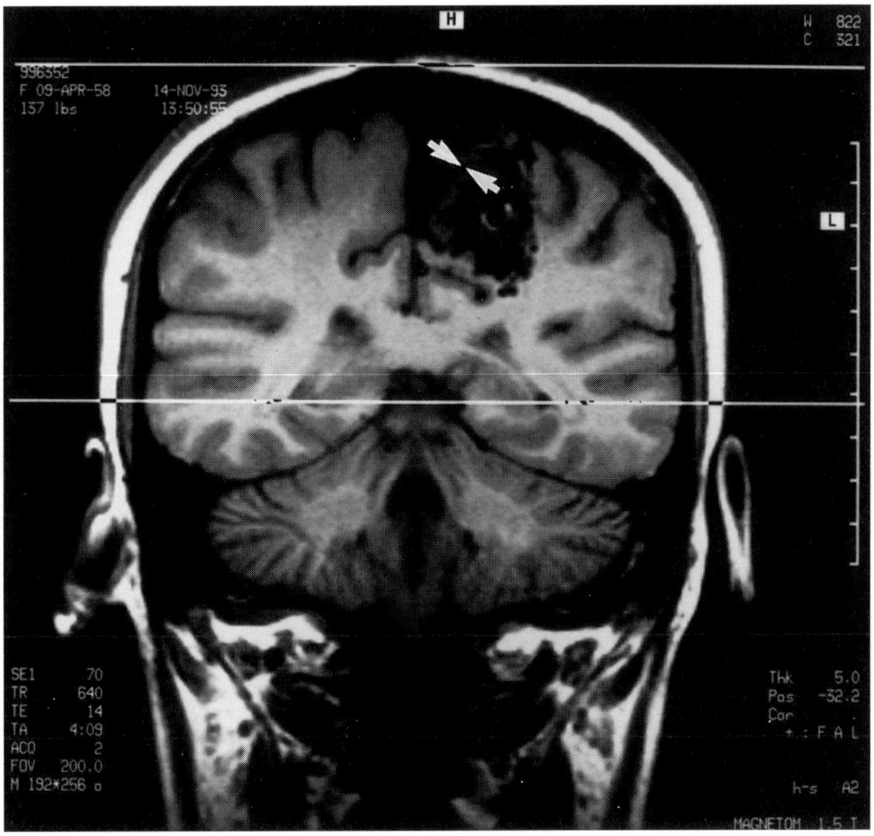

Figure 16A. This sensorimotor AVM had four compartments, but only two compartments are seen in this film. The medial and lateral compartments are separated by a low flow void that appeared to be a partition-like divider (arrows). *Continued*

of these treatment modes is considered appropriate for large AVMs in any location, including the functional areas.

The authors believe that surgical intervention for AVMs in the sensorimotor, speech, and visual areas is feasible, with acceptably low mortality and morbidity rates and a positive prognosis for a useful life. In contrast, results from the use of embolization and irradiation for AVMs in these regions have not been clearly established.

Surgical treatment or embolization of AVMs in the capsulostriatothalamic areas has been reported.[56,100,101,124] However, radiosurgery may play an important role in treating AVMs in these areas, particularly when such AVMs are diffuse.

The statistics for patients with AVMs in the brain stem, and their mode of treatment, are limited.[25,56] Surgical intervention has been advocated for those AVMs located in the superficial layers of the brain stem, or those surrounded by a hematoma. Indications for embolization and radiosurgery must be determined on an individual basis. Cavernous hemangiomas do not have angiographically demonstrable feeding arteries or draining veins, and resist radiosurgery and embolization for their elimination. Surgical resection of cavernous hemangiomas in the brain stem has recently become effective in preventing hemorrhage and for securing a useful life in many patients.

Factors Involved in the Surgical Treatment of AVMs

To rationalize any mode of treatment for AVM patients, the following two assumptions must be fulfilled. First, the safety and benefit of each treatment must statistically supersede the advantage of conservative treatment. Such statistical considerations include: (1) a comparison of the mortality and morbidity of the natural history versus those related to treatment, (2) a comparison of the incidence of AVM bleeding relative to patient age, (3) the condition of the AVM (size and location), (4) the timing of surgery, and (5) the incidence of seizures. The second assumption is that the advantage of treatment must be individualized according to the AVM location, size, arterial and venous connections, and the patient's condition.

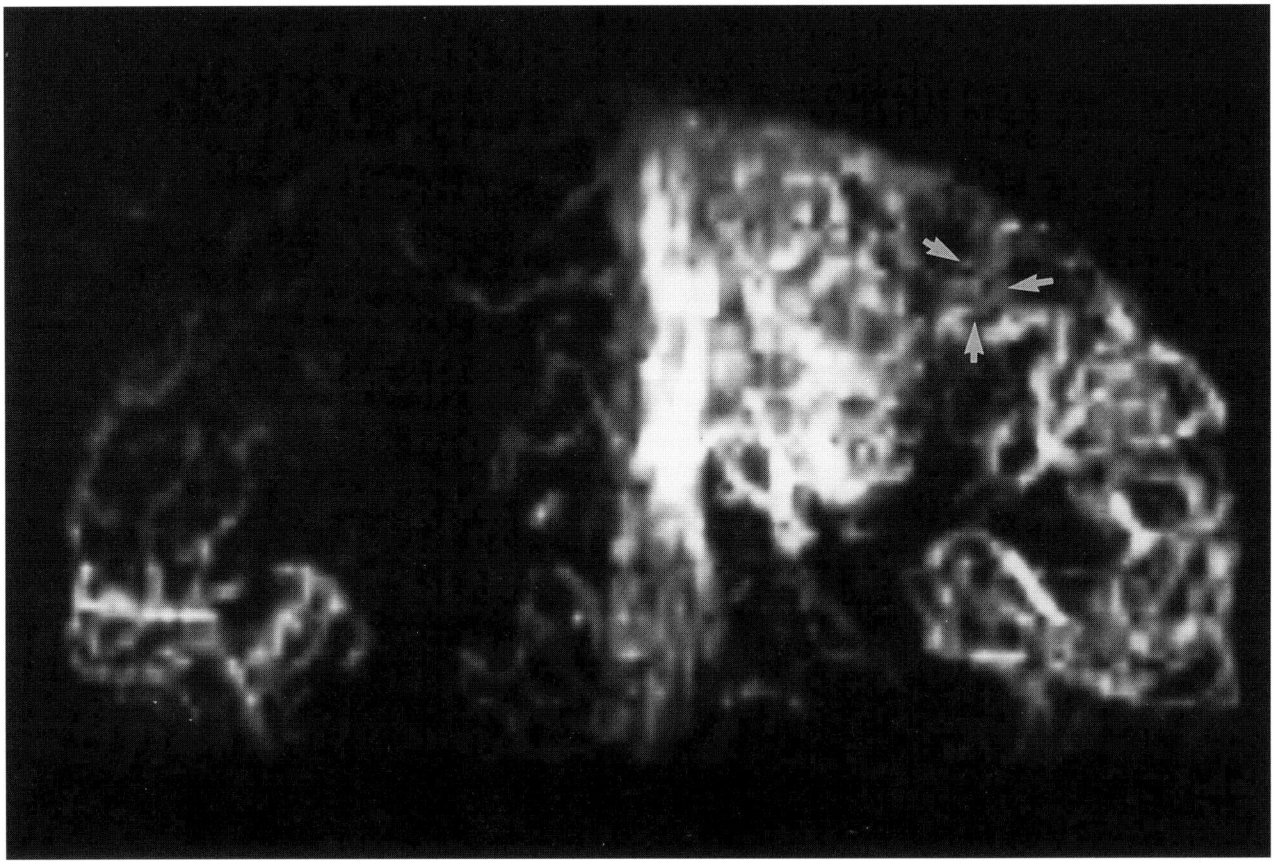

Figure 16B. An MRA of the same AVM showing a cluster of fine vessels (arrows) lateral to the lateral compartment, either a satellite AVM or crowded juxtanidal veins that were not identified in MRI.

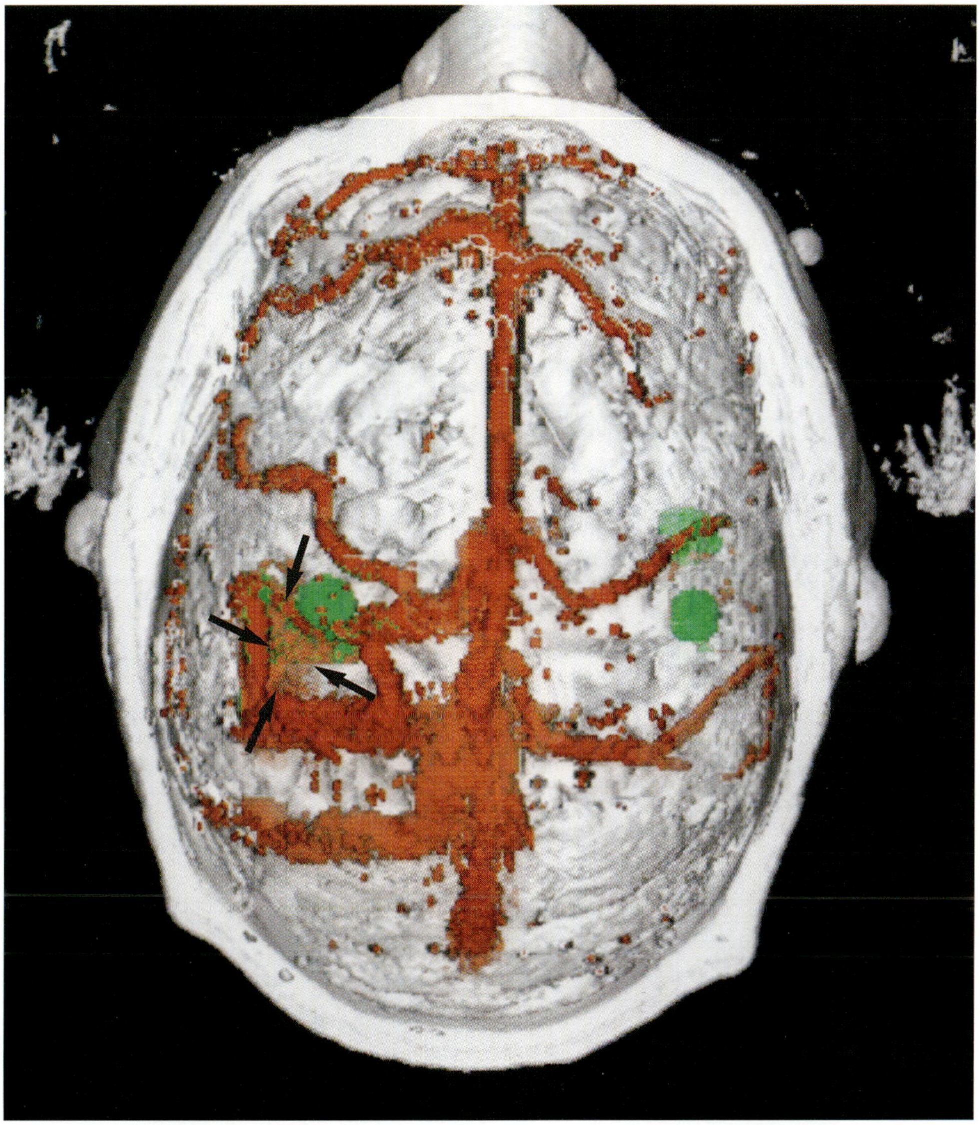

Figure 17. Magnetic source imaging (MSI) depicts a noninvasive representation of various parts of the body in motor and sensory area. This 3-D image shows a sensory arm region by a green square overlying the subcortical AVM (arrows), which is surrounded by dilated cortical vein (red areas). Note the arm region is in contact with the AVM.

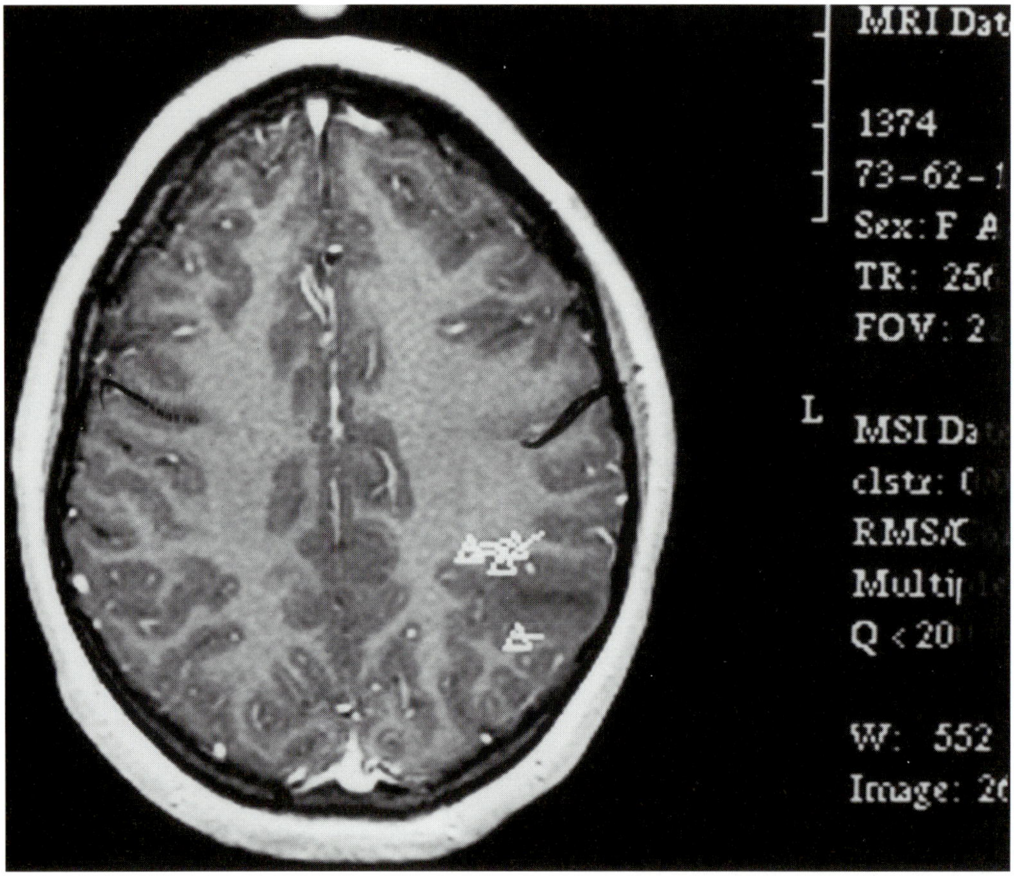

Figure 18. Triangles indicate precise locations of sharp waves in MSI, signifying seizure foci.[34]

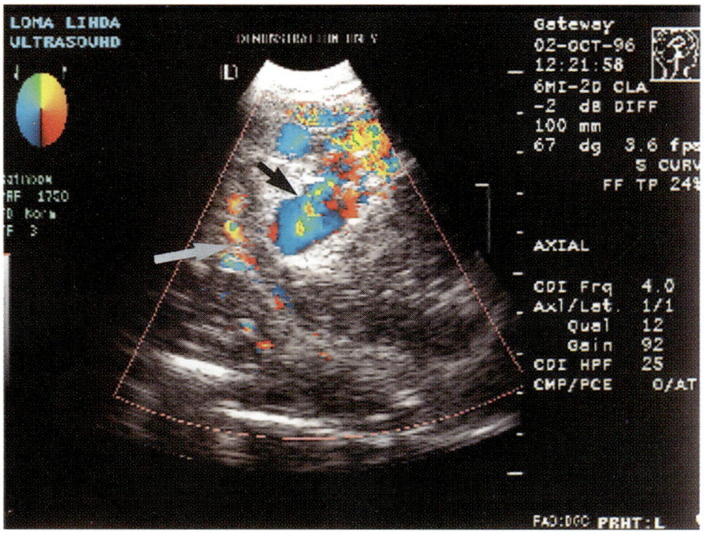

Figure 19. Color Doppler ultrasonography is an effective study for identifying the AVM core, feeding arteries (white arrow), and draining veins (black arrow). The imaging allows the surgeon to accurately follow the draining vein, particularly a tortuous vein in the sulcus. The size, depth of the superficial side, and the depth of the deep side of the AVM are calculated. Since shunting arterioles are too small to be identified without a microscope, the surgeon must locate these shunting arterioles crowded near the feeding artery without exposing this artery which passes inside the brain.

Mortality and Morbidity

Natural history studies have shown that approximately 15%–20% of AVM patients perish within 15 years, and 40% of the survivors develop mild to severe neurological signs, including weakness, numbness, and speech or visual difficulty.[11,16,29,32,38,42,50,58,68,69,71,82,96,108] Inference can be made that morbidity and probably mortality rates in patients with AVMs in functional areas would be significantly higher than those in silent areas.

Surgical resection of AVMs can be justified despite its mortality (<5%) and morbidity (4%) rates.[21,40,44] The rationale for surgical treatment in AVM patients came about by comparing the risks of surgery versus the risks of allowing the AVM to remain untreated. If the same circumstances for aneurysm patients are examined, statistics clearly indicate that surgery is justified. For example, a natural history study of patients harboring a ruptured aneurysm shows a 50% mortality rate within 2 months of the initial hemorrhage.[106] In contrast, the surgical mortality during prompt treatment of grades 1 and 2 aneurysms is only 1%–5%. Unquestionably, if it is deemed technically feasible and risk factors are properly considered, surgical intervention for an aneurysm is warranted. Although the justification for surgical resection of AVMs is not as dramatic as for aneurysms,[20,24,35,44,53,65,72,89,100–102,110,111,113,115] the statistics similarly show that surgery is justified. The authors' current series had a mortality rate of only 0.7% and a morbidity rate of 4% (only mild neurological deficit or slight worsening of symptoms) for surgical resection of AVMs located in the functional area. Considering the 15%–20% mortality and the 25%–40% morbidity in patients with AVMs in all locations over 15 years, the data showing the mortality and morbidity of AVMs in functional areas are in favor of surgical rather than palliative treatment. With current knowledge, procedures, diagnostic studies, and technology, the surgical benefits clearly outweigh the risk of surgery, especially when considering the results of conservative treatment.

Patient Age

Among the risk factors considered in making decisions about AVM treatment is the patient's age. The reason for this consideration is that the highest incidence of bleeding is in the youngest age group. It is suggested that with conservative treatment only, 50% of teenagers survive without neurological deficits through the first 15 years after detection of the AVM. The person must live through each successive 15-year period with the same risk he/she had during the first 15-year period. The inference can be made that the younger the patient with an AVM, the higher the incidence of neurological deficit as he/she lives longer.

AVM Size and Location

Other risk factors are AVM size and location, especially if the AVM is located in a functional area. Earlier studies have confirmed that larger AVMs offer greater surgical risk.[102,103,111] Early studies also suggested that AVM location was the primary surgical concern. For example, several authors have stated that en bloc resection in functional areas will likely lead to neurological deficits.[2,44,77,80,90,93,108] Such concerns are similar to those for resection of an epileptic focus or glioma infiltrating the functional areas.[83]

In contrast, Tönnis[110] emphasized that the size of an AVM is the major factor for risks involved in resection. His conclusion was based on the total removal of AVMs in 123 cases with intracranial AVMs, 96 (86%) of which were in the functional area. He stated that the location of an AVM in the functional area did not, in itself, contraindicate direct intervention. Rather, contraindications were the presence of a large AVM and an elderly age of the patient; either or both of these factors could produce serious complications.

Timing of Surgery

The timing of AVM surgery is an important concern. Bleeding does not require emergency surgical intervention. Only a small AVM identified on CT or MRI may be resected at the time of decompressive evacuation of a large hematoma immediately after AVM rupture. Likewise, occult AVMs that are only microscopically recognized can be removed at the time of operation for hematoma removal. The advantages of delaying direct intervention over emergency surgery for a ruptured AVM include:

1. Angiographic detail can be better outlined preoperatively and the appropriate surgical approach combined with other modes of treatment can be better planned.
2. Dissection of AVMs can be done with less damage to surrounding brain structure and function. This is because early after bleeding, the brain is fragile and edematous. Over time, it becomes firmer and more resistant to surgical insult, and it is easier to develop cleavage between these structures.
3. Rebleeding from an AVM can be prevented or minimized by maintaining normal blood pressure or inducing hypotension pharmacologically (mean arte-

rial pressure [MAP] 60–80 mm Hg). Control of MAP utilizes the hemodynamic characteristics of AVMs, that is, the pulsation of the AVM becomes minimum when a MAP is decreased to 60 mm Hg. Even with a slightly higher pressure, the dampening effects of arterial pressure inside the AVM core and in the draining veins lower the incidence of bleeding.

Incidence of Seizures

More than 50% of patients with AVMs develop generalized or focal seizures. Focal seizures are typical in patients with AVMs in functional areas. Indications for surgical removal of AVMs in these patients are failure of seizure control with medication, worsening of seizures (frequency and severity), progressive neurological deficits associated with seizures, and seizures associated with paroxysmal throbbing headaches. Based on the authors' surgical experience, these signs and symptoms are indicative of hemorrhages from an AVM.

Patients with AVMs in the temporal lobe often present with temporal lobe seizures. Those with AVMs in the dominant superior temporal lobe show speech difficulty simultaneously with or after seizures. Based on publishedsurgical statistics,[35,119] many or all of the AVMs had evidence of hemorrhage, even though presenting symptoms were seizures or throbbing headaches.

Controversy still exists whether a seizure disorder itself constitutes an indication for elimination of an AVM. Some believe that an AVM in patients with a history of occasional seizures should not be aggressively treated. Their conclusion derives from the following findings: (1) not all of these patients become seizure-free after AVM elimination, and (2) often seizure foci (on electroencephalography (EEG) were found in areas remote from the AVM or on the contralateral side.

From the authors' experience, surgical procedures to resect the AVMs in seizure patients are justified because: (1) all patients had evidence of hemorrhage around the AVM at operation, and (2) seizure foci demonstrated by EEG or MSI, regardless of presence of foci close to or remote from the AVM or both, often diminished or disappeared after surgery.

Grading System

A grading system for decision-making in AVM surgery[99,102] is a practical method of evaluating surgical safety. Spetzler and Martin graded the risk for AVM surgery (grades 1–6) by totaling the risk of each of various categories, such as location, size, venous drainage, and age of the patient. The significance of location (functional area) was graded low. Apparently, this grading system was based mainly on mortality, rather than on morbidity risks.

Based on the authors' experience, points assigned for AVM grading by Spetzler require modification when AVMs in functional areas are graded. The AVMs extending subcortically and partially underneath the sensorimotor or speech area may be assigned point 1. Those totally surrounded by sensory, motor, and speech-related neurons or giant AVMs (>6 cm from our measurement) should be assigned point 2. The readers must be reminded that the diameter of the AVMs that we present is a calculated diameter of the sphere with the volume equal to the AVM volume; therefore, a 6-cm diameter of our AVMs is considerably larger than AVMs with 6 cm as the largest diameter (other diameters are usually smaller). When the AVM undermines the functional cortices and extends to the neighboring brain structure in two or more directions, the grading should be point 3.

AVM Surgery

History of AVM Surgery

AVM Surgery in General

In the 1920s and 1930s, the pioneers of modern neurosurgery[17–19,91] attempted to resect AVMs with surgical techniques similar to those used for brain tumors. Such surgery was not usually successful since a common occurrence of such AVM dissection was unexpected uncontrollable bleeding. The difficulty in understanding the hemodynamics of AVMs discouraged such surgery for this anomaly. Cerebral angiography, developed by Moniz[70] in 1927, was the first contribution to the hemodynamic imaging of normal as well as abnormal vasculature, including AVMs. However, it was not until 1957 when Olivecrona and Ladenheim[77] published a monograph describing their en bloc resection technique that AVM surgery in the silent area became relatively safe and acceptable as a standard technique. Although the operative mortality of patients with AVMs in the silent area was 9% and the serious postoperative morbidity rate was 4%, these figures represented an astonishingly low complication rate at that time.

A key advance in AVM surgery was the introduction of microsurgery by Yasargil[129] in 1969 and the invention of bipolar forceps cautery by Malis.[62] These technological advances allowed precise AVM surgery, which reduced the mortality rate of AVM resection to 5% or less by the 1980s,[21,40,

[44,58,69,75,89,95,104,107,113,114] and further stimulated the development of surgical techniques for AVMs in functional areas.

Surgery for AVMs in Functional Areas

Perhaps the greatest concern in AVM surgery is that 35%–70% of AVM patients harbor this anomaly in functional areas.[53,82,111] Although there is no established natural history of these AVM patients, the mortality and morbidity rates for these patients without treatment is expected to be much higher and more serious than those for patients with AVMs in the silent area. Unfortunately there is a paucity of literature addressing whether surgical intervention in the functional areas should be a goal of treatment for such AVMs. This paucity is likely due to the reluctance of neurosurgeons to accept the high risk inherent in surgery of these AVMs.

Prior to Microsurgical Technique Development: AVM surgery in functional areas was done predominantly by en bloc resection and its modifications prior to the development of microsurgical procedures. This procedure involved removing brain tissue surrounding the AVM[30,77,81,92,93] and clipping the feeding arteries, which were angiographically demonstrable. As a result, the procedure compromised circulation in many vascular branches distributed throughout the brain tissue surrounding the AVM. Nevertheless, this was a procedure practiced by Olivecrona and many other neurosurgeons at that time; however, Olivecrona[77] warned against applying this technique to AVMs located in functional (sensorimotor, speech, and visual) areas. His appropriate advice was based on technical difficulties, which limited the neurosurgeons' capacity to preserve the function of these areas.

Throughout the pre-microsurgery era, AVM surgery in functional areas was debated by many surgeons. For example, Krayenbühl and Yasargil (personal communication, 1967) recommended surgical intervention for lesions located in the functional area only when severe neurological deficits were present. Houdart[48] considered the risk of AVM surgery in the motor area to be greater than the natural history of neurologically disabling deficits.

Despite concerns about preserving brain function, resection of AVMs in functional areas was performed. Pool[93] described total resection of small AVMs in the sensorimotor area. Removal of AVMs in the motor and speech areas was also reported by Kunicki[54] and by Zoltan.[133] Of Zoltan's 38 patients, 28 patients (74%) remained in good health, 5 (13%) died, and 5 (13%) had temporary hemiplegia. These authors attributed the success of AVM resection in motor, sensory, and speech areas, in general, to the fact that vessels comprising the anomaly were not essential to the cerebral circulation, and the parenchyma within and immediately adjacent to the AVM was not "functional" brain tissue. Others postulated that the AVMs surgically treated by these surgeons were not located in the functional areas, or there was evidence of transfer of function to another area.[7,23]

Kunc[53] published the first detailed report on direct resection of AVMs in or near the motor or speech areas. In 15 of 18 patients, there were severe neurological deficits before surgery. Using magnifying glasses, he removed the AVM in all 18 patients, resulting in only one case of permanent postoperative disability and one death due to a later rupture of a partially removed AVM. However, no new technical development was described in detail except for the removal of AVMs close to the border between the AVM and its surrounding tissue. Although the sizes of the AVMs were small or medium by current classifications, this report is notable for its consideration that the site of an AVM may constitute a greater risk factor for morbidity than its size.

After the Development of Microsurgery: After the development of microneurosurgery by Malis and Yasargil[62,129] in 1969, Drake,[24] Mullan,[72] and Wilson[113] separately in 1979 and DaPian[20] in 1980 described AVM surgery in functional areas and discussed the intricacies involved in this surgical treatment and its complications. Based on his experience with 16 cases, Drake [24] concluded that medium and large AVMs located in the speech and rolandic areas and even small AVMs in the basal ganglia constituted increased risk for neurological complications. Heros[44] has an opinion similar to that of Drake.

New Technical Development for Resection in the Functional Areas: In 1982, a surgical procedure designed specifically for AVMs located in functional areas was described.[115] This procedure was designed and performed according to the newly described AVM hemodynamic anatomy. In 18 cases, there was no mortality and only one case of homonymous hemianopia as a significant morbidity. All patients returned to normal activity. Other recent reports of resection of AVMs in functional areas have been published,[13,65,86,100–102,112,125] specifically in the visual area[65] and in the capsulostriatothalamic area.[56,100,101]

Despite these achievements, for many years it was believed to be impossible to resect AVMs in the sensorimotor and speech areas without causing excessive neurological deficits.[44] Even now, many are skeptical about such AVM resection, based on the known risks inherent in surgery to excise tumors (e.g., falx meningiomas totally covered by functional cortices in the convexity) or epileptogenic foci in functional areas by en bloc resection.

More recently, important advances in the understanding of the hemodynamics of AVMs and of brain structures surrounding AVMs, as well as surgical techniques designed specifically for AVMs, have prompted more positive evaluations of AVM surgery in functional areas.[119] However, the following areas of concern remain:

1. Blood vessels of AVMs are intermingled with functional brain tissue.
2. Brain tissue has to be removed to reach the AVMs, which are almost always located subcortically.
3. Feeding arteries that appear from subcortical depth to the cortical surface travel into the subcortical depth again, sending many branches to functional cortices before directly connecting to the AVM core.
4. In large AVMs, the courses of feeding arteries relative to the AVM are often unpredictable, based on the knowledge obtained from angiograms; connections of juxtanidal veins and draining veins to cortical veins over the convexity and mesial surface of the hemisphere are extremely complex.

Surgical Techniques

Anesthesia

Chapter 4 is dedicated to anesthesia for AVM surgery in or adjacent to the functional area.

SSEP recordings[12,119,121] are of great value in determining the location of the sensory cortex and motor cortex (interpreted from phase reversal from sensory cortex), detecting abnormalities in sensory pathways, functional impairment of cerebral function due to excessive hypotension, or increased intracranial pressure from hematoma formation or impaired cerebrospinal fluid (CSF) circulation. Bipolar stimulation of the median, ulnar, tibial, or common peroneal nerve is a common method to elicit responses in the sensory cortex through a monopolar electrode placed directly on the cortical surface or parietal scalp corresponding to the area of the homuncular presentation of stimulated body. For correlation of MSI and SSEP,[33,34] median nerve stimulation is adapted. Cortical stimulation for motor, sensory, and speech areas is described in detail in another chapter. We do not use cortical stimulation[8,36,64] under local anesthesia because our surgical techniques avoid removal of the neurons involved in motor, sensory, and speech functions. General anesthesia prevents patients from becoming excited from headaches, nausea and vomiting, fear, awareness or misunderstanding of what is going on in the surgery suite, and most importantly, any event that may cause a sudden rise in the blood pressure. Unexpected rupture of the AVM and brain swelling interferes with the smooth performance of the operation.

Controlled hypotension, although rarely necessary for AVMs in the silent area, is vital for safe dissection of AVMs in the functional areas.[24,115,119] It minimizes bleeding during dissection of the wall of aneurysmal dilatations, and during the exposure of the deep side of the AVM core and draining veins connected to venous sinuses. Mean arterial blood pressure (MABP) below 60 mm Hg, induced by intravenous titration of sodium nitroprusside (Nipride)[120] markedly reduces AVM pulsation and minimizes rupture of AVM vessels. Controlled hypotension utilizes the fact that blood "steal"[27,55,67] into the AVM is diverted back into the cerebrovascular bed while the mean pressure is lowered to 60 mm Hg or below.[89,120] When bleeding occurs from venous loops, however, pulsatile expansion of the entire AVM core develops, and it may be necessary to dampen pulsatile pressure by lowering MABP to between 40 mm Hg and 50 mm Hg. Fortunately, studies of SSEPs and reduction/oxidation activity of cytochrome oxidase indicate that brain metabolism and electrophysiology are not significantly compromised until MABP falls below 40 mm Hg.[120,122] Even this MABP is not an absolute threshold since in 4 of our 56 patients, unexpected bleeding decreased MABP to between 25 mm Hg and 30 mm Hg for approximately 45 minutes, but these patients recovered without apparent physical or neurological consequences.

Patient Positioning (Figure 20)

Patients should be positioned on the table without strain to the head and neck, extremities, chest, or abdomen. The patient's position should provide sufficient space for a microscope and other instruments to be accommodated in the area. Stimulating electrodes for SSEP recordings may be inserted to the median, ulnar, tibial, or common peroneal nerve, but should not interfere with arterial and venous catheter lines. Any pressure or strain to the vascular system in the head and neck must be prevented to avoid kinking the internal jugular vein at the base of the skull. The shoulder may be pulled down gently, with one end of the tape placed on the shoulder and the

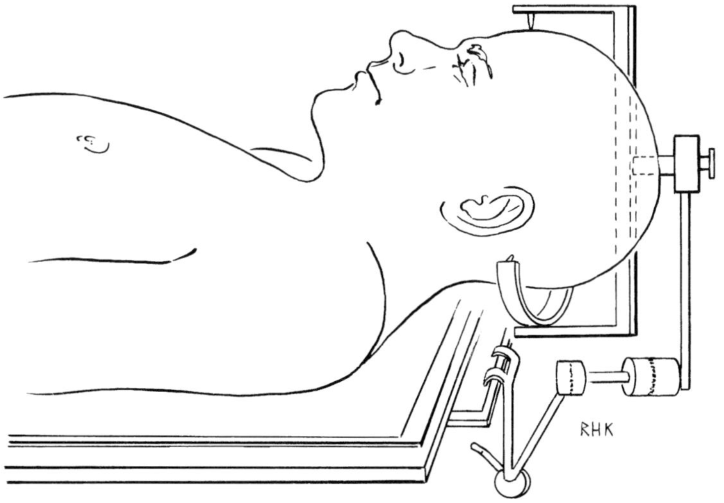

Figure 20. The patient must be positioned so that there is no strain on any part of the body, especially the carotid and vertebral arteries and the jugular veins. The Mayfield clamp is used to stabilize the head against the operating table. This head immobilization secures the stability of the retractors, which are held to the head ring or operating table bar.

other end on the side of the table, while the patient is placed in the lateral or half lateral–half supine position.

Careful positioning of the patient avoids hard traction on the shoulder and stretching of the upper trunk of the brachial plexus, which can result in temporary or permanent paralysis (Erb-Duchenne type). The chest and abdomen must be free of compression, which causes increased intrathoracic or abdominal pressure and consequently results in an increase in intracranial venous pressure.

The operating table may be bent in the middle, so the patient's head may be elevated above the heart, and the legs may be raised above the horizontal level. This position reduces intracranial pressure and cerebral venous pressure appropriately and reduces inadvertent blood loss from the AVM. Elevation of the head by tilting the table in a reverse Trendelenburg's position should be avoided because orthostatic hypotension may be precipitated by even a smal amount of sudden blood loss under anesthesia, particularly while controlled hypotension is being used.

The head may be immobilized in a Mayfield clamp to prevent unexpected head movement during microsurgery, particularly while the AVM core or draining vein is being dissected (Figure 20). This immobilizer may be attached to the Greenberg retraction apparatus (Codman Co.), a circular frame that surrounds the craniotomy (e.g., Budde halo [Codman Co.]), or the Yasargil-Leyla retractor (Aesculap), in order to maintain stability of the head and instrumentation during dissection of the AVM. It is usually most convenient to have the craniotomy site or the entrance through the cortical surface placed at the highest part of the head. Exceptions may be practiced in unusual cases, such as: (1) when a small AVM is located near the mesial surface and the brain can be retracted away from the falx, the head may be tilted to the side of the lesion so that the brain can sag with gravity, thus negating the use of a retractor; and (2) during dissection of an AVM from the cortex and immediate subcortical layer, the retractor must be placed underneath the motor cortex from the premotor area. In such a case, the head may be tilted slightly backward, so that the brain will fall posteriorly as the sensorimotor cortices are gently retracted outward, away from the AVM (Figure 21).

AVMs located in the occipital area may be approached through an occipital craniotomy, with the patient in the prone position and the head and neck in the neutral position and immobilized with a Mayfield clamp. The authors do not place the patient in the sitting position because the pulsatile effect to the AVM venous loops does not change in this position unless MAP is reduced to 60 mm Hg. The authors prefer to reduce AVM pulsation by controlled, rather than by orthostatic, hypotension.

Surgical Procedures in General

The craniotomy must be large enough to cover the entire diameter of each of two dimensions of the AVM (e.g., sagittal and coronal or vertical diameters). The dura is opened circumferentially in a rectangular

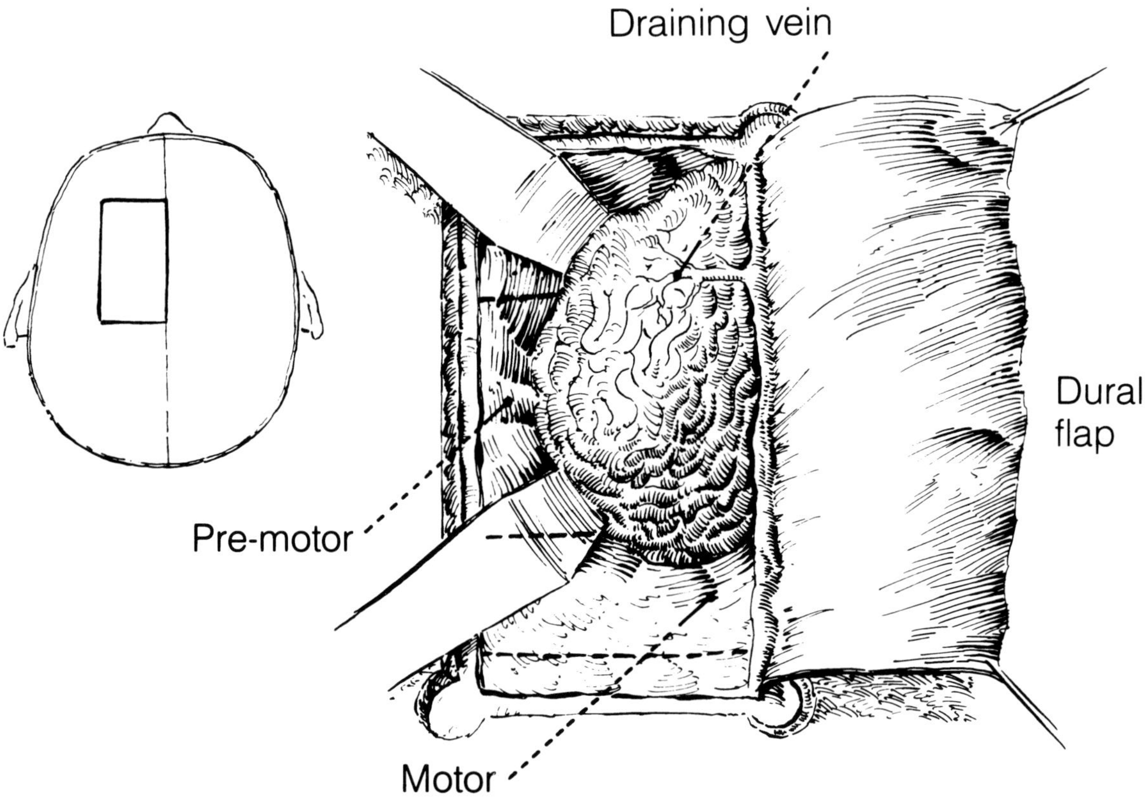

Figure 21. The craniotomy must be large enough to expose the entire two diameters of the AVM. This allows the surgeon adequate vision for dissection of the AVM. A craniotomy and dural opening that is too small interferes with insertion of retractors to surround the AVM core. Dissection of the AVM underneath the sensorimotor cortex through an opening in the premotor area requires the extension of the head and neck to allow the cortex to sag posteriorly by its own weight.

or semicircular shape (Figure 21). This opening should be outside the area crowded with the cortical veins that are dilated with arterial blood.

If the dura is adherent to an area of cortical veins dilated with arterial blood, separation of this dural portion from the cortex must be avoided. Cauterization of these cortical veins may result in propagation of thrombosis to the vein of Trolard and vein of Labbé, which may cause temporary or permanent neurological deficit. In such a circumstance, the dural flap may be incised in a radial fashion to isolate a circular island of the dura adherent to the dilated cortical veins.

Bleeding from small core vessels (<500 μm) with arterial blood is often resistant to effective coagulation by electrocautery, probably because of fragility of anomalous veins under arterial pressure. It is best to place a small piece of Surgicel on the bleeding vessels, cover them with a cottonoid patty of an appropriate size, and apply gentle pressure with a suction tip (#3 or #5 gauge). Continuous irrigation with normal saline solution enhances hemostasis.

The pia mater must be kept intact. Otherwise, there may be interference to the surgical procedure by blood quickly filling the subarachnoid space or infiltrating subpially when bleeding occurs from the AVM or cortical veins dilated under arterial pressure.

Access to the AVM Core: Either the transcortical or the transsulcal approach is acceptable if the entry is located in the nonfunctional area. The transcortical approach has been practiced by the senior author for medially located AVMs or deep gray matter AVMs. However, the AVM totally surrounded by functional gray and white matter must be approached by following the major draining vein that travels in the sulcus.

Operative Hemostasis: One of the important techniques to successful resection of AVMs is to promptly control bleeding from the core and surrounding vessels before blood flooding occurs in the area and interferes with cauterization of bleeding vessels, or infiltrates into the brain tissue. Bleeding during careful cauterization of small vessels can occur at any time, even with copious amounts of saline irrigation. This is because thin-walled venules can rupture before coagulation is adequately completed. Bipolar coagulating forceps that are insulated, except for the fine tips, should be quickly placed around the venules for prompt cauterization. Sometimes rupture occurs at the junction of the venules to a venous loop of the core. This situation can result in a larger hole in the venous loop. When this happens, the venous loop wall, not the entire loop, should be grasped around the hole using the bipolar forceps, and coagulation should be done. If coagulation does not effectively control bleeding from the venous loop, the hole becomes increasingly larger as blood flow increases, and the entire AVM core also increases in size proportionately.[115] In order to break this vicious circle, a small piece of Surgicel must be placed on the point of bleeding to achieve hemostasis, and then a cottonoid patty is immediately placed on top of the Surgicel and suction is applied. This will control the bleeding in 2–3 minutes, or at most, within 15 minutes.

It is recommended that dissection be continued in other areas, instead of waiting for hemostasis to be completed at the previous point of bleeding. Application of Gelfoam soaked with thrombin is effective only for control of bleeding under venous pressure, but not for bleeding from shunting arterioles, venules, or venous loops under arterial pressure.

Bleeding from a shunting arteriole occurs only when these arterioles are sectioned before coagula is adequately formed inside the arteriole or when the AVM core or surrounding brain tissue is retracted with slightly excessive force to pull an arteriole off a venous loop. Bleeding from shunting arterioles should be handled in the same manner as bleeding from the venules. After cauterization and sectioning, shunting arterioles remain in situ, whereas the venules retract into the brain tissue. Usually, adequate coagulation of communicating venules of 100 μm in diameter requires approximately 2 seconds, while coagulation of shunting arterioles of the same diameter requires 5 seconds or longer. In comparison, cauterization time for adequate coagulation of normal venules and arterioles of the same diameter is 0.5 seconds and 1.5 seconds, respectively.

Although communicating venules of 50–200 μm must be individually cauterized and sectioned, those of <50 μm are simultaneously coagulated in a bundle. Extremely small venules (20 μm) are sectioned only by cautery, and contract and disappear into the surrounding brain tissue and cause no bleeding.

An operating room camera and a television screen are advantageous to the scrub nurse since they can provide information quickly about the need to apply homeostatic material and cottonoid patties whenever an AVM rupture is recognized. Recently, the use of the neuroendoscope has provided greater magnification and illumination of shunting arterioles and communicating venules, and visual identification of these small vessels and cauterization have become more accurate (see Chapter 2, Section 5).

Coagulation Mechanism and Blood Volume Control: Blood loss should be replaced whenever the surgeon feels that it is necessary. In the author's opinion, blood transfusion should be started if the blood loss reaches 500 cc before the AVM resection begins, and should be administered slowly. When a large amount of vigorous bleeding occurs, the blood transfusion should be temporarily halted until hemostasis is completed. The surgeon will realize that one unit of blood transfusion given during rapid bleeding of a large amount accelerates the blood loss to two to three times the amount of the transfusion.

The reason for accelerated blood loss is explained by two mechanisms: (1) blood flow to the brain is 20% of the total cardiac output, and blood flow through the AVM of 4–5 cm diameter is equal to the blood flow of the entire brain in the normal individual. The circulation of the brain with an AVM of this size is maintained at approximately 81%–90% of normal.[115,122] The preferential flow to the AVM naturally continues during AVM bleeding. (2) The AVM flow follows the Poisollo-Hagon law:

$$BF = \frac{(Pa - Pb)\,\pi r4}{1\eta}$$

where Pa = proximal blood pressure
Pb = distal blood pressure in the blood vessels
r = radius
l = length
η = viscosity.

When any part of the AVM ruptures, Pb is equal to O, and Pa-Pb becomes greater. Since the AVM lacks autoregulation, the radius of core venous loops does not change, but rather often becomes greater as blood flow increases.[115,125]

Coagulation mechanism must be maintained at the normal level. Prothrombin time, partial prothrombin time, and platelet count are tested before surgery, and during surgery if hemostasis becomes more difficult. Platelet dysfunction must be tested if an unknown hemorraghic tendency is noted. Overloading of crystalloid without adequate blood transfusion during or after blood loss causes low hematocrit. Blood cells lose an ability to stick together, if the hematocrit is lower than 28 (hemoglobin less than 9 g/dL).

Retraction: Retractors may be applied on the AVM and on surrounding brain tissue. It is preferable to retract the AVM core rather than brain tissue, which should be protected from compression ischemia. To prevent AVM rupture during retraction, the intravascular pressure of the venous loops is minimized by administration of anesthetic agents (e.g., isofluorane) or by controlled hypotension. A metal retractor may be applied gently on a Bicol (Synthetic Collagen) sheet or cottonoid pledget, which is placed on the AVM loops. Retraction of the core vessels and the surrounding brain allows visual identification of the shunting arterioles and communicating venules during dissection on the deep side of the core, around the aneurysmal dilatation, or underneath the cortex covering the AVM core. Further, the authors have recently found the curved endoscope (Murphy-Endoscope) to be beneficial in safely interrupting these vessels. Retraction with a metal retractor applied directly on the brain or AVM should be avoided in order to prevent rupture of the core venous loops or cutting brain tissue with the edges of the retractor.

Ischemia due to excessive brain retraction can be avoided by an experienced surgeon and assistants who sense excessive retraction pressure. To secure appropriate retraction, additional monitoring can be used, such as: (1) pressure recording between the self-retaining retractor and the brain,[1] (2) SSEP recordings,[121] and (3) continuous thermistor cerebral blood flow recording.[14,119] With these monitoring techniques, the surgeon may be warned of changes in parameters that reflect neurological dysfunction.

During isolation of the major draining vein, it may become necessary to gently retract the brain covered by a cottonoid pledget in the deeper area of the sulcus, to expose the transition of the draining vein to the AVM core. Careful retraction of the brain tissue allows for appropriate stretching of the communicating venules for coagulation and sectioning. After all communicating venules are interrupted, the retractor may be removed from the sulcus; the cottonoid patties placed on the sulcal cortex will keep the sulcus widened in a conical shape.

If, however, retraction is likely to be prolonged for many hours, Bicol sheets must be placed directly on the cortex. This prevents bleeding from the cortical surface, which sometimes occurs upon removal of cottonoid patties that have been placed directly on the cortex for hours.

Multistaged Operation: Multistaged operations are required for resection of most large AVMs and some medium AVMs in the functional area. Removal of AVMs in multiple stages[24,86,103,113,115] has the following advantages:[115,119]

1. *Improved control of bleeding.* Thrombosis propagates from the coagulated arterioles and venules into the AVM core, making the active part of the AVM bloodless at the second operation.

2. *Ease of vascular identification.* Between stages, angiograms demonstrate feeding arteries and draining veins to nonthrombosed AVM portions more discretely.

3. *Microcirculatory rearrangement.* Adjustment of cerebral tissue surrounding the AVM to a new circulatory environment is established between staged operations, and an appropriate interval for the second stage of the operation seems to be 4–8 weeks after the first.

4. *Prevention of cerebral edema.* Cerebral retraction, tissue manipulation, and electrical coagulation is minimized, so recovery of cerebral function occurs quickly. We have not encountered intraoperative or postoperative malignant edema, which was reported by Spetzler, et al.[103]

5. *No postoperative bleeding from the circumscribed compartment.* This is compared with a reported high incidence of rebleeding after partial AVM removal,[77] which is likely due to reopening cauterized and sectioned venous loops. Two of our patients suffered intraventricular rebleeding between stages, apparently originating from the undissected area of AVMs in the thalamus and choroid plexus but not from the dissected compartment. External ventricular drainage effectively controlled this complication.

En Bloc Resection in the Silent Areas

En bloc resection has been performed with reference to the following principles (Figure 22):

1. En bloc resection[9] should start with clipping of the feeding arteries that are highly demonstrable by angiography. Access to feeding arteries, which always travel under the cortex as they approach the core, requires removal of brain tissue first.

2. The next step should be removal of a thin layer of brain tissue around the AVM, without exposing the core venous loops.

3. After circumscribing the AVM core, bloc resection should be ended by clipping and sectioning the draining veins.

Upon observation of a specimen from en bloc resected AVMs (Figures 23A-C), one may wonder how the AVM can be resected alone without removing surrounding brain tissue, as shown in Figure 1B.

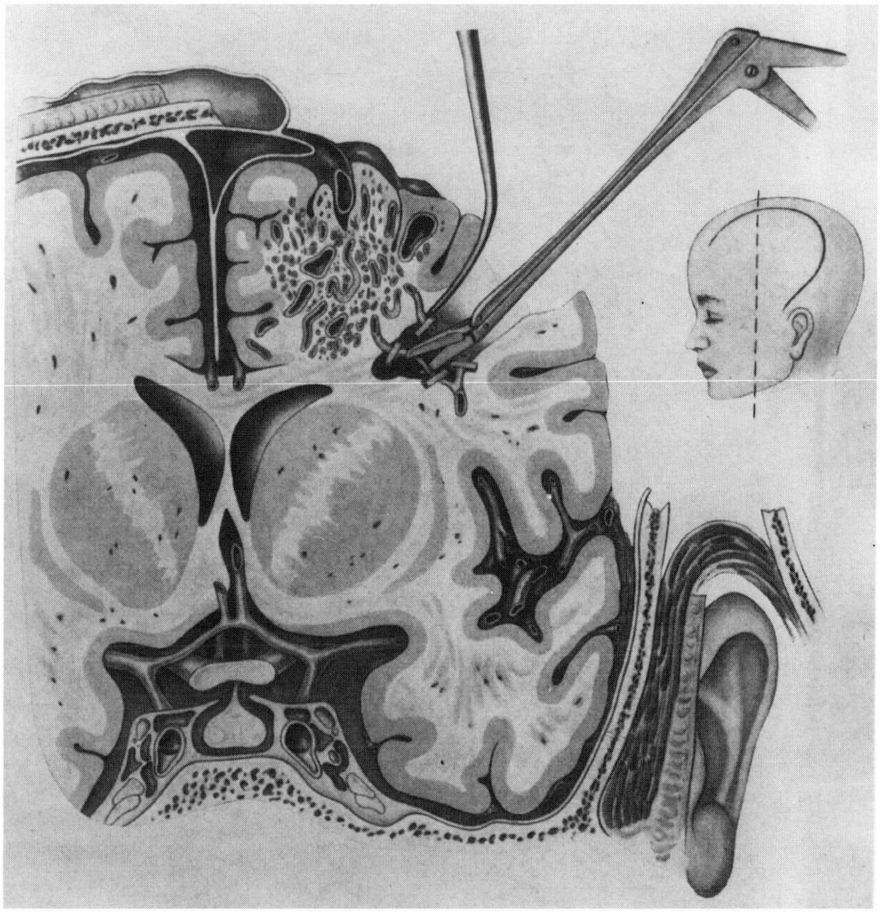

Figure 22. The schematic drawing of en bloc resection of the AVM by Olivecrona and Ladenheim is familiar to neurosurgeons. This technique should not be used for AVM resection in functional areas. Figure used with permission of Springer Verlag.

Surgical Technique for AVMs in Functional Areas

Successful resection of AVMs located subcortically to the functional cortices requires specific surgical principles: (1) avoidance of removal of functional brain tissue, (2) preservation of microcirculation to the functional brain, (3) maintenance of the circulation through the draining veins until the completion of the AVM dissection, (4) protection of the functional cerebral cortices overlying the AVM and the neuronal fibers originating from them (no excavation is formed after resection of the functional cortex), and (5) circulatory observation of the cortical veins that are dilated with arterial blood but that are not a part of the AVM core.

In order to fulfill these principles, surgeons must refrain from the traditional techniques used for AVMs in the silent area.

1. *En bloc resection.* In Figures 24A (operative field) and Figures 24B and C (angiogram), the AVM is located in the motor and sensory areas. If it were located in the silent area, cortical incision around these red cortical veins and en bloc resection can be done safely. However, the same procedure in the sensorimotor area is likely to cause hemiplegia in the patient.

2. *Clipping feeding arteries.* There is no feeding artery visible from the cortical surface. The exposure of the feeding artery necessitates brain tissue removal. Clipping of an angiographically demonstrable feeding artery necessarily causes obliteration of its cerebral branches and ischemia in their territories.

3. *Isolating the draining vein.* The dictum "never touch the draining vein until the end of AVM dissection" is no longer applicable. Now, it is not only safe to isolate the draining vein using microsurgical techniques, but is essential to avoid brain tissue removal in reaching the AVM core.

4. *Adjacent brain tissue.* In the past, the surgical

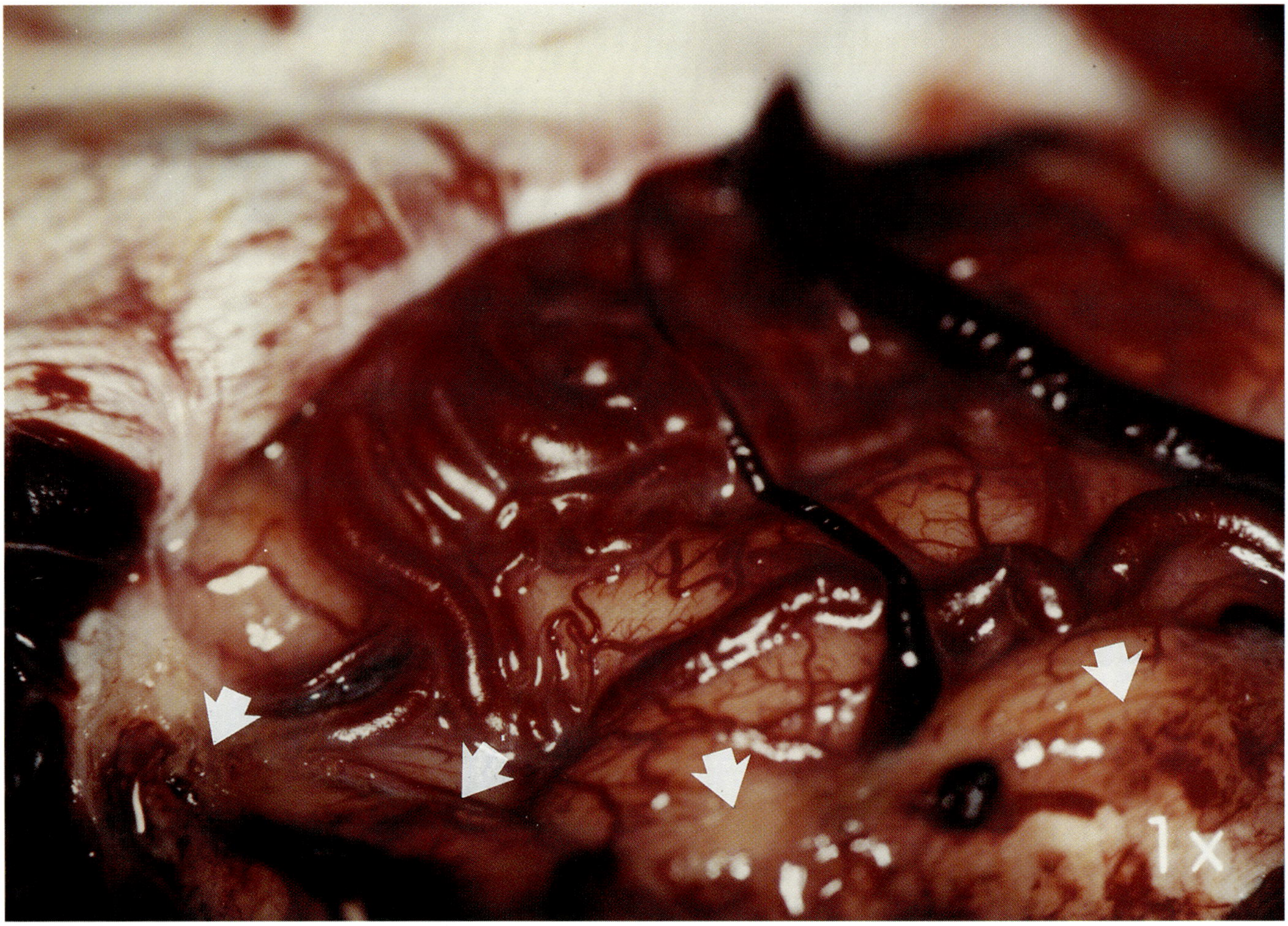

Figure 23A. En bloc resection of a frontal parasagittal AVM in a patient who presented with paroxysmal throbbing headaches is shown to circumscribe the AVM core removing a thin layer of brain tissue. Arrows indicate the edge of the brain tissue removal. Arterial blood flowed through the cortical vein located in the upper right corner before dissection began. *Continued*

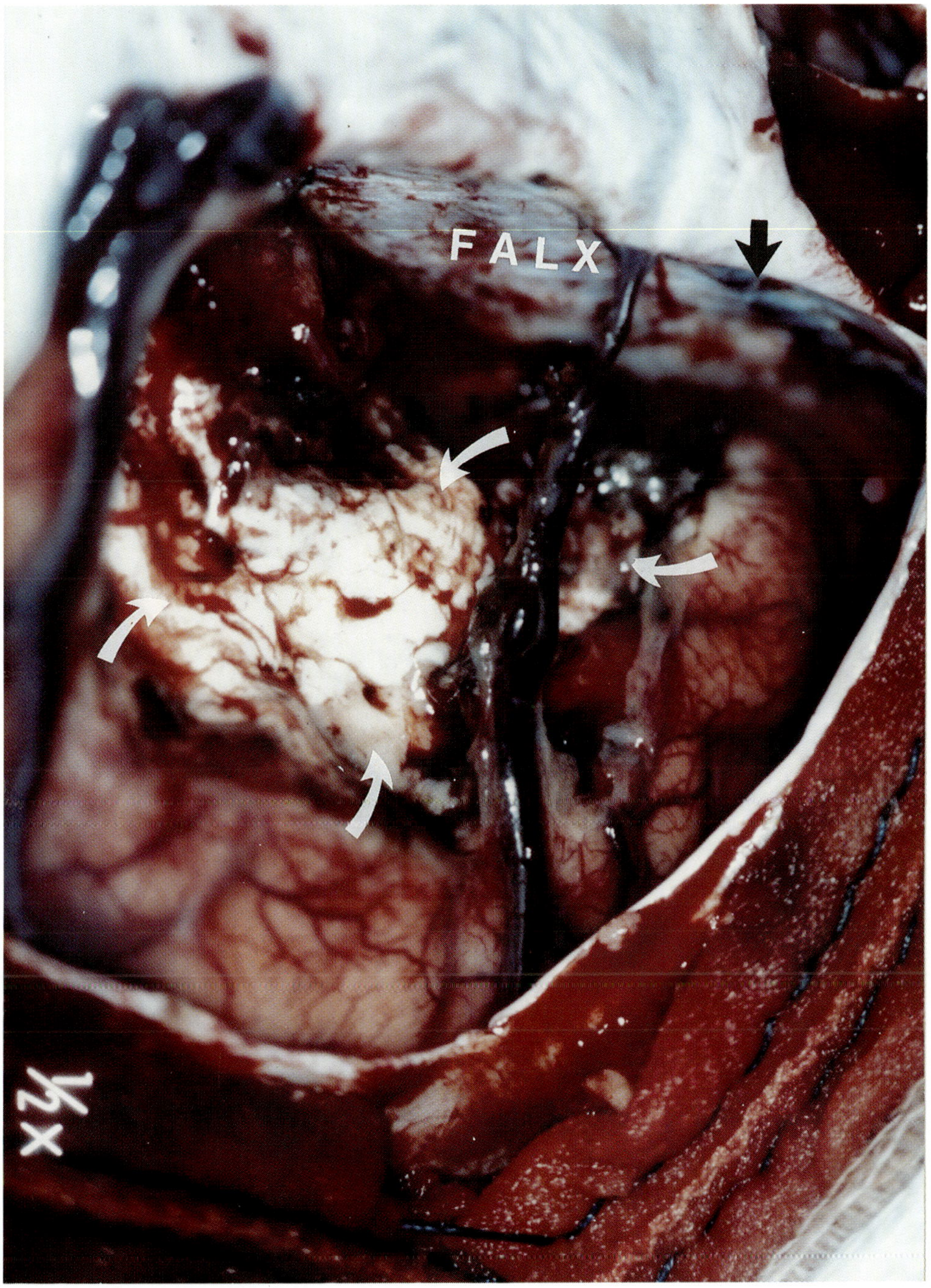

Figure 23B. A cavity of the brain (with white matter exposed) is always present after en bloc resection. Curved arrows are directed from the cortical edge into the cavity. The superior sagittal sinus is shown by a black arrow. *Continued*

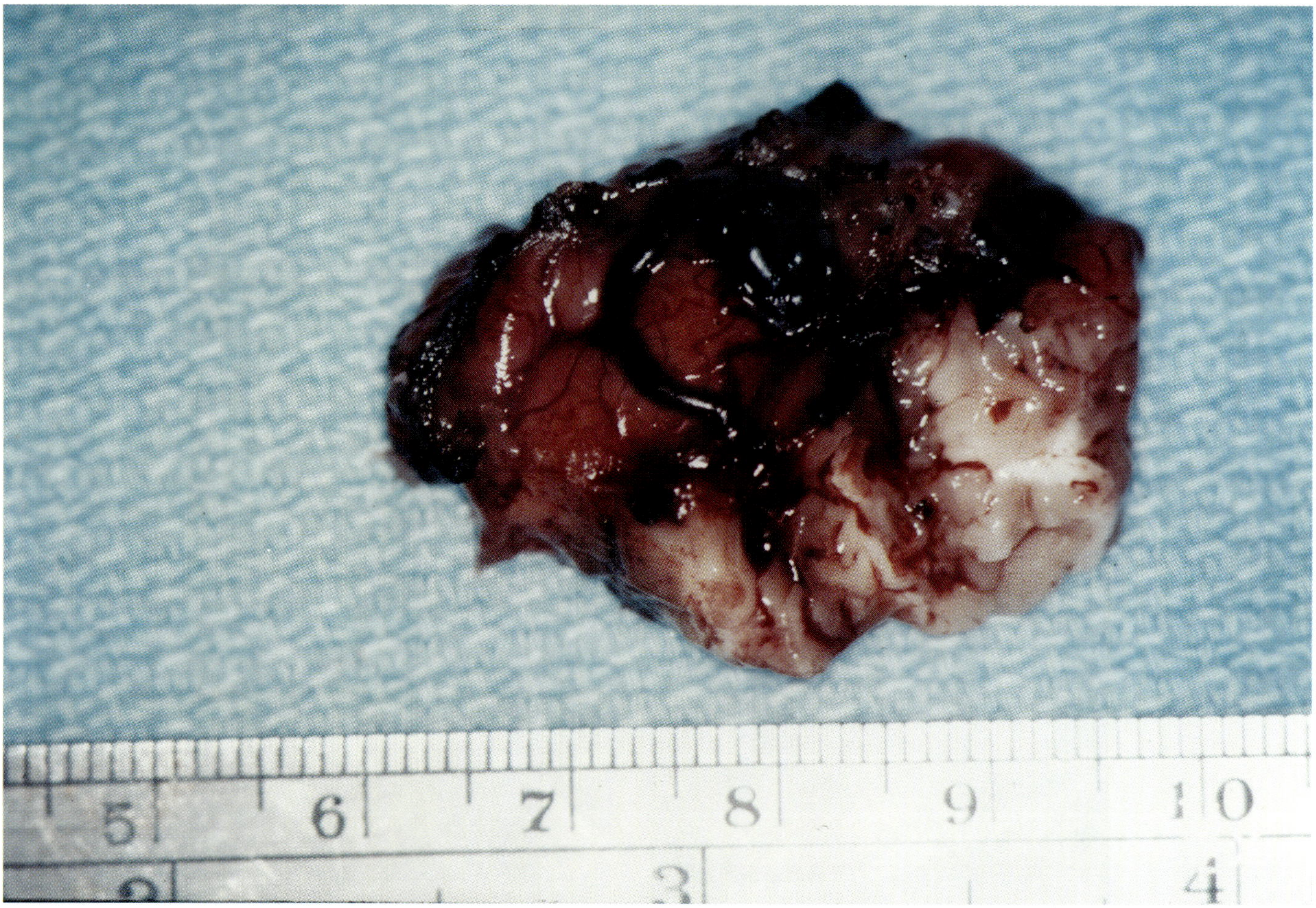

Figure 23C. An excised specimen of the AVM surrounded by brain tissue is very different from the specimen removed by the author's technique shown in Figure 1B. It is impossible to identify shunting arterioles and communicating venules using the en bloc resection technique.

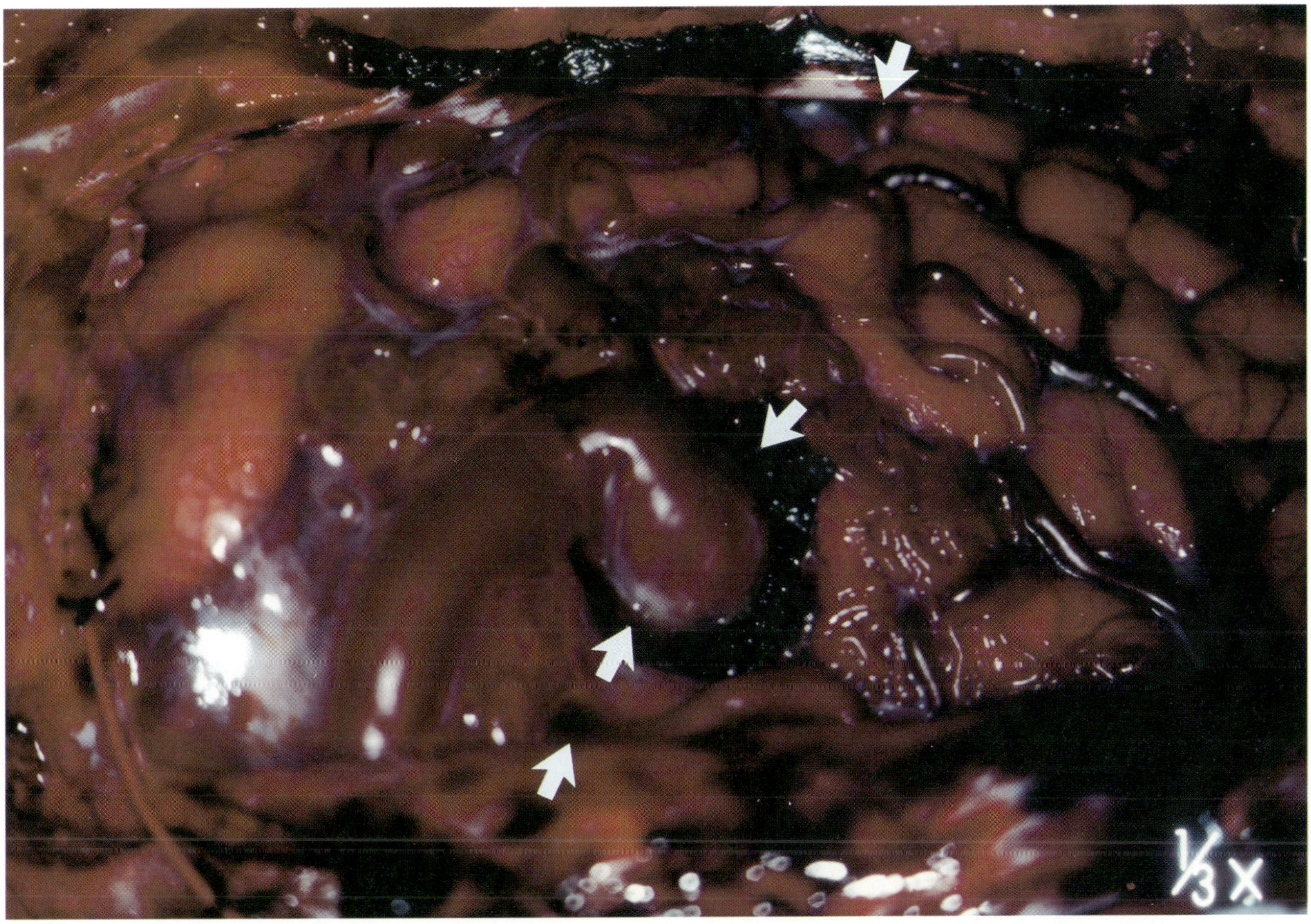

Figure 24A. The AVM core located underneath the sensorimotor cortex has rich communication with cortical veins: large cortical veins with the major draining vein and small ones with the AVM core through juxtanidal veins. These dilated veins and venules filled with arterial blood are not part of the AVM core. The AVM core must be dissected underneath the cortex (refer to text). The arrows indicate the central sulcus and the junction of the major draining vein and a large cortical vein. The motor cortex is located anterior to the junction (to the right), the sensory cortex posterior to the junction (to the left). A strip of Surgicel was placed around the junction for hemostasis. *Continued*

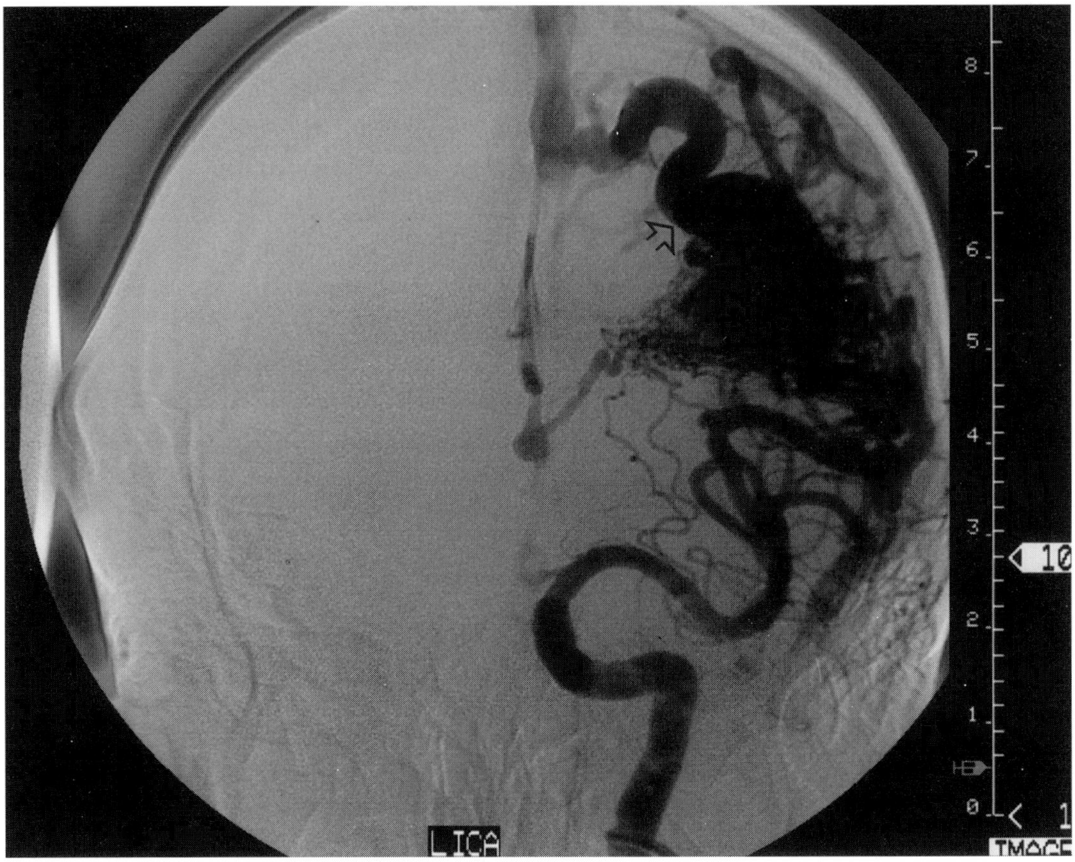

Figure 24B. Preoperative angiogram, lateral view, from the same patient. Arrow indicates the major draining vein. *Continued*

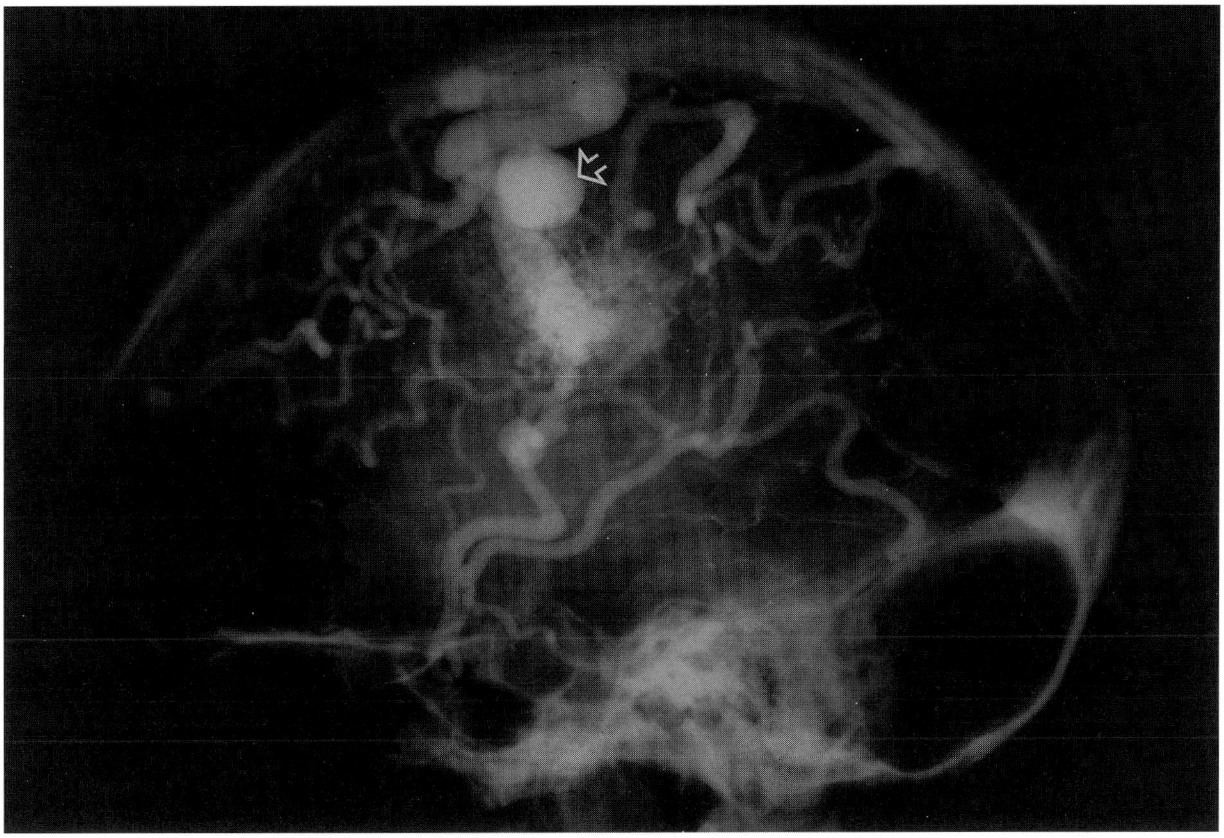

Figure 24C. AP view; arrow indicates the major draining vein.

technique for AVMs included the teaching "A thin layer of brain tissue can be removed without causing neurological deficits. The assumption is that glial tissue completely surrounds the AVM core as a result of blood steal-induced ischemia." From the author's experience, the majority of brain tissue adjacent to a large AVM's core is functionally and structurally normal.

AVMs are almost always hidden underneath the cortex, except for rare cases in which an AVM core extends to a small area of the cortical surface. Microdissection of the AVM core is essential to successful resection. The basic surgical techniques for dissecting the core are:

1. Accessing the AVM core by following the major draining vein, without removing brain tissue.
2. Superselective interruption of shunting arterioles and communication venules that are connected to the AVM core.
3. Forming cleavage between the core loops and surrounding brain tissue.
4. Shrinking core venous loops by cauterization.
5. Interruption of the major draining vein.
6. Delivery of the shrunken core through a small cortical entrance or through the sulcus opening.
7. Clear identification of the junction between each major draining vein and the cortical veins, because occlusion of some cortical veins can cause temporary or permanent neurological damage.
8. Cauterization of the major draining vein should not extend beyond the junction to the superior and inferior anastomotic veins (veins of Trolard and Labbé). Surgical occlusion of the vein of Trolard often causes temporary or permanent hemiplegia. Occlusion of the vein of Labbé in the dominant hemisphere may cause receptive aphasia or cognitive dysfunction due to venous infarction around these veins.[130,131]

Step 1: The first step in AVM surgery in functional areas is isolation of the major draining vein. It is essential to gain access to the AVM core without removing brain tissue. First, the superficial end of the major draining vein must be identified before the major draining vein is isolated. Usually, cortical veins containing arterial blood travel in a radial fashion with the major draining vein in the center (Figure 25). The external end of the major draining vein has the highest blood oxygenation, in comparison to the dilated

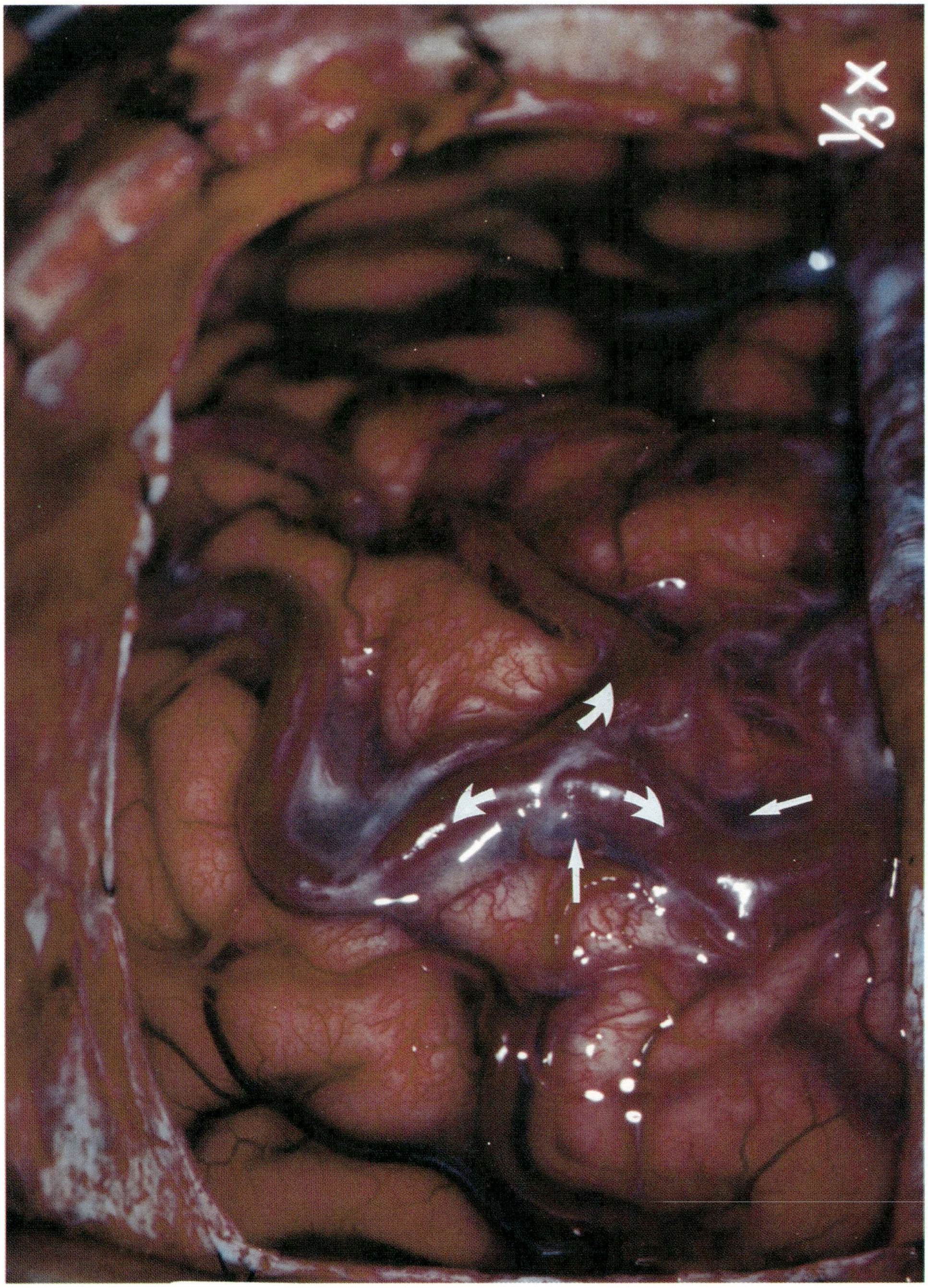

Figure 25. An AVM underneath the sensorimotor area. Three curved arrows indicate the direction of oxygenated blood flow from the external end of the major draining vein in a radial fashion into the cortical veins. The straight arrows indicate the left central sulcus. Base of the dural flap on the right covers the sagittal sinus (refer to illustrative case 2). How to find the junction is explained in the text.

cortical veins. This radial flow pattern of highly oxygenated blood helps to determine the draining vein. These veins should be matched with the radiographic findings to confirm the external end of the draining vein. It should be noted, however, that these methods for identifying the draining vein may be fallible. Therefore, it may become necessary to dissect several cortical veins from the surrounding brain tissue until the external end of the draining vein is found in the sulcus. The distance for isolation of these cortical veins can be minimized by using color Doppler ultrasonography to identify and localize the major draining vein. The external end of the major draining vein is more quickly and accurately identified when an angiographic hologram is reviewed and the major draining vein is followed, using a pointer, from its junction to the AVM core until it reaches the cortical surface. The dilated cortical veins connecting to the draining vein are now clearly demonstrated.

After an incision of the arachnoid membrane around the superficial end of the draining vein is completed (Figures 26A and B), the vein is followed inside the sulcus toward the AVM core. Venules (200–300 μm) connecting the draining vein and the cortical venules or veins in the sulcus are cauterized with an insulated bipolar cautery and then sectioned (Figures 27A and B). If an extremely large draining vein fills the sulcus, which is usually enlarged by the pressure of the vein, MAP should be lowered to 60 mm Hg. At this level of blood pressure, the pulsatile pressure of this vein is minimized and its rupture is prevented. It cannot be overemphasized that the continuity of the major draining vein should be maintained until the last stage of AVM resection.

Retrograde isolation of the major draining vein was practiced earlier by others.[20,63,87,88] They claimed that the advantage of using the sectioned draining vein as a handle is to easily gain access to feeding arteries although detailed techniques were not described. However, the exposure of feeding arteries, except for superficially located type 1 final feeding arteries, requires removal of brain tissue. The main purpose of the senior author's technique for isolation of the major draining vein is to open a pathway to the AVM core *without* removing brain tissue. Although manipulation of the major draining vein was at one time considered a hazard, the procedure has been shown to be safe if conducted by an experienced surgeon under microscopic magnification.

Step 2: The shunting arterioles and communicating venules are coagulated with insulated long forceps and sectioned with long microscissors (Figures 28A and B). As the venous loops are retracted with forceps, the surrounding brain will pull away to form a cleavage. To accomplish this delicate procedure, a narrow retractor (3–5 mm) should be gently placed on either the core venous loops or the surrounding brain tissue, which are covered by Bicol sheets or cottonoid patties. Once retraction becomes effective in determining the direction of core dissection, the retractors may be removed. By this time, the surgical field has become a conical or cylindrical shape. Bipolar forceps and a suction tip (#3 or #5 gauge) function as retractors, while being used at the same time for suction and cautery. Constant usage of retractors is seldom necessary except during dissection of the deep side of the AVM.

Intraoperative color Doppler ultrasonography, correlated with angiographic findings, allows the surgeon to identify the feeding artery in ultrasonographic imaging as it approaches the AVM core in the area where shunting arterioles are crowded. Interruption of a number of shunting arterioles (50–250 μm in diameter) and type 2 final feeding arteries (300 μm) in this area effectively diminishes AVM pulsation. Cleavage formation continues around the AVM core until the core vessels are totally isolated (Figure 28C). Type 2 final feeding arteries are encountered more often in larger AVMs than in smaller ones.

When the AVM core is isolated from the surrounding brain and its vascularity, the pulsation of the AVM core is markedly attenuated. The surgeon can then cauterize a small segment of the core venous loops with bipolar forceps one at a time without causing rupture of these vessels, until the entire AVM core is shrunken to a small cluster of vessels. This is in contrast to the easy rupturing of these vessels and vigorous bleeding before they are disconnected from shunting arterioles (as experienced by neurosurgeons before the days of en bloc resection technique).

Step 3: When the core becomes shrunken, the collecting veins that were often hidden between the core venous loops become visible. The collecting veins are seen to interconnect the core venous loops and the major draining vein (Figure 29). Shunting arterioles and communicating venules connected to the collecting veins are now interrupted, and the already freed major draining vein is coagulated and sectioned within the sulcus. The isolated AVM core should be rotated to facilitate identification of any other draining and collecting veins. After the other draining veins, if present, are sectioned, the entire shrunken AVM (Figure 30A) is removed from the subcortical space through a small opening of the sulcus (about 2 cm in diameter). Hemostasis must be confirmed along the AVM cavity wall before routine wound closure (Figure 30B).

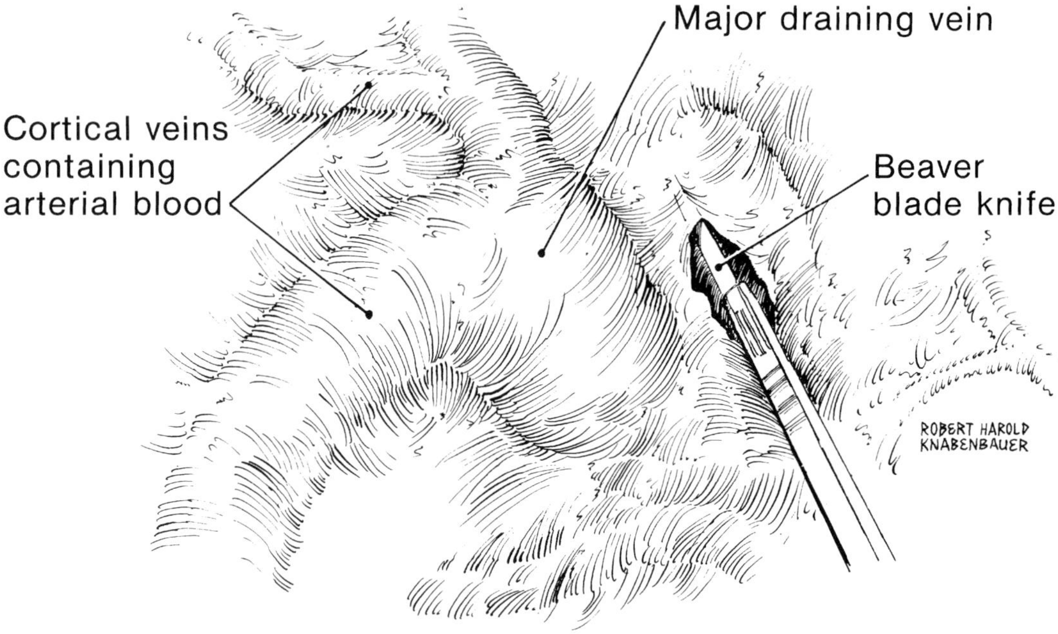

Figure 26. Steps of AVM surgery. **A.** An incision of the arachnoid membrane around the external end of the major draining vein. Figure used by permission of the Journal of Neurosurgery.[119] *Continued*

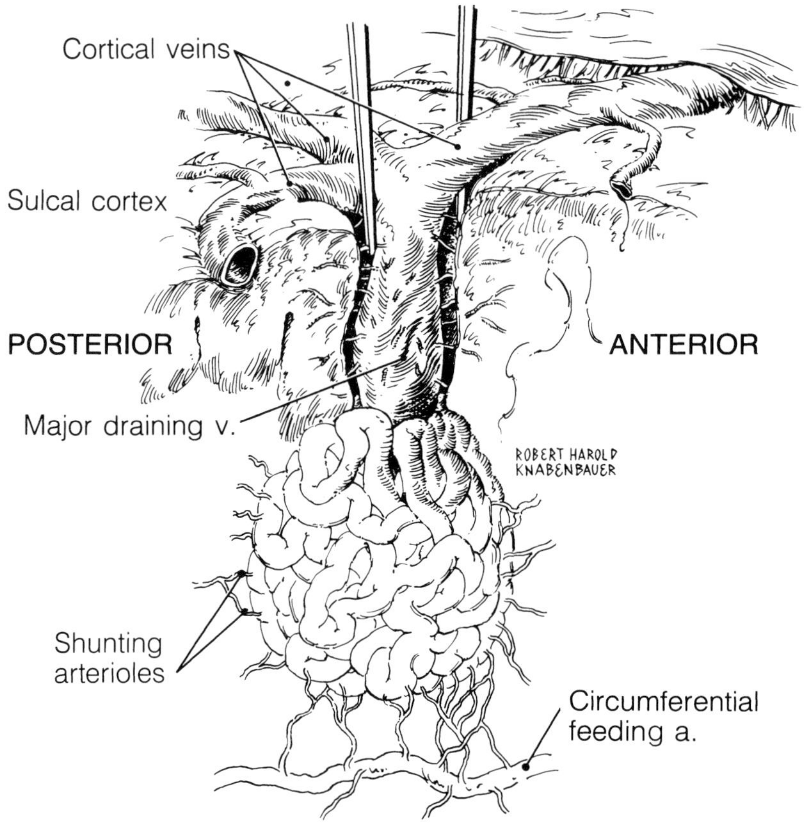

Figure 26B. A 3-D view of the AVM core, the major draining vein, and cortical veins dilated by direct flow of arterial blood from the draining vein.

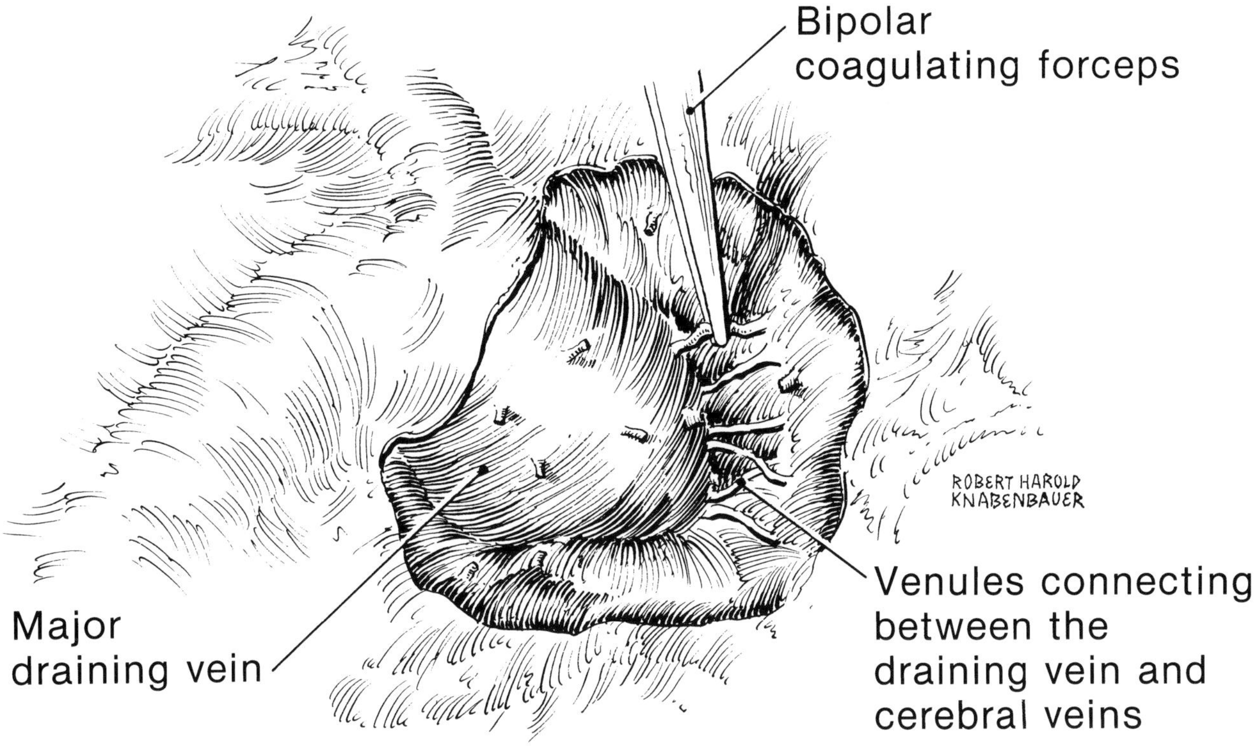

Figure 27A. Cauterized and sectioned communicating venules are connected to the draining vein and sulcal cortical veins. Figure used with permission of the Journal of Neurosurgery.[119] *Continued*

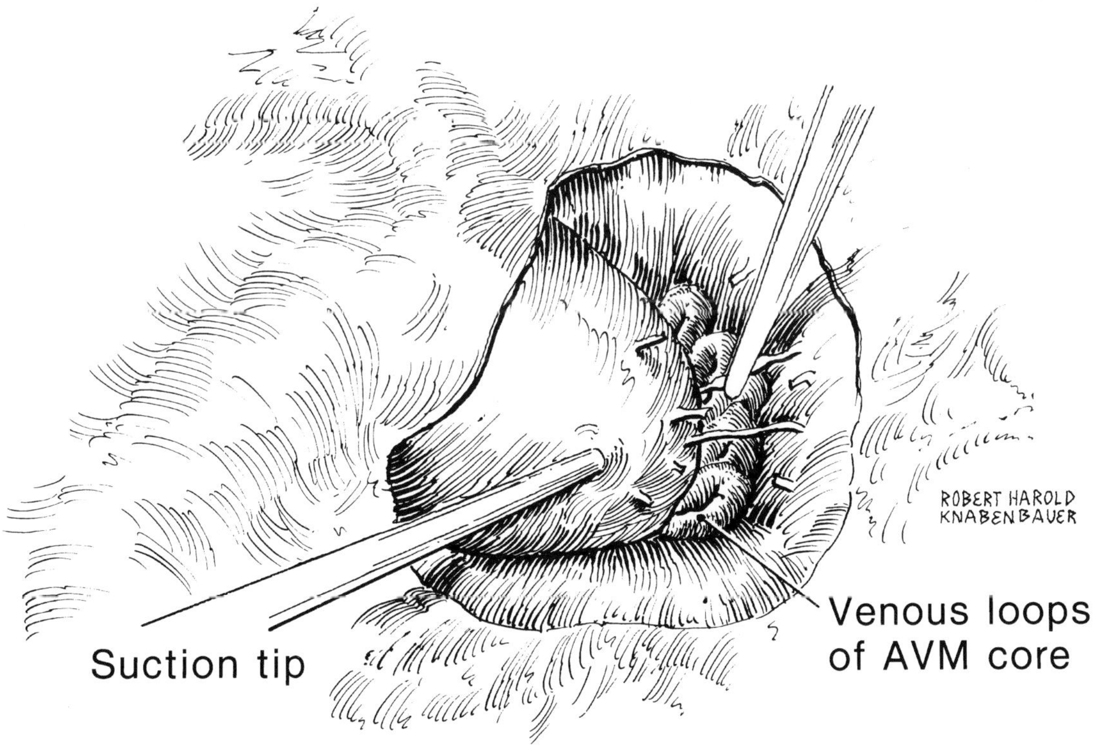

Figure 27B. Isolation of the draining vein allows exposure of the AVM core. Collecting veins are covered by crowded core vessels and are not seen at this stage (refer to text). Figure used with permission of the Journal of Neurosurgery.[119]

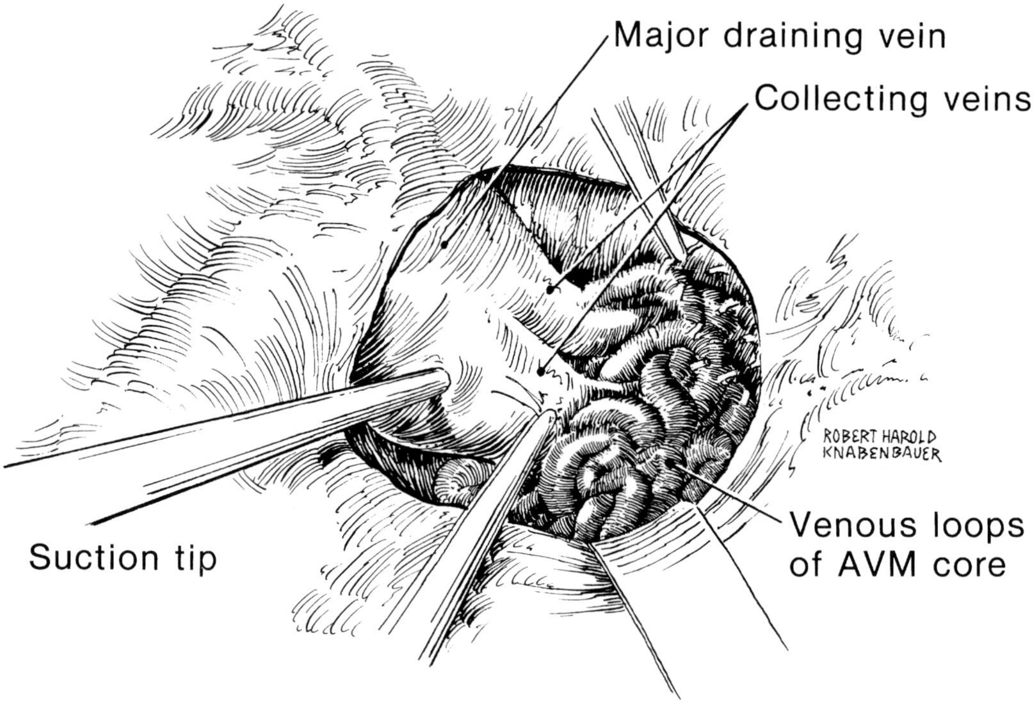

Figure 28A. Interruption of shunting arterioles and communicating venules, which allows cleavage formation between the core vessels and surrounding brain tissue. Toward the end of the core isolation, collecting veins come into view. Figure used with permission of the Journal of Neurosurgery.[119] *Continued*

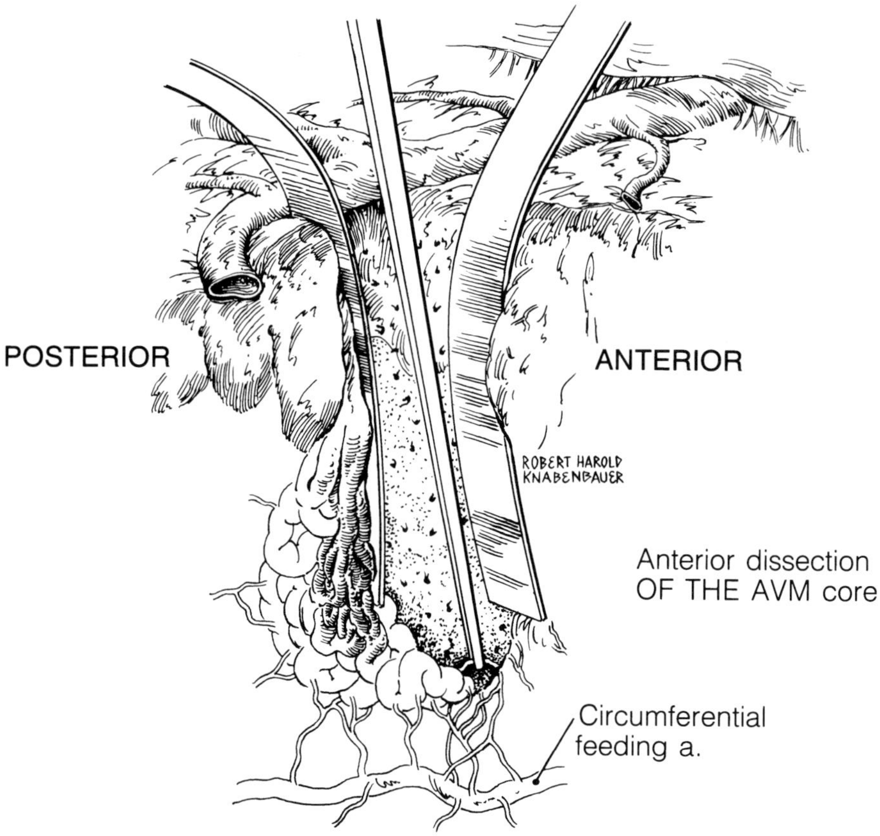

Figure 28B. Dissection of the anterior aspect of the AVM core. *Continued*

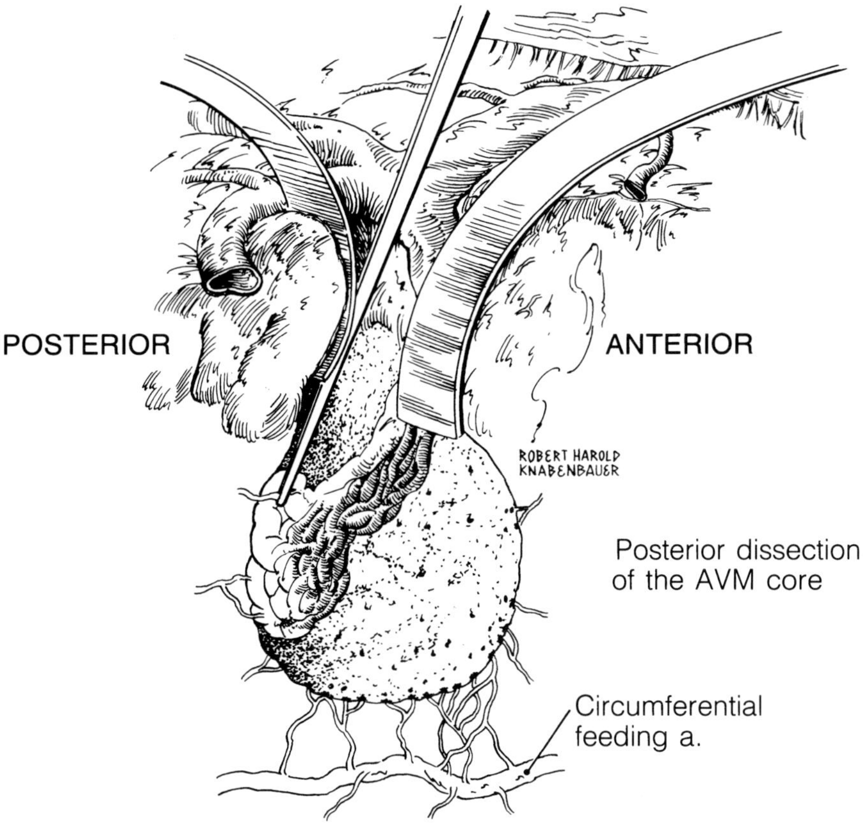

Figure 28C. Dissection of posterior aspect of the AVM.

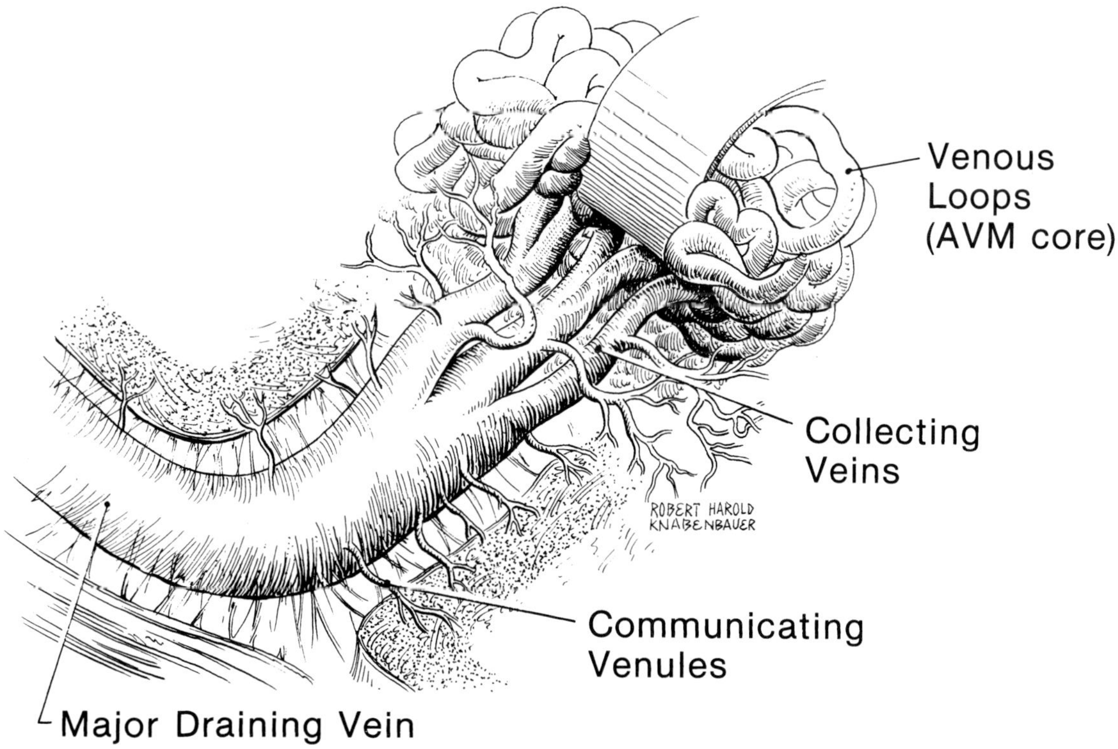

Figure 29. Collecting veins are fully exposed after circumferential dissection of the core. Each of the core loops is ready to be cauterized. The collecting veins are connected to both shunting arterioles (omitted in this drawing) and communicating venules.

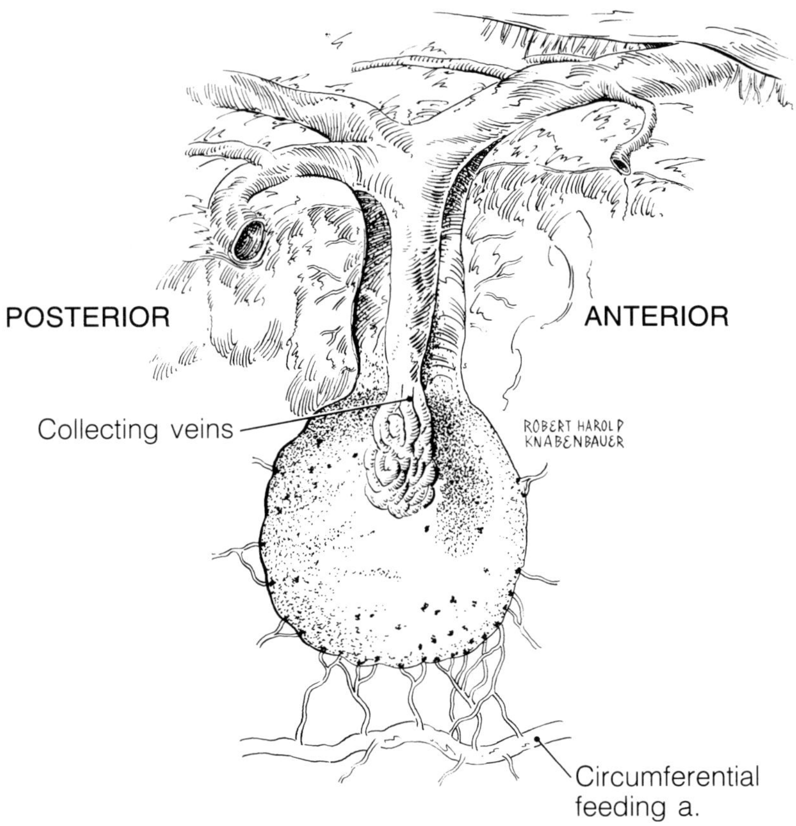

Figure 30A. The shrunken AVM after cauterization of all core vessels. *Continued*

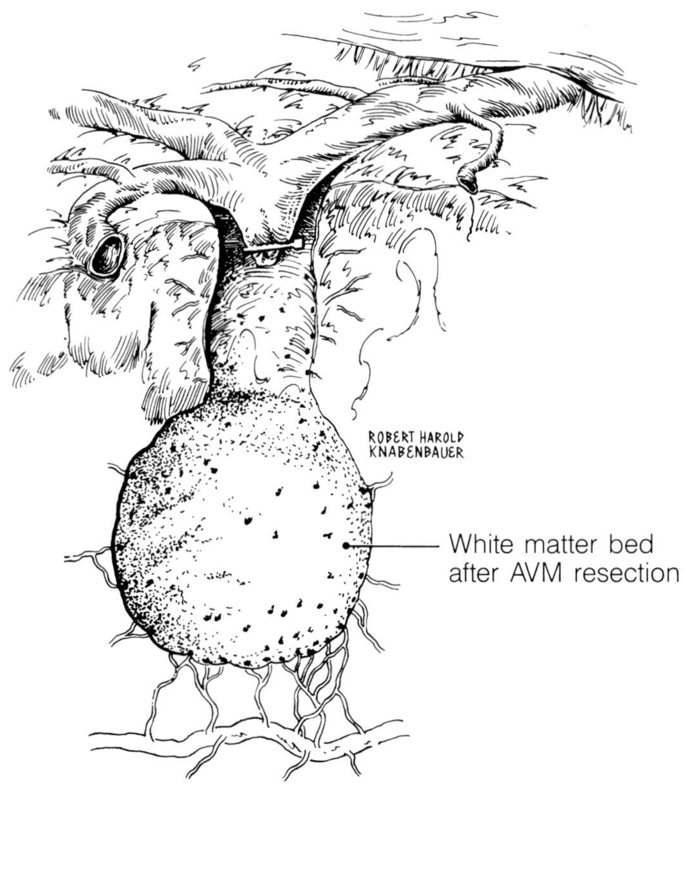

Figure 30B. The phase after interruption of the major draining vein and removal of the AVM core. Hemostasis of the cavity wall is done meticulously by cauterizing small open vessels and Surgicel strips are also applied for this purpose.

Resection of Multicompartment AVMs

The concept of AVM compartments and identification of different compartments on imaging studies have contributed to the advancement in AVM resection in functional areas. The techniques that the senior author developed consist of the separate isolation of each compartment.

Surgical procedures for large AVMs require a thorough knowledge of AVM compartments and the unique techniques for resection. It is essential to identify the location and shape of each AVM compartment, the distribution of feeding arteries to each compartment, and the draining veins from each compartment. This identification should be made using all available imaging techniques. Especially useful for this purpose are stereoscopic or superselective cerebral angiography, MRI, and MRA (three-dimensional if available), CT angiography, intraoperative color Doppler, and recently developed angiographic holograms.

Surgical procedures vary depending on the location and size of the AVM compartments, the borders between compartments, and the arterial feeders and draining veins of each compartment. However, the basic surgical technique of isolating each compartment is similar to the resection of one-compartment AVMs. Each of these surgical procedures consists of: (1) providing access to one of the AVM compartments, (2) interrupting the shunting arterioles and communicating venules, (3) forming cleavage between the core vessels and brain, and (4) cauterizing each compartment until it becomes shrunken to a small mass. In each compartmental procedure, functional cortex and the cortical veins dilated with arterial blood must be preserved. This basic technique prevents a large excavation of the brain, as is expected after en bloc resection.

Surgical Procedures for Multicompartment AVMs in the Sensorimotor Area

For clarity of the technical detail, AVMs in the sensorimotor area are described first. Large AVMs (about 5 cm diameter) may be entirely surrounded by the sensory and motor cortices and white matter fibers originating from them. The AVMs in this location usually have the major draining vein traveling through the rolandic fissure, and its external end connects to the vein of Trolard (Figure 31) and often to the vein of Labbé. Other AVMs may be located partly anterior or posterior to the sensorimotor area and

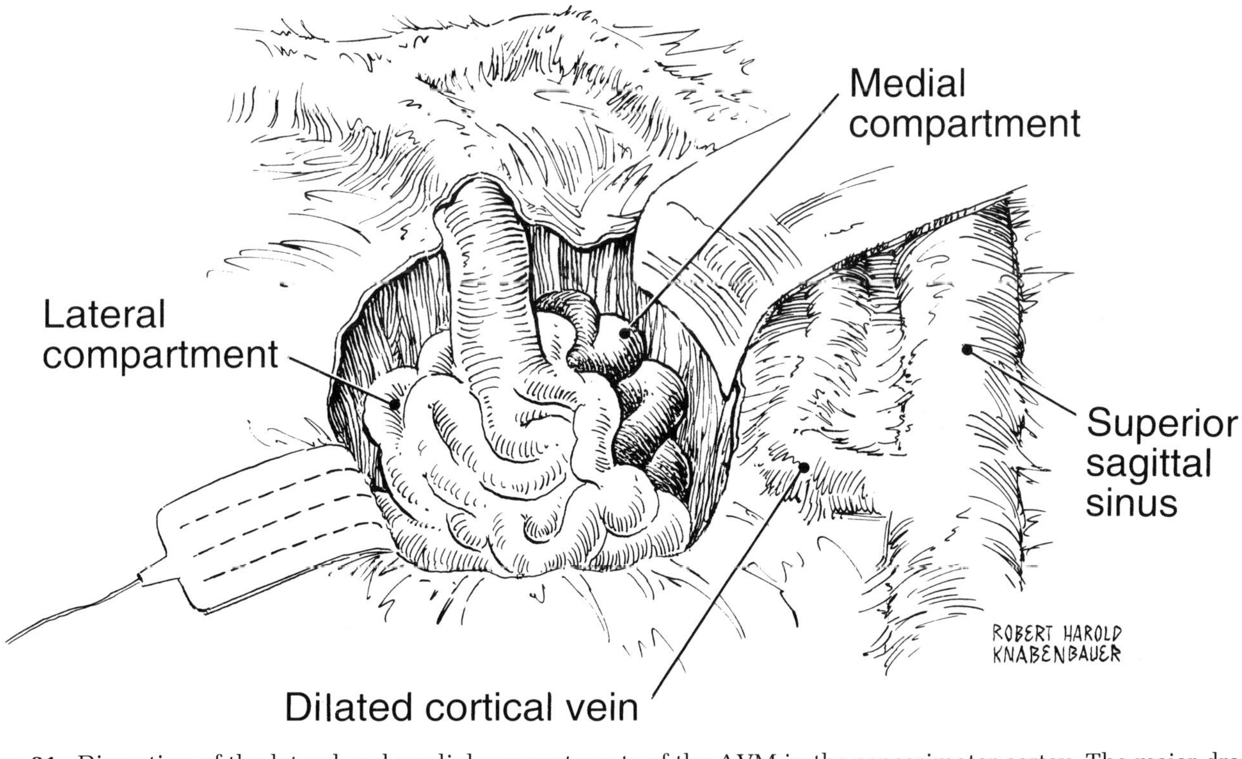

Figure 31. Dissection of the lateral and medial compartments of the AVM in the sensorimotor cortex. The major draining vein has been isolated in the central sulcus. The AVM core, surrounded by motor and sensory neurons, is exposed. The anterior lateral surface of the medial compartment comes into clear view as isolation of the lateral compartment progresses.

partly underneath these cortices. Giant AVMs (>9 cm in anteroposterior diameter) may be located underneath the sensorimotor cortices, and extend anteriorly to the motor cortex and posteriorly to the posterior parietal area.

The most efficient and safe way to approach these AVMs is to follow the major draining vein that is connected to the lateral (convexity) cortical veins. It may be more difficult to identify and isolate the major draining vein than for a one-compartment AVM for the following reasons:

1. Numerous cortical veins and venules are usually dilated with well-oxygenated blood in the area, obscuring the identity of the major draining vein whose blood may not be oxygenated much higher than the cortical veins (Figures 24A and B).

2. The communicating venules that connect the major draining vein and the sulcal cortical veins are extremely crowded and crisscross in the sulcus. Meticulous cauterization and sectioning of these venules is required to reach the lateral compartment without removing brain tissue.

At this point, the lateral compartment can be isolated from surrounding brain tissue anteriorly and inferiorly, then laterally and superiorly underneath the cortex, then posteriorly, and finally medially to the border of the lateral and medial compartments (Figure 32A). When pulsation of the lateral compartment diminishes, each venous loop is cauterized individually until the lateral compartment becomes a small mass of shrunken vessels (Figure 32B).

The lateral or superior dissection requires the insertion of a retractor much deeper underneath the sensorimotor cortices than for one-compartment AVMs (Figures 33A-C). The head must be tilted with the chin held up in a head-neck extended position, so that the sensorimotor area sags backward instead of resisting retraction.

Recognition and identification of the major draining veins of the medial compartment is fundamental. They usually originate from the medial aspect and join the mesial cortical veins until a large one connects to the superior sagittal sinus. Occasionally, one originates from the lateral aspect of the compartment and then continues to the convexity cortical veins.

The majority of shunting arterioles connected to the medial compartment originate from the anterior cerebral artery or its branches, one of which forms a circumferential feeding artery. Isolation of the medial compartment is done along its medial aspect, starting anteriorly and then directed posteriorly. Interruption of shunting arterioles and communicating venules must be done subcortically beneath the mesial cortex. As the arterioles and venules are interrupted, the feeding artery gradually moves away from the AVM core toward the mesial cortex (see Chapter 10, Section 4). Dissection of the medial compartment can be performed safely without difficulty in hemostasis, in spite of the claims that profuse bleeding is usually a great hazard and presurgical embolization is needed to facilitate hemostasis (Fukushima T, Stein BM, Steinberg G, personal communication, 1996). After dissection of the lateral anterior, inferior, and medial aspects of the medial compartment, the pulsation of the compartment diminishes. At this time, cauterization of the venous loops of the medial compartment can be done safely until this compartment shrinks to a small cluster of vessels.

It is advisable to dissect the medial compartment beneath the cortex (Figure 32B). Should the pia and arachnoid be penetrated, the dissection should return to the subcortical layer without removing brain tissue. If the AVM is approached from the mesial surface of the hemisphere, the surgeon will find numerous veins and venules dilated with arterial blood on the cortical surface. These veins are passively dilated by communication with the medial compartment, similar to the convexity cortical veins, and are easily ruptured. Rupture of these small and large veins bridging from the mesial cortex to the falx causes difficulty in controlling bleeding. Additionally, exposure of large medially located AVMs from the mesial hemispheric cortex may require interruption of a large bridging vein connected to the superior sagittal sinus. This procedure alone can cause risks for hemiplegia and congestion of the AVM and cerebral vasculature. Therefore, retraction of the mesial hemispheric cortex should be avoided.

Interruption (clipping or cauterization and sectioning) of angiographically demonstrated feeding arteries does not diminish AVM pulsation unless all of the shunting arterioles are interrupted. Furthermore, clipping of feeding arteries may inadvertently also include veins since they travel adjacent to each other. The accumulated effects of obstruction of many small mesial veins before interruption of shunting arterioles may lead to an increase in intravascular pressure of the AVM core and subsequently to its rupture or brain swelling.

The posterior compartment is usually the last one to be isolated for AVMs in the sensorimotor area. The isolation of the posterior compartment begins at its border with the already shrunken lateral compartment and then extends to the border with the shrunken medial compartment. Since the posterior compartment is located medially, the isolation of this compartment is accomplished similarly to that of the medial compartment. The draining veins from this

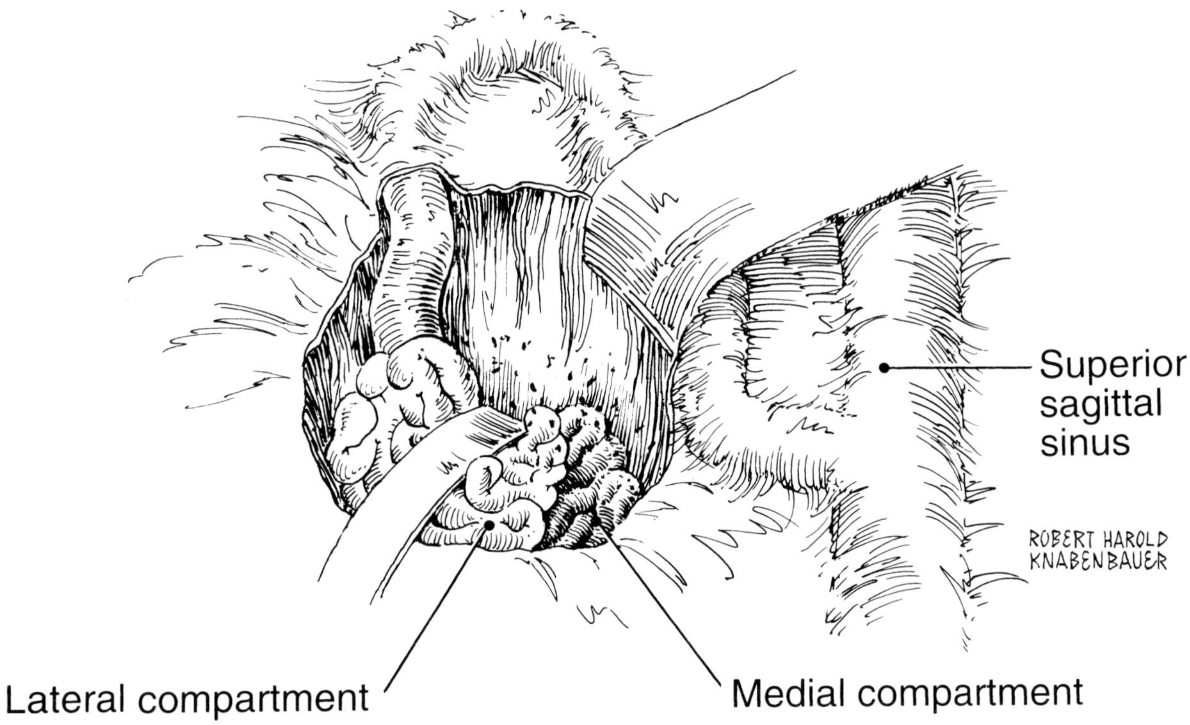

Figure 32A. The lateral compartment has been isolated circumferentially except for the medial aspect that has contact with or is connected to the medial compartment. *Continued*

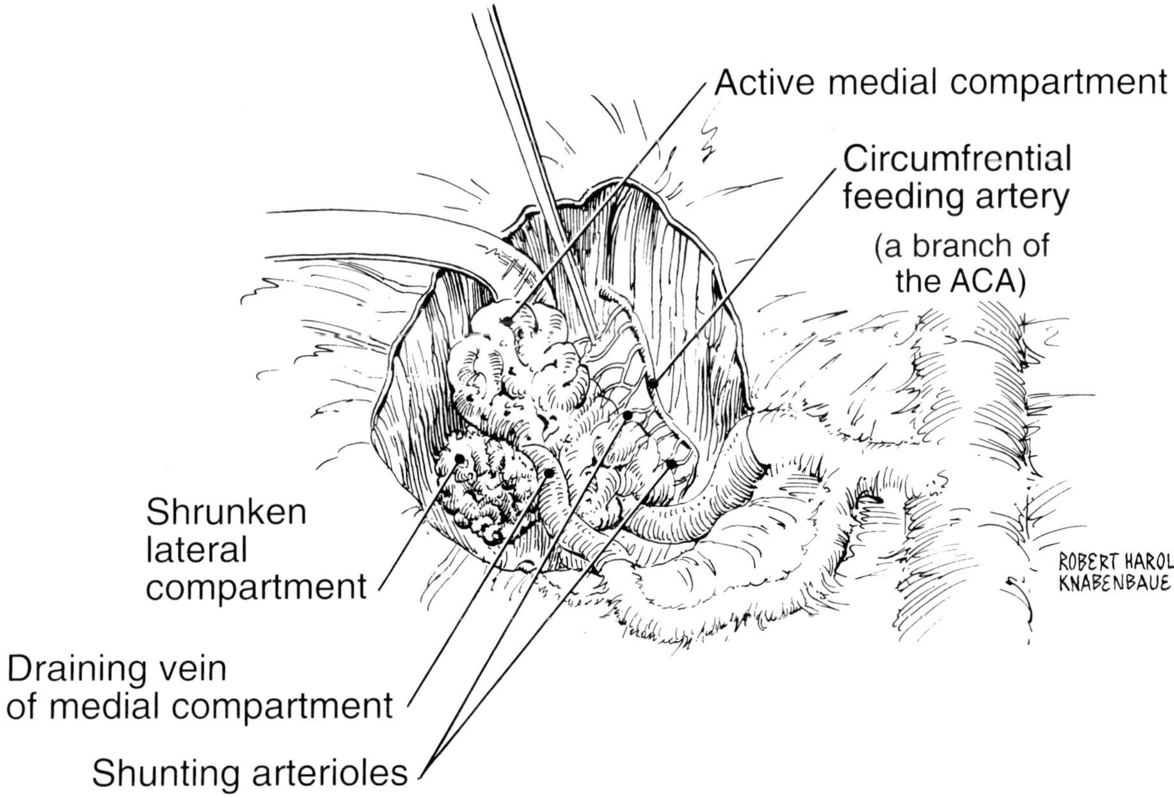

Figure 32B. The medial compartment, dissected after the lateral compartment, was cauterized and shrunken. Its medial aspect must be dissected underneath the mesial surface of the hemisphere.

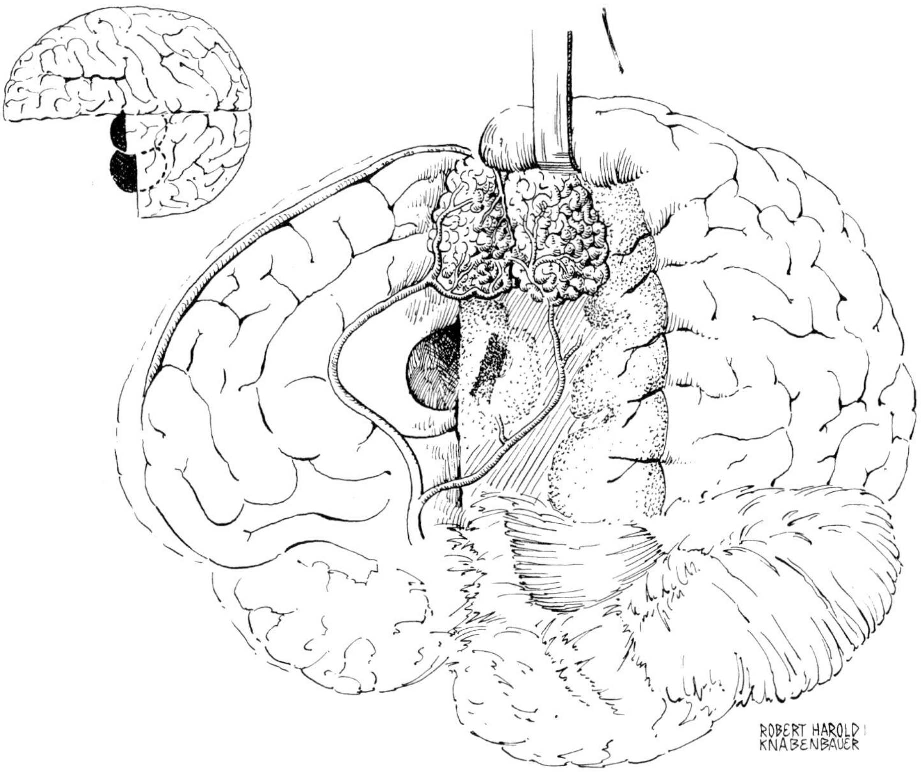

Figure 33A. A schematic drawing of the medial and lateral compartments after removal of the anterior quadrant of the left hemisphere. The arterial phase is emphasized in this drawing, with the lateral compartment supplied by the middle cerebral artery branches and the medial compartment supplied by the anterior cerebral artery. A retractor is inserted underneath the sensorimotor cortices for the AVM dissection. *Continued*

compartment must be kept intact until the end of the AVM isolation. The venous loops of this compartment are then cauterized segment by segment until the compartment is shrunken. The draining veins, some surfacing near the sagittal sinus and others at the hemispheric convexity, are cauterized and sectioned before they join the cortical veins. The major draining vein from the lateral compartment and that from the medial and posterior compartments may come together immediately lateral to the superior sagittal sinus. They may be obliterated at this junction without occluding the cortical veins. Smaller draining veins joining these two major draining veins are also obliterated at their junction.

The type 1 final feeding artery, which usually originates from the anterior cerebral artery, often travels on the mesial surface of the hemisphere as it approaches a venous loop that is located adjacent to the draining vein. This artery may be clipped or cauterized and sectioned immediately before the interruption of the draining veins.

If a giant AVM extends from the prefrontal to the posterior parietal area, undermining the sensorimotor area, dissection of the posterior compartment from the premotor area can be done by retracting the sensorimotor cortices outward and the core inward. The posterior compartment may be separately approached from its posterior aspect by following the major draining vein, if it surfaces at the lateral convexity.

When lifting the shrunken lateral compartment, not infrequently an active draining vein may suddenly come into view (see Figure 4B). This vein is found to originate from and travel along the lateral aspect of the medial compartment and to surface at the superficial cortex of the hemispheric vertex. The arterial blood in this vein is drained into the superficial cortical veins and further into the nearby sinus. The circulation of this hidden draining vein between compartments should not be occluded until the venous loops of the medial compartment are obliterated and shrunken.

While dissecting larger AVMs, one may encounter multiple areas of hemosiderin-laden brain tissue adjacent to the AVM core. These are evidence of previous hemorrhage from the AVM loops.

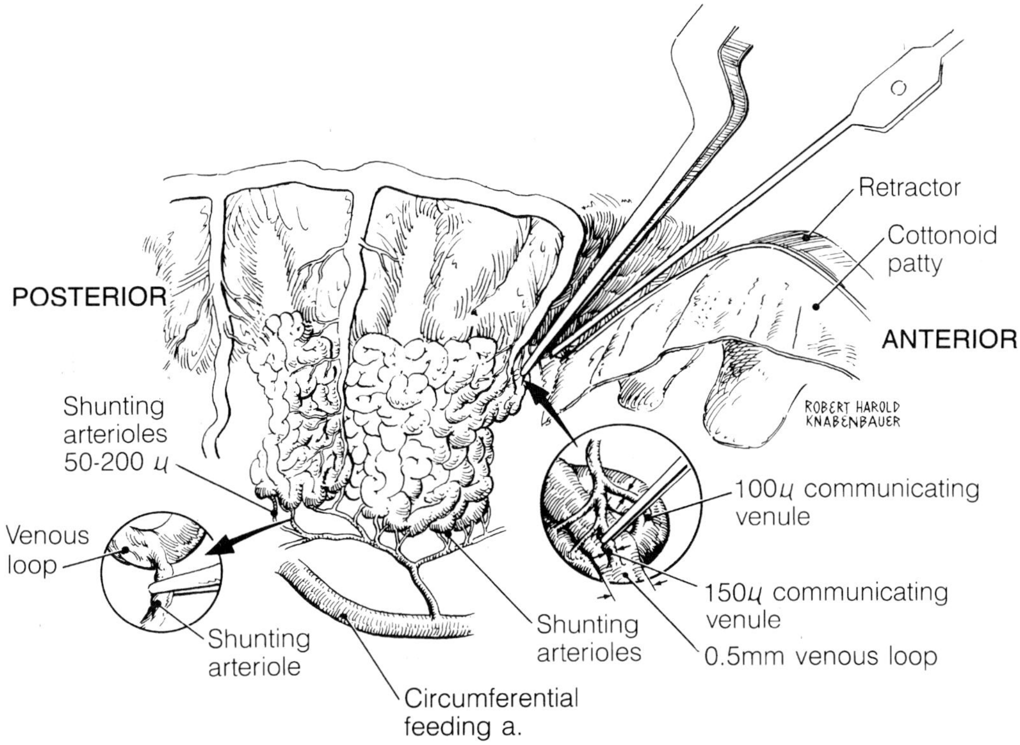

Figure 33B. The AVM core and sensorimotor cortex in the sagittal section. Dissection begins from the anterosuperior edge of the AVM. *Continued*

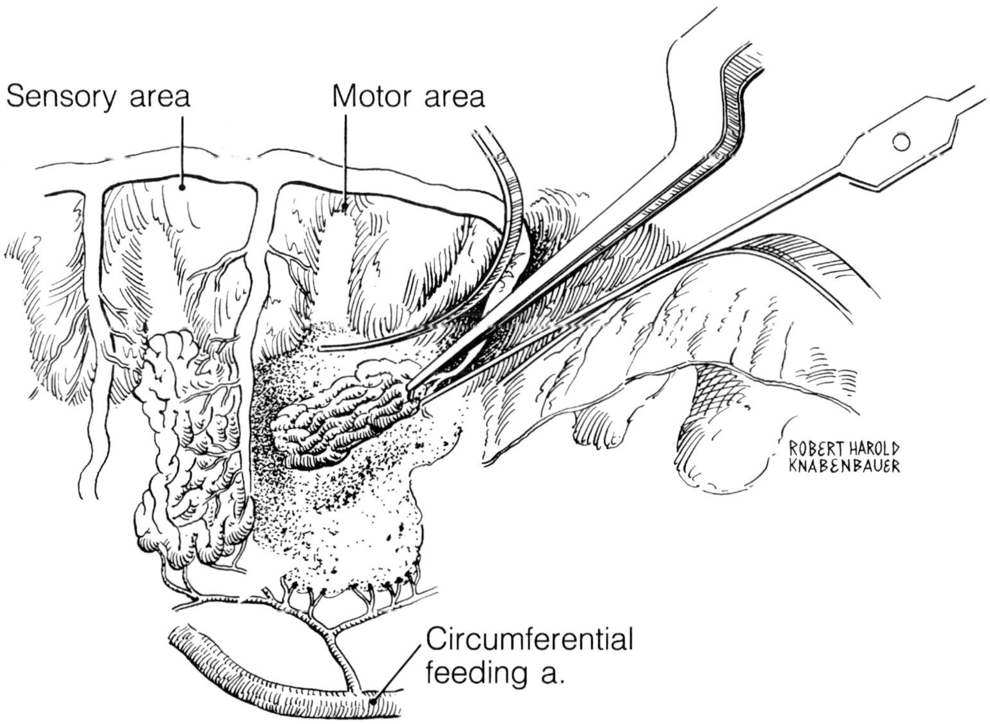

Figure 33C. The medial compartment has been dissected and shrunken. It remains in situ until the posterior compartment is dissected. Sometimes, if the bleeding is under perfect control, shrunken lateral and medial compartments can be removed before the posterior compartment is dissected.

Surgical Procedure for AVMs in the Superior Temporal Gyrus

Large AVMs in the superior temporal gyrus are composed of several compartments: (1) a large lateral compartment, (2) a smaller anterior compartment, and (3) the posterior compartment. The first two compartments are supplied by the middle cerebral artery and the posterior compartment by the posterior cerebral artery branches, and partially by the middle cerebral artery branches.

Large AVMs in the superior temporal gyrus are approached via a frontotemporal or temporoparietal craniotomy (Figure 34). One of the major draining veins originates from the lateral aspect of the AVM core and usually travels in the superior sulcus, sometimes in the inferior sulcus. The external end of this draining vein is usually connected to a few cortical veins, one of which is posteriorly connected to the vein of Labbé. After a modified rectangular dural flap is folded back superiorly or inferiorly, the junction of the major draining vein and the dilated cortical veins passively dilated with arterial blood is located (Figure 35). As previously described, the major draining vein is followed in the sulcus. After exposure of this vein to a depth of about 2 cm from the external end, this draining vein is found connected to the lateral aspect of the AVM core (Figure 36). Dissection of the core may extend from the lateral aspect to the anterior aspect, to the inferior aspect, and then to the posterior aspect.

The posterosuperior portion of the core is difficult to expose during earlier AVM dissection because this portion extends deep under the cortex and its exposure in the early stage of dissection requires forceful retraction of the surrounding brain, and shunting arterioles are crowded around its medial aspect as terminal branches of the posterior cerebral artery. Likewise, the anteroinferior aspect of the core is difficult to dissect without forceful downward retraction of the brain below the AVM core. The alternative to dissection through the same entry is to gain access to the anterior aspect of the core. Gentle retraction of the anterosuperior temporal lobe below the sphenoidal ridge allows for exposure of another major draining vein, which surfaces in the anteromedial temporal lobe (Figure 37A). This draining vein usually has junctions to bridging veins that are connected to the sphenoparietal sinus and rarely to the cavernous sinus. These bridging veins are cauterized and sectioned as the dural arteries feeding the AVM are cauterized and sectioned along the medial sphenoidal ridge. The draining vein is followed in its own sulcus until the core is reached.

At this point, the lateral, inferior, and anterior aspects, as well as the anteromedial aspect of the core are isolated. The anterior portion of the core (anterior compartment supplied by the anterior temporal artery) is coagulated loop by loop so that the shrunken venous loops can be transferred into the first sulcal opening. Next, the superior, posterior, and posteromedial aspects are dissected.

The isolation of the superior aspect of the AVM core begins from the anterosuperior dissection, parallel to the anterior sylvian fissure, but not into the fissure itself. As the dissection from the brain tissue extends posteriorly, the AVM is found approaching the sylvian vein.

The next step is to isolate the AVM core from the sylvian vein in preparation for the superior dissection of the AVM (Figures 10A and 37B). Numerous small draining veins (<1 mm) are found bridging the

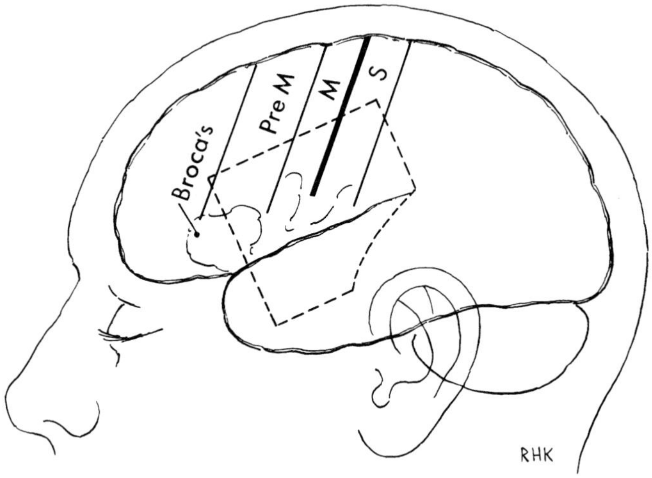

Figure 34. Planning of dural opening is drawn with an interrupted line.

laterosuperior edge of the AVM core and sylvian vein. An almost equal number of feeding arteries, originating from the sylvian group of the middle cerebral artery and corresponding to type 2 final feeding arteries, are connected to the superior aspect of the core. These arteries and veins are crowded and travel parallel to each other. They are so close together that sectioning each individual vessel tends to cause rupture of the adjacent vessels. To reach those vessels, the arachnoid and the pia must be opened in the same plane, as groups of a few of these arteries and veins are cauterized and sectioned together at a time. After the sylvian vein is isolated and the sylvian fissure is opened, the AVM is dissected from the superior aspect through the sylvian fissure underneath the superior temporal gyrus.

The large lateral compartment is supplied by the sylvian group of the middle cerebral artery branches. Venous loops of this compartment are difficult to coagulate. The retractor may be inserted on the superior aspect of the AVM. Its medial aspect can be dissected from the superior aspect downward to the medially located draining vessels.

After the isolation of the lateral, anterior, anteromedial, inferior, superior, and superomedial aspects of the AVM core, the pulsatile expansion of the AVM core is diminished except for the posterior portion. The venous loops are cauterized to extend coagulation to include the anterior one-half or two-thirds of the AVM core.

The AVM core can now be rotated superiorly, inferiorly, and posteriorly through the sylvian fissure opening. All major draining veins, except for those medially and posteriorly located, are cauterized and sectioned. The posterior aspect of the core is the last to be dissected. The posterior or middle temporal lobe is retracted around the AVM core, as shunting arterioles derived from the posterior cerebral artery branches, as well as communicating venules, are interrupted (Figure 38). The posterior portion of the AVM is cauterized segment by segment. The shrunken AVM core can be rotated anteriorly, and interruption of all posteriorly and medially located draining veins is completed. Finally, the draining veins connected to the vein of Galen or its tributaries are cauterized and sectioned.

Some superior temporal gyrus AVMs extend into the posterior frontal lobe across the sylvian fissure. The frontal lobe portion of the AVM may be isolated underneath the superficial cortex. During this isolation, the branches of the middle cerebral artery that pass through the sylvian fissure and the sylvian vein must be protected. If protection of the opercula is difficult, the frontal portion of the AVM may be ap-

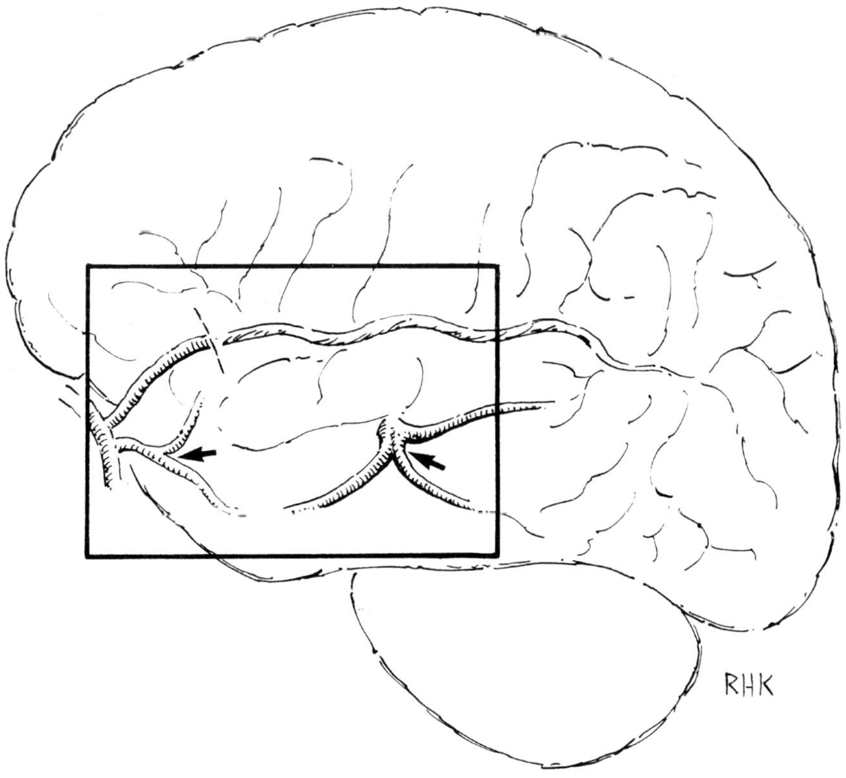

Figure 35. The sylvian vein and the external end of the two draining veins are connected to cortical veins (arrows) in the rectangular dural opening.

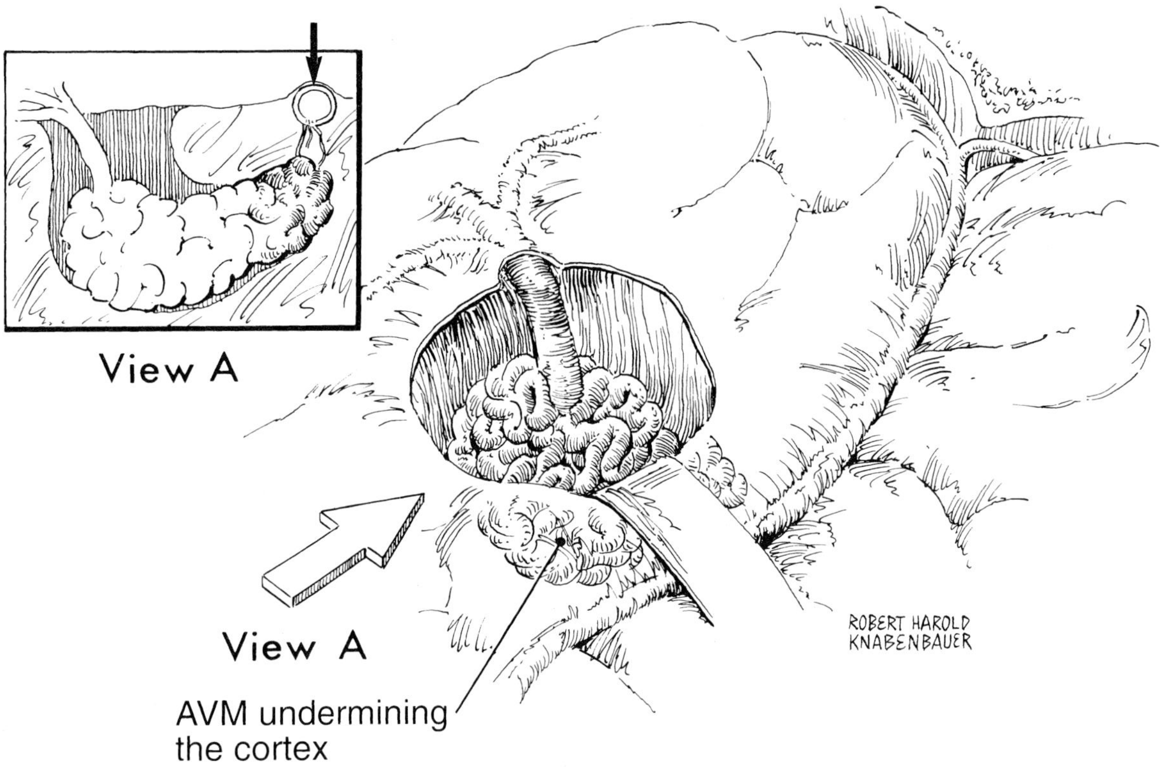

Figure 36. The lateral compartment was accessed by following the posterior draining vein, and the lateral and inferior aspects were dissected. The inset shows the coronal transection of the superior temporal lobe and the AVM with the sylvian vein (arrow) shown in the right upper corner. This figure depicts the posterior frontal area down to the lobe.

proached along the draining vein located above the sylvian vein. Techniques for dissection of the AVM portion above the sylvian fissure are similar to those for the dissection of each compartment in the sensorimotor area.

The resection of a large AVM in the superior temporal gyrus forms a significant post-resection cavity. However, the author's procedure saves the gyrus, underlying white matter, and the covering pia and arachnoid. Neither a large excavation of the brain nor a large arachnoid opening is formed after AVM resection. The arachnoid membrane later regenerates around the sylvian vein and closes the gap between this vein and the superior temporal gyrus. The cavity that remains after core removal is filled by a fibrous tissue similar to the arachnoid structure and fluid identical to cerebrospinal fluid. Therefore, the cavity fluid does not move freely, as does ventricular fluid. This cavity should not be interpreted as encephalomalacia on an MRI study, as is often reported by radiologists.

Resection of AVMs in the Occipital Lobe

The surgical access to AVMs located subcortically in the visual cortex should be through the convexity occipital cortex for the following reasons:

1. The striate cortex should not be removed or damaged during an approach to the AVM.

2. The draining vein travels in the sulcus of the mesioinferior occipital lobe directly from the AVM to the cortical surface in the coronal plane. Therefore, it is impossible to isolate this vein in the sulcus, unless the striate cortex is forcefully retracted so that its surface faces the surgeon's visual direction. Such retraction on the striate cortex is damaging to the primary visual cortex (area 17) neurons, and probably area 18 and 19 neurons.

It is more appropriate to approach mesioinferiorly located AVMs from the convexity. However, draining veins are usually more tortuous in the sulcus and there is a longer distance from the external end of the draining vein and its junction with the AVM core than those seen in the sensorimotor or other areas. For these anatomical reasons it is not as easy to find the major draining vein connected to an AVM in the occipital convexity as in AVMs in the sensorimotor area and other locations. There are several cortical veins dilated with arterial blood on the occipital cortex, and they are not aligned in a radial fashion around the major draining vein. The surgeon

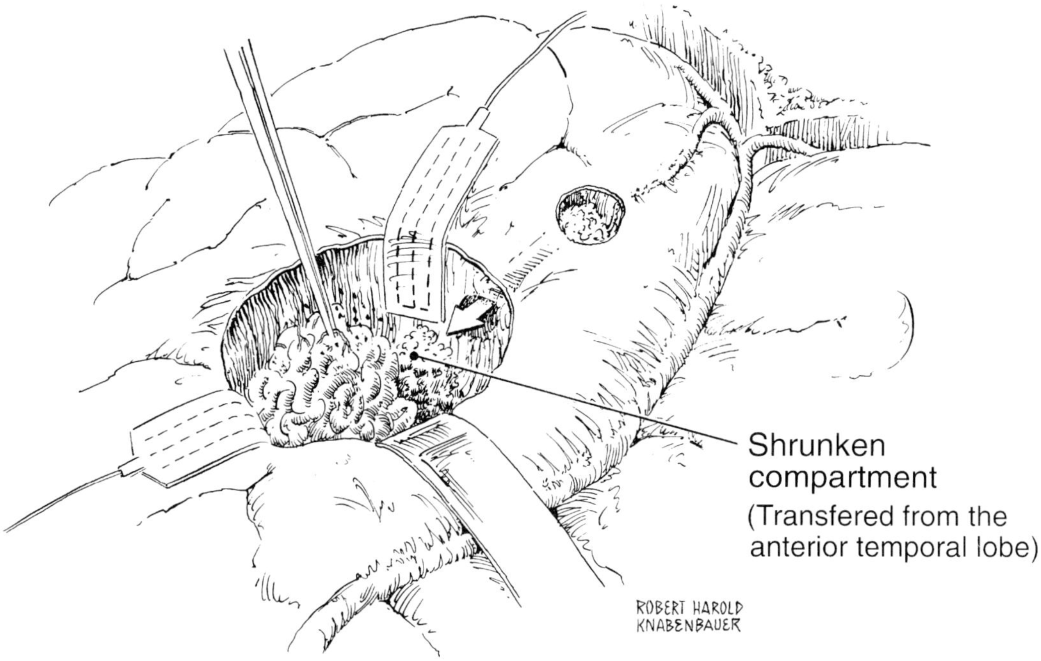

Figure 37A. The anterior compartment was reached through the sulcus where another draining vein traveled, and was isolated and coagulated. The shrunken portion of the anterior compartment was transferred into the posterior opening. *Continued*

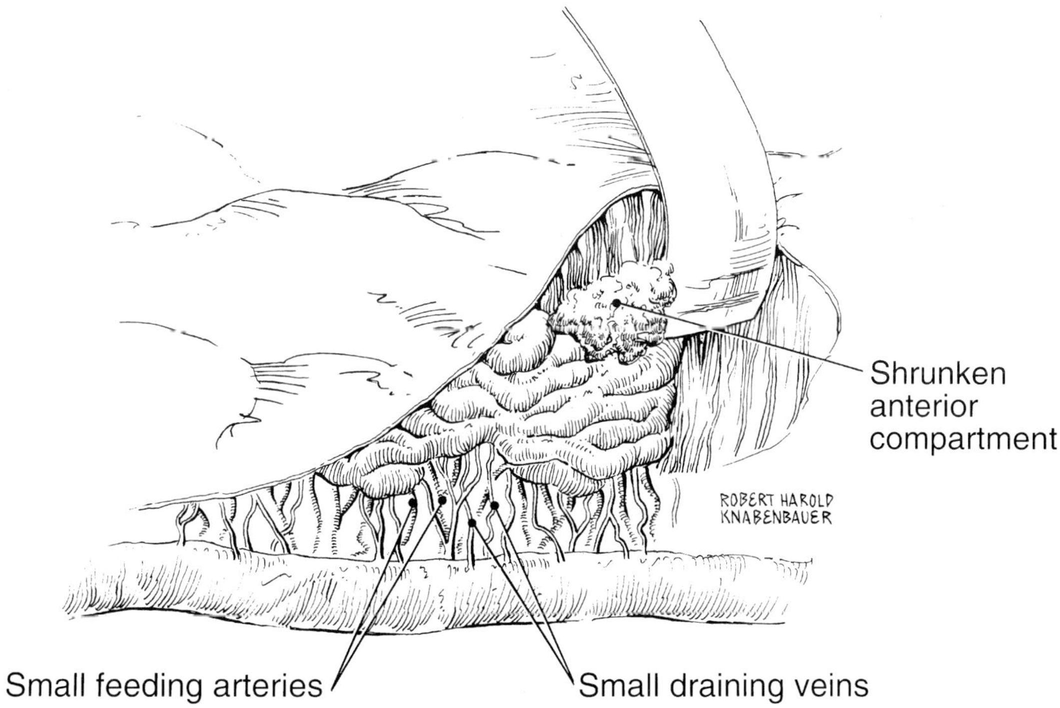

Figure 37B. The anterosuperior dissection of the anterior and lateral compartment exposes the sylvian vein from medioinferiorly. Small feeding arteries to the AVM and small draining veins to the sylvian veins are parallel to each other (refer to text).

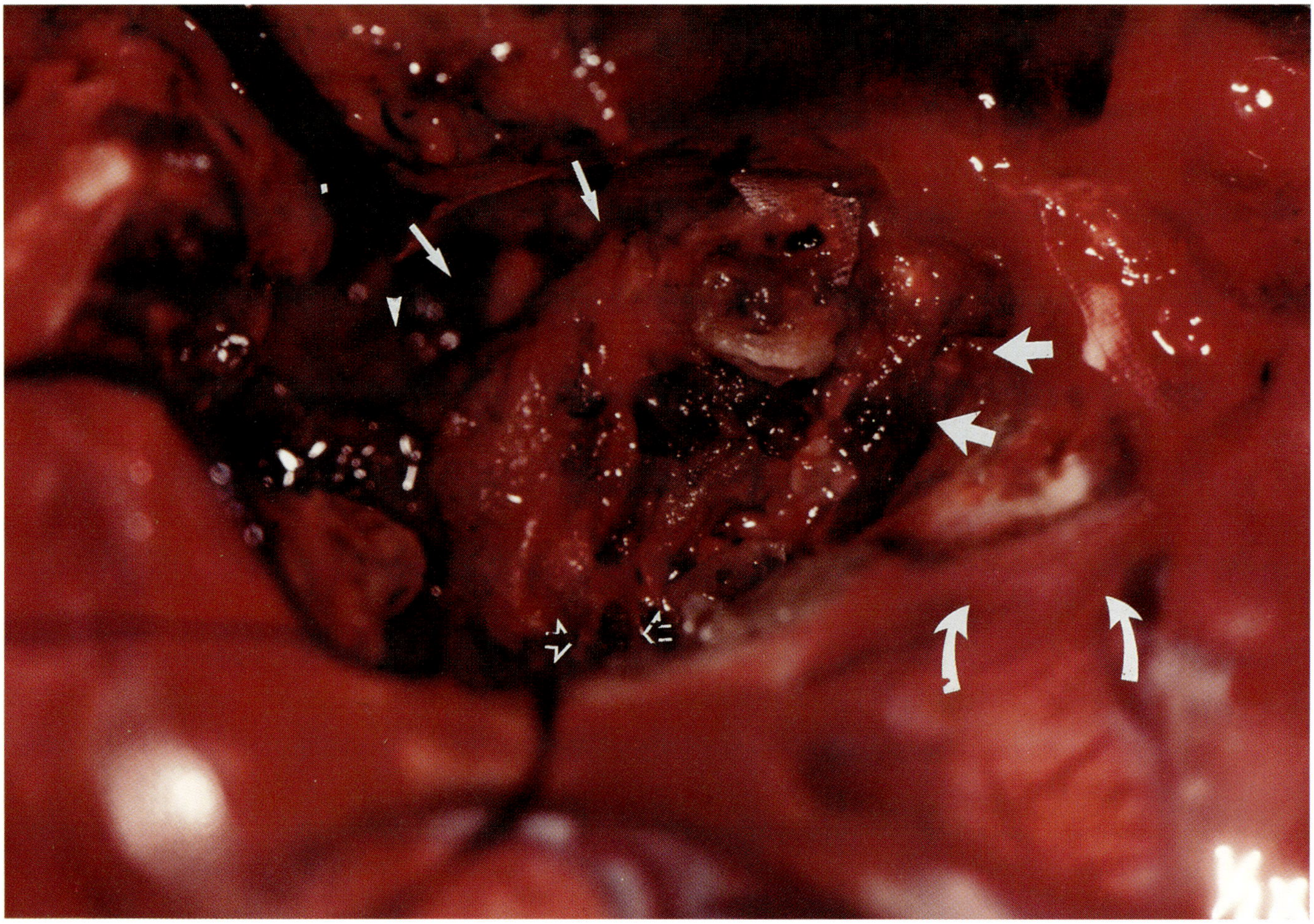

Figure 38. A photograph of the surgical field of the superior temporal gyrus AVM. The AVM was dissected all around its circumference, including superolaterally along the sylvian vein (large arrows), and posteroinferiorly (thin arrows). Medially located draining veins will be transected (arrowhead). Two small draining veins are seen connected to the sylvian vein (open arrows). Curved arrows indicate the sylvian drain which has already been isolated.

may have to follow several veins dilated with arterial blood into the sulci until the true draining vein is found. Other veins dilated with arterial blood are attenuated as they travel in the sulci and are not found to be directly connected to the AVM core. It is important to retract the sulcal cortex very gently while the draining vein is being isolated, or the geniculocalcarine radiation can be damaged easily. Angiographic holograms are valuable tools for identifying and following the major draining vein. When the proper draining vein is found, the AVM core can be reached and isolated by the technique of interrupting shunting arterioles and communicating venules, as previously described. Attention must be directed to meticulous subcortical dissection of the AVM venous loops from the striate cortex.

Resection of AVMs in the Dominant Parietal Lobe

As discussed in the section on symptomatology, surgical complications for resection of dominant parietal lobe AVMs may cause physical as well as intellectual disability. For this reason surgical procedures must be performed meticulously to avoid brain damage and to preserve microcirculation of both arterial and venous phases. Surgical approach to this AVM is similar to those in the sensorimotor areas: (1) following the major draining vein in the sulcus to gain access to the AVM core, or (2) stereotactic approach either with the use of stereotactic instrumentation or free-hand stereotaxy with the aid of color Doppler ultrasonography. The latter is used only when there is no major draining vein available to follow from the convexity side, usually for AVMs deep in the medial side of the posterior parietal lobe. A cortical entry is chosen 3 cm lateral to the midline in the posterior portion of the parietal lobe (7–8 cm above the inion). The probe is directed toward the AVM until it reaches the target point (closest point to the AVM core relative to the cortical entry). Dissection of large AVMs using the multicompartmental procedure is described in the section on surgical procedures for resection of multicompartmental AVMs in the sensorimotor area.

Resection of Capsulocaudatothalamic AVMs

Total resection of AVMs in the basal ganglia, internal capsule, and thalamus have been reported.[56,100,101] The structure of totally removed AVMs from these areas is likely to be of a compact type.[56,119] Access to these AVMs requires transcallosal, (DeAlveira A, personal communication, 1998), transcallosal-transventricular,[56,101] stereotactic transcortical,[126] and transylvanian-insular[100] approaches. Surgical procedures for diffuse AVMs is limited to the cauterization of the individual AVM vessels. Radiosurgery[105] is favorable for obliterating the diffuse AVMs to protect functional area neurons. Embolization has been successfully used in some patients to obliterate AVMs in the capsulocaudatothalamic area without causing neurological deficit (Moret J, personal communication, 1990).

From the author's experience, the approach through the frontal or occipitoparietal cortex directly to the compact AVM is preferred. Dissection technique is similar to that described earlier for subcortical AVM resection by interrupting shunting arterioles directly connected to the AVM core. The diffuse AVMs can be approached through the frontal or occipitoparietal cortex entering the anterior or posterior portion of the lateral ventricle.[56] Then the diffuse AVM can be cauterized from the distal to the proximal portion. Obliteration from the proximal part of the feeding arteries seems to cause more neurological deficit than the approach from the distal part. Large diffuse AVMs can be cauterized from the distal side in the caudate nucleus, putamen, and upper thalamus to reduce the AVM size to 2.5 cm of less in diameter.

The morbidity that results from any mode of treatment for the capsulocaudatothalamic AVMs is not negligible for the following reasons: (1) motor, sensory, and visual pathways and the thalamic nuclei are crowded into this small area; (2) obliteration of small feeding arteries can cause circulatory impairment in these functionally important structures; and (3) statistics of treatment have not divided the AVMs into compact and diffuse types. So far, no distinction has been made between compact and diffuse AVMs in evaluating the results of any mode of treatment in the subject area.

Resection of Brain Stem AVMs

The most common presentation of patients with brain stem AVMs is signs and symptoms secondary to hemorrhage. These include evidence of damage to motor, somatosensory, and acoustic sensory pathways or one or multiple involvement of brain stem nuclei. Surgical intervention is limited only to superficially located compact AVMs or those surrounded by a hematoma (relatively large for this area). Various approaches to brain stem AVMs[56] are similar to those for brain stem cavernoma, which are described in detail in Chapter 6. The essential technique includes interruption of shunting arterioles around the AVM core and resecting it as a small mass without removing functional brain tissue.

Large AVMs in the cerebellum extending into the brain stem can best be treated by surgical obliteration of the entire cerebellar portion and partial obliteration of the brain stem AVM, followed by radiosurgery (the reader may refer to illustrative cases).

Embolization or any intravascular intervention is likely to cause high morbidity. Radiosurgery of small AVMs may be effective in some cases.[25]

Stereotactic Approach to AVMs Located Mesially or Deep in White Matter

Safe resection of compact AVMs located in the functional area has been described in the previous sections. However, there is an exception to this technical rule. When the AVM is located in the medial hemisphere, its feeding arteries are usually the anterior cerebral artery or the posterior cerebral artery and their branches. The draining veins arising from the AVM core end in the mesial surface of the hemisphere by connecting to the surface veins. Numerous veins bridging the mesial surface and the falx are dilated with arterial blood. This arterial blood then drains into the superior or inferior sagittal sinus or into the internal cerebral vein and the vein of Galen. Under these circumstances, approaches from the mesial hemispheric surface to the medially located large AVMs should be avoided as previously described. Insertion of a probe through a predetermined trajectory by the stereotactic method through the silent area prevents unnecessary damage to the functional area neurons. Important vascular structures such as the AVM core, feeding arteries, and draining veins are excluded from the trajectory of the probe.[94,126]

Stereotactic localization of the AVM requires plain x-ray superimposed on either angiograms, CT scan with contrast, or MRI. The trajectory of the stereotactic probe is determined for the safe access to and dissection of the AVM. The target point is determined to avoid damage to the neuronal pathways of the functional areas. Similarly, the trajectory of the stereotactic probe must pass through the silent area cortex and white matter. This process is in preparation for the dissection of the AVM with superselective interruption of the shunting arterioles and communicating venules. It is also equally important to avoid the feeding arteries including the anterior, middle, and posterior cerebral arteries and their large branches, as well as the lenticulostriate artery.

Stereotactic Instrumentation: Various stereotactic instruments are now available such as Leksell, Todd-Wells, Brown-Roberts-Wells (BRW), and Austin's socket ball instrument.[126] The socket ball instrument has been used for conventional skull films (Figures 39A and B) and the BRW for CT scan imaging. The authors have used either angiographic skull films or CT scan with contrast coordinated with computer localization of the entry and target points. The illustrative cases in a later section include the stereotactically approached AVMs (Figure 40).

Conventional X-ray Imaging: The conventional imaging method utilizes the plain films taken at the time of stereotactic surgery, superimposed on the previously obtained angiogram. The x-ray films with Towne's view, i.e., modified anteroposterior (AP) view and lateral views must be imaged exactly the same as those of the angiography (Figures 39A and B).

A burr hole is placed 12 cm behind the glabella, 1 cm anterior to the coronal suture, and 2.5 or 3.0 cm lateral to the midline. The socket and ball type stereo (tactic) instrument is applied to the trephine. The line parallel to the midline is drawn through the center of the (expected) burr hole. In the AP view, this parallel line meets with the anterior-superior portion of the AVM. This point is selected as the target. An appropriate point of the AVM may be selected as a target (near the midplane in the medially located AVMs). The distance from the target to the coordinate in the lateral view is determined in the following manner.

The fiducial for the angiogram superimposed films includes the orbitomeatal plane, the planum sphenoidale, and its posterior edge or dorsum sellae for the lateral view, and midplane and anterior clinoid processes (same plane as the posterior planum sphenoidale) for Towne's view. Thus the distance of the target from the midline (AP view) and that from the planum sphenoidale (lateral view) is measured. The planum sphenoidale plane is drawn in the lateral film, and then a line perpendicular to this plane passing through the posterior edge of this planum is drawn. The vertical distance between the target and the planum and the horizontal distance between the target and the vertical line drawn above are determined. The target is thus shown in the lateral film, and the trajectory is estimated in coordination with the target location by the Towne's view.

CT Imaging: Brown-Roberts-Wells (BRW) stereotactic system was used in connection with General Electric (GE) CTi 9800 (Milwaukee, WI), and HL Ad-

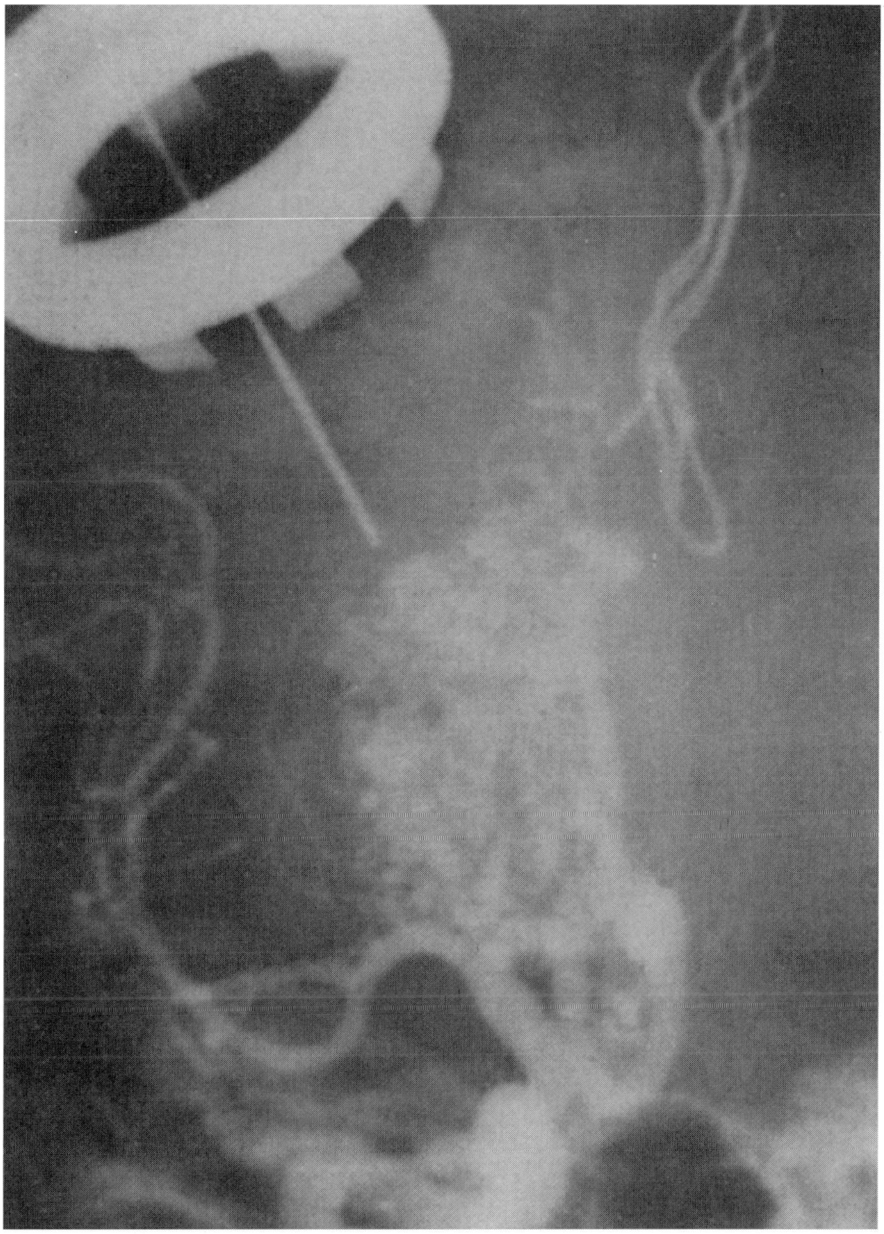

Figure 39. An angiographic AP view **(A)** and angiographic lateral view **(B)** of an AVM located in the medial part of functional area. It was reached by stereotactic approach. The stereotactic probe was inserted from the silent area through a trajectory predetermined by stereotactic instrumentation. The target point was selected along the anterosuperior aspect of the AVM at the border between the functional and nonfunctional areas. The stereotactic instrument is removed except for the probe, and a thin layer of brain tissue is removed around the probe. The AVM dissection starts from the target point. *Continued*

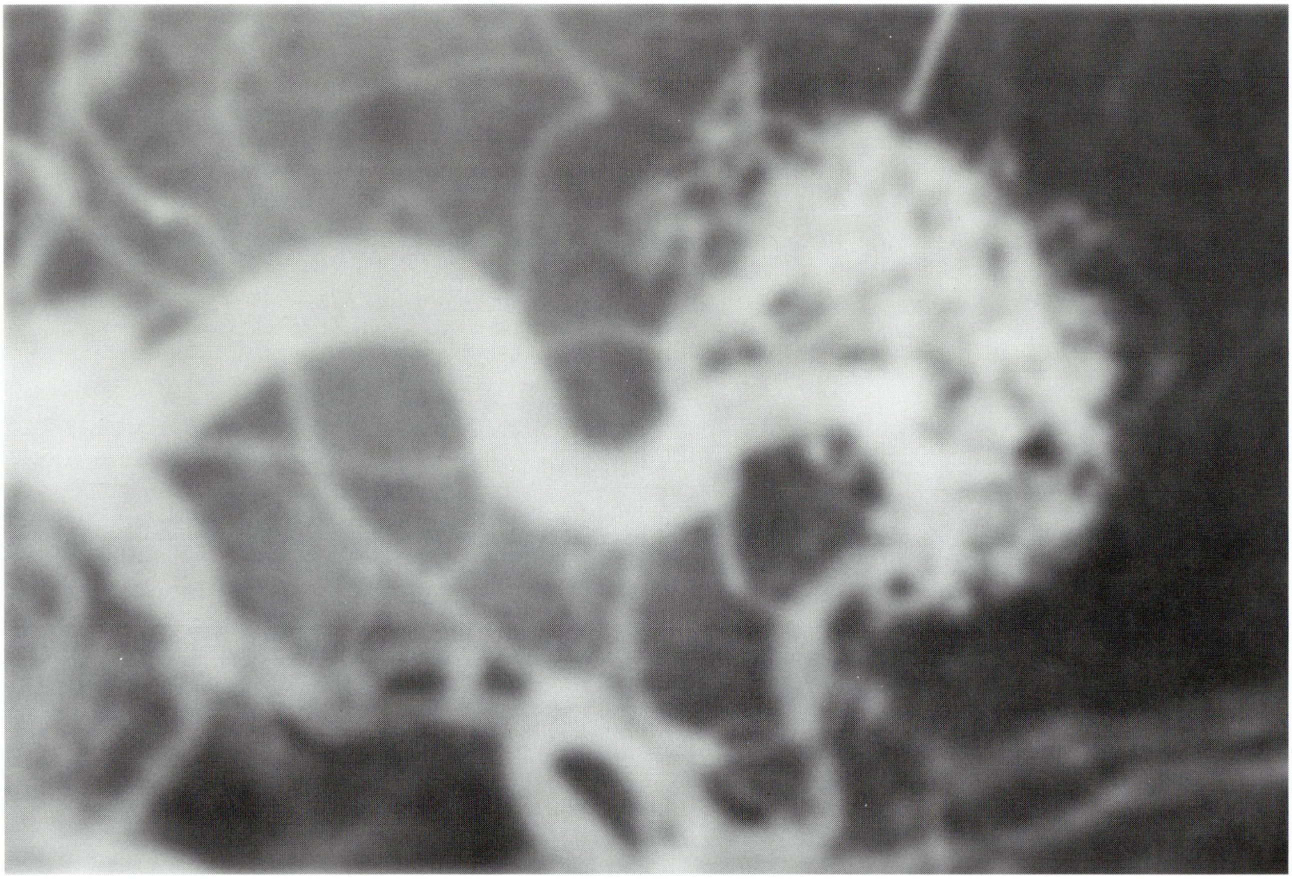

Figure 39B. Lateral view of an AVM located in the medial part of the functional area.

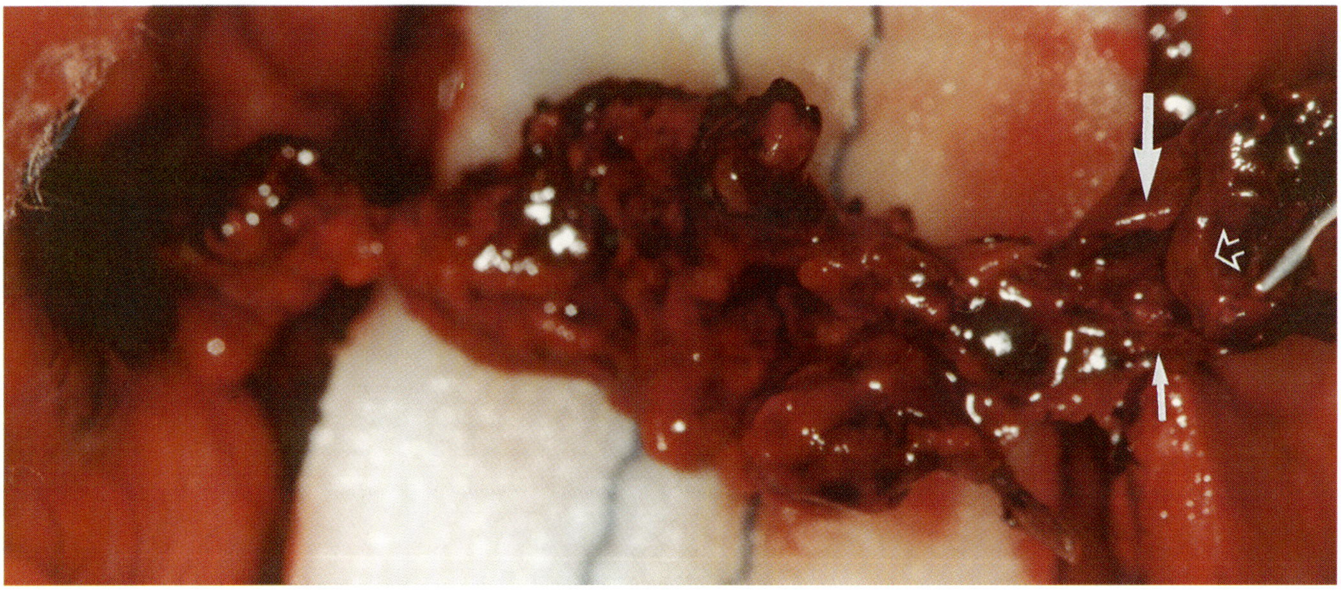

Figure 40. This photograph shows a shrunken AVM that was brought to the cortical surface and placed on a cottonoid patty. Collecting veins (small arrow) are seen at the right still connected to the draining vein (arrowhead). A feeding artery (branch of the anterior cerebral artery) is shown by the large arrow.

vantage computed tomographic imaging systems for data collection. Data processing was completed with a programmable calculator system (HX-20, Epson West, Placentia, CA).

The BRW ring was applied to the patient's head as the base ring, which was secured to the calvarium by carbon fiber post and nylon-steel set pins. A localizer unit interfaces with the base ring to allow the production of extracranial reference points on a CT scan slice (usually with axial plane) that may be spatially related to the intracranial target. A Kirshner wire was inserted into the brain through a calvarial burr hole or opened craniotomy in the direction of trajectory to the point 2 mm short of the target depth. Full insertion was avoided to prevent puncture through any of the AVM vessels. An arc system was exchanged for a localizer unit at the scanning and allowed multiple angle setting for appropriate projections to the target points in rigid fixation, and a phantom base allowed extracranial simulation of the cranial entry and intracranial points. These components permitted point access within 1 mm of the target. This target was determined by the AVM contour demonstrated by CT scan imaging with contrast. When the tip of the probe was confirmed to be at the target point, a thin layer of brain tissue was removed around the probe until the target was reached and then the probe was removed. Resection of the compact AVM was performed using the routine technique.

Neuronavigational Approach: Several stereotactic instrumentations are available without placing conventional stereotactic instruments to the head. These include Vector Vision (image guided surgery system, Brain LAB USA, Inc., Palo Alto, CA), Elekta (electronically controlled viewing wand, and Ricker (Depuy). Both the Zeiss Company and the Leitz Company manufacture a microscope-incorporated navigator that is useful for selecting the trajectory with the desired cortical entrance. Recent development of intraoperative MRI, which develops images instantly as the probe is placed either outside or inside the cranial cavity, has provided for accurate placement of the probe to the target. This technology demonstrates the plane that includes the entire trajectory of the probe and the surrounding cerebral and vascular structures (Mandybur GT, communication, 1998).

Surgical Results for AVMs Resected in Functional Areas

Overall Results

The surgical results presented are derived from the 135 patients at the authors' institution who underwent superselective isolation of AVMs in functional areas of the brain between 1974 and 1996. The age of the patients ranged from 3 weeks to 76 years (average 34.2 years). Postoperative follow-up periods range from 2 years to 24 years.

Primary locations of AVMs included: sensorimotor area in 79 patients, speech area in 21, occipital visual area in 22, capsulocaudatothalamic area in 7, brain stem in 5, superior temporal gyrus in 2. Large and giant AVMs had extension beyond the designated primary area; for example, 22 patients with superior temporal gyrus involvement had AVMs that extended from the sensorimotor and speech areas. Size of the AVMs included small (<8.2 cm^3, equivalent to 2.5 cm diameter sphere) in 24 patients, medium (8.2 to 65.5 cm^3, equivalent to 2.5 to 5 cm sphere) in 68 patients, large (≥ 65.5 cm^3, equivalent to a 5 cm sphere) in 35 patients, and giant (>113.3 cm^3, equivalent to 6 cm sphere) in 9 patients. Major draining vein or veins were located on the lateral convexity surface in 13 patients, mesial cortical surface in 30 patients, and both lateral and medial hemispheric surfaces in 92. Arterial supplies were from: MCA (26), ACA (9), PCA (2), MCA + ACA (34), MCA + PCA (20), MCA + ACA + PCA (52), SCA + AICA + PAICA (2), AICA + PAICA (2), and SCA + MCA (1).

At operation all cases showed evidence of preoperative hemorrhage in the form of hematoma, liquefied blood, arachnoid adhesions, and hemosiderin-laden brain tissue often associated with glial scar. Thus, there was no statistical difference in the incidence of hemorrhage between small, medium, large, or giant AVMs; however, multiple small hemorrhages were found more frequently around large or giant AVMs than smaller ones. There was a trend that the patients who presented with hemorrhagic ictus had a high incidence of harboring smaller AVMs (<4 cm) and those who presented with seizures had larger AVMs (5–6 cm) (see Figures 13A and B).

Partial elimination of large AVMs (by cautery coagulation) to a size <3 cm in diameter was followed by gamma knife radiosurgery in the following patients: 2 with capsulocaudatothalamic AVMs and 1 with a cerebellar-brain stem AVM. Partial isolation of a giant AVM in the sensorimotor area will be followed by intravascular embolization and proton beam radiation because the patient remains severely hemiparetic from the preoperative period and another surgery risk is considered unwarranted.

Preoperative neurological conditions of patients were normal in 25 patients, mild deficits in 42, moderate deficits in 32, and severe deficits in 36. Postoperative conditions were normal in 88 patients, mild deficits in 27, moderate deficits in 14, and severe deficits in 6. One-third of the patients had transient mild neurological deficits.

Of 25 patients with preoperatively normal neurological findings, 23 remained normal and 2 developed mild deficits. Of the 2 who had neurological deficits, 1 patient developed left leg monoparesis, which requires a short brace for long-distance walking, and the other with a giant AVM developed left hemianesthesia, which subsided to involve only a part of the hand and foot (this case is also included in the following section, *Results for AVMs in the Superior Temporal Gyrus*).

Of the 42 patients with preoperatively mild deficits (motor, sensory, speech, or visual) that interfered only with practical occupational skills, 33 patients regained normal function postoperatively although 1 patient (occipital AVM) developed homonymous hemianopia, 8 remained with mild deficits, and 1 with a giant AVM developed mild hemiparesis and decreased hand skill but became free of intractable seizures.

Of the 32 patients with moderate deficits (definite but no disabling motor, sensory, or speech, or cognitive deficits), 22 became neurologically normal, 9 improved to mild deficits, and 1 infant died of pneumonia.

Of the 36 patients with severe neurological deficits (hemiplegia or severe hemiparesis, sensory and speech difficulties), 8 became normal postoperatively, 8 improved to mild deficits, 13 improved to moderate deficits, and 4 remained with severe deficits (3 capable of self-care, 1 dependent). Of 2 comatose patients (included in the serious deficit group), 1 patient regained normal function and the other regained consciousness with mild deficits. Temporary postoperative deficits were noted in one-third of patients with large or giant AVMs.

The one death, not directly related to AVM surgery, occurred in a 5-month-old girl with postoperative awakening and movement of all extremities. She then developed bronchial obstruction due to tracheal tube kinking and subsequently developed irreversible severe pneumonia.

Of 69 patients with a history of seizures, 56 (81%) are seizure-free without anticonvulsants; 13 patients have good seizure control with medication using significantly less medication than used prior to surgery. The latter group had violent generalized seizures (initiated by focal) preoperatively. The necessity of postoperative use of anticonvulsants was not related to the size of the AVMs.

Preoperative and postoperative occupational capacities were as follows: Preoperatively no one held a full-time occupation; 6 patients remained in part-time work; 53 were out of work; 62 were disabled (no chance of work); and 14 were totally dependent. Postoperatively, 88 patients (1 with monoparesis and 1 with homonymous hemianopia) have regained full-time occupation; 25 hold part-time jobs; 3 remain out of work requiring convalescence or occupational training; 6 continue to be disabled although neurologically improved; 2 are still dependent; and 1 died.

Results for AVMs in the Superior Temporal Gyrus

Of the 22 patients with AVMs in the superior temporal gyrus, the AVM extended into Broca's area in 10 patients, Wernicke's area in 3 patients, and the capsulostriatothalamic area in 7 patients. Each of the AVMs extended into the lower sensorimotor area. All 22 patients regained neurological functions or improved beyond the preoperative neurological status, except for 1 who developed postoperative hemianesthesia after coagulation of a diffuse AVM in the thalamic portion but regained normal activities. All 7 patients who presented with seizures are seizure-free without anticonvulsants, and the 3 patients with a history of hemorrhagic ictus and seizures gained seizure control with smaller dosage of anticonvulsants. Two patients had temporary worsening of expressive dysphasia, which subsided over 3–6 months to the preoperative minimum speech difficulty. Two patients who presented with severe hemiparesis and dysphasia as a result of a large hematoma have improved to mild hemiparesis and dysphasia in 2 years. One of these 2 patients is ambulating with a cane and one without a cane.

There are several reports on surgery of temporal lobe AVMs.[43,61,132] Resection of the superior temporal gyrus AVM was described earlier by the authors.[116,117] This procedure can be performed with minimum morbidity if approached systematically and done meticulously. It is important to follow the order of dissection as described in the surgical procedure, particularly for small feeding arteries and draining veins along the sylvian vein, to prevent postoperative cerebral swelling.

Temporary worsening of the expressive speech difficulty can be caused by excessive retraction in the frontal operculum during AVM dissection. Diffuse AVMs in the lower thalamus should be coagulated and then treated with irradiation.

Seizure control was excellent in all cases. This corresponds to the postoperative results reported by others.[132] Overall results of AVM resection in the superior temporal gyrus, which extends to speech and sensorimotor areas (underneath the cortex) or the capsulocaudatothalamic area (with a compact type), are promising.

Results for AVMs in the Occipital Area

Of 22 total patients with AVMs in the occipital areas, 11 had AVMs in the mesial occipital lobe, including the striate area (4 of these on the left), and another 11 had AVMs in the convexity occipital area (6 of these on the left). After surgical isolation and coagulation of a large mesioinferior occipital AVM, 1 patient developed homonymous hemianopia due to postoperative propagation of the thrombosis that extended into the calcarine branch (posterior cerebral artery).

Results for AVMs in the Capsulocaudatothalamic Area

Seven patients underwent resection of AVMs confined to the capsulocaudatothalamic area. Five had episodes of hemorrhage, 1 presented with progressive weakness, and 1 had mental and physical (hemiparesis, incoordination) deterioration. Four patients with compact AVMs (2 large and 2 medium) underwent total resection and recovered without neurological deficits except for temporary hemiparesis in 2. Another 3 patients had diffuse AVMs. Two of these with large AVMs had obliteration to reduce the size to 2.5 cm in diameter for gamma knife radiation. One patient had subtotal surgical obliteration with cauterization several years after neutron irradiation. All patients live a normal life except for one who goes to regular school with limited activity (refer to illustrative case 10).

Results for AVMs in the Brain Stem

Five patients presented with a history of hemorrhage. One patient had an AVM in the anterior lateral pons with facial palsy, 3 had an extension to the cerebellum, and 1 had an extension to the medial temporal lobe. Two patients had total resection of small AVMs, and 1 had total resection of a medium AVM extending into the cerebellum. One patient, dependent on mother's care because of severe ocular movement impairment, incoordination, and gait difficulty, had a large AVM 5 cm in diameter (cerebellar, brain stem). Surgical cauterization was performed, starting in the vermis to obliterate shunting arterioles and communicating venules medial to pairs of superior cerebellar arteries, and anterior and posterior inferior cerebellar arteries, to shrink the AVM to the size of 2.0 cm for later treatment with gamma knife. A large AVM extending into the medial temporal lobe was treated with proton beam irradiation after surgical subtotal resection. Four patients live normal lives, and 1 ambulates with a wheelchair and takes care of herself.

Illustrative Cases

Individual cases have different histories, approaches to AVMs, and postoperative conditions. In this section, preoperative, intraoperative, and postoperative conditions of several representative cases are summarized.

Case 1: Single Compartment Sensorimotor AVM

On the day of admission in January 1981, this 51-year-old woman had three episodes of jerking of the right arm, one extending to the right leg and another progressing to a generalized seizure that rendered her unconscious. The family reported an earlier incidence of jerking of her entire body 2 years prior to admission. No neurological deficits were found.

Imaging Findings

Angiography showed 4 cm (vertical) $\times$ 3.5 cm (lateral) $\times$ 2.5 cm (AP) AVM, 18 cm^3 in volume (Figures 41A-C). The AVM was located in the central area surrounded by the motor cortex anteriorly and the sensory cortex posteriorly, partly exposed to the hemispheric surface through the widened central sulcus. Similarly, a small draining vein was connected anteriorly with three smaller cortical veins (Figure 42A). The external end of the major draining vein was connected to the junction of three cortical veins dilated with arterial blood (Figure 42A). There were two circumferential feeding arteries, one anterior and the other posterior to the AVM core. Both were concealed in brain tissue and only one of the branches of the posterior feeding artery was exposed.

Operative Procedure

After a 5 $\times$ 4 cm craniotomy and dural opening, a part of the AVM was located in the central sulcus. An arachnoid incision along the posterior lateral surface of the AVM allowed exposure of the external end of the major draining vein. This vein was followed 2 cm deep to its junction to the AVM core. Shunting arterioles and communicating venules of 50 μm to 200 μm, and occasionally 250 μm, were interrupted to isolate the posterior aspect of the core. The sensory cortex, verified by SSEP recordings, was preserved intact. Anterior shunting arterioles were more crowded with shorter distances between them than posterior shunting arterioles. The motor cortex was retracted anteriorly and the AVM was retracted posteriorly and superiorly, and kept intact (Figure 42B). Shunting arterioles and communicating venules

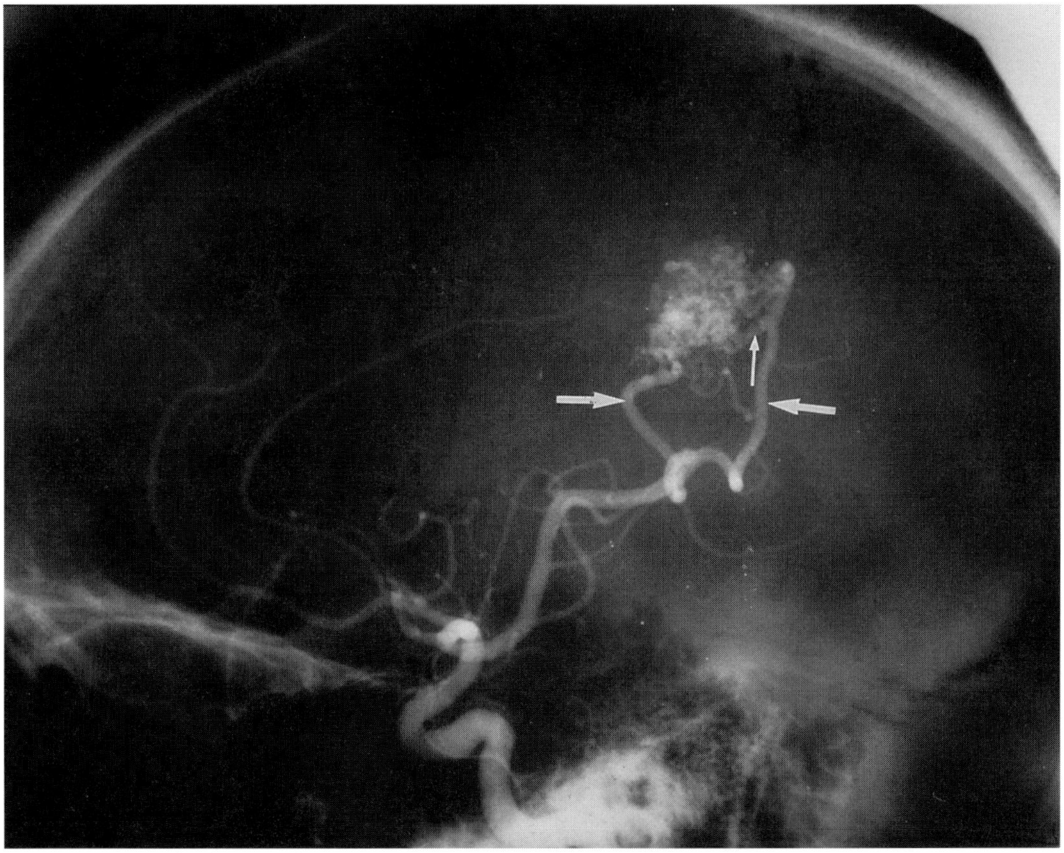

Figure 41A. A lateral angiogram of an AVM underneath the left sensorimotor area extending into the widened rolandic fissure. It revealed two feeding arteries (arrows), one located anteriorly and the other posteriorly to the AVM core. The posterior feeding artery was circumferential with four identifiable branches (one marked by a thin arrow) terminating as shunting arterioles (see illustrative case 1). *Continued*

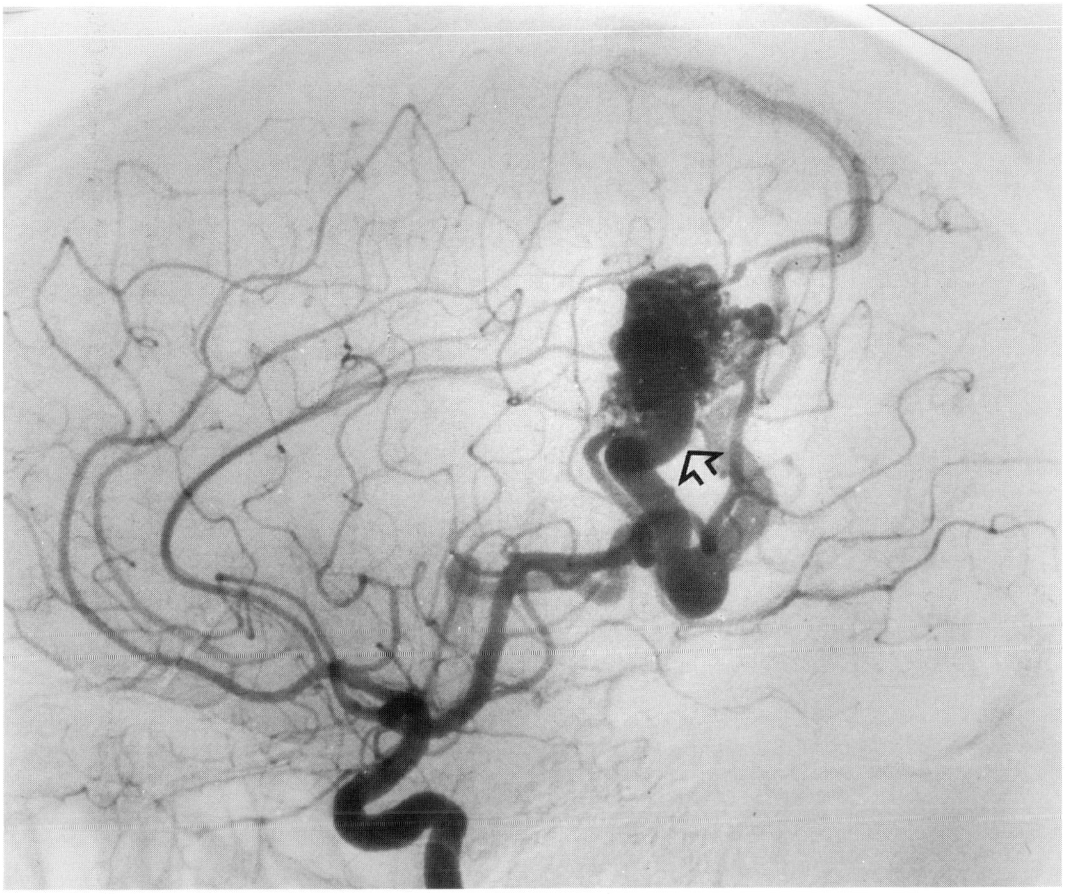

Figure 41B. The later phase of the lateral angiogram shows the major draining vein (arrow) originating from the AVM core deep in the sulcus (see illustrative case 1). *Continued*

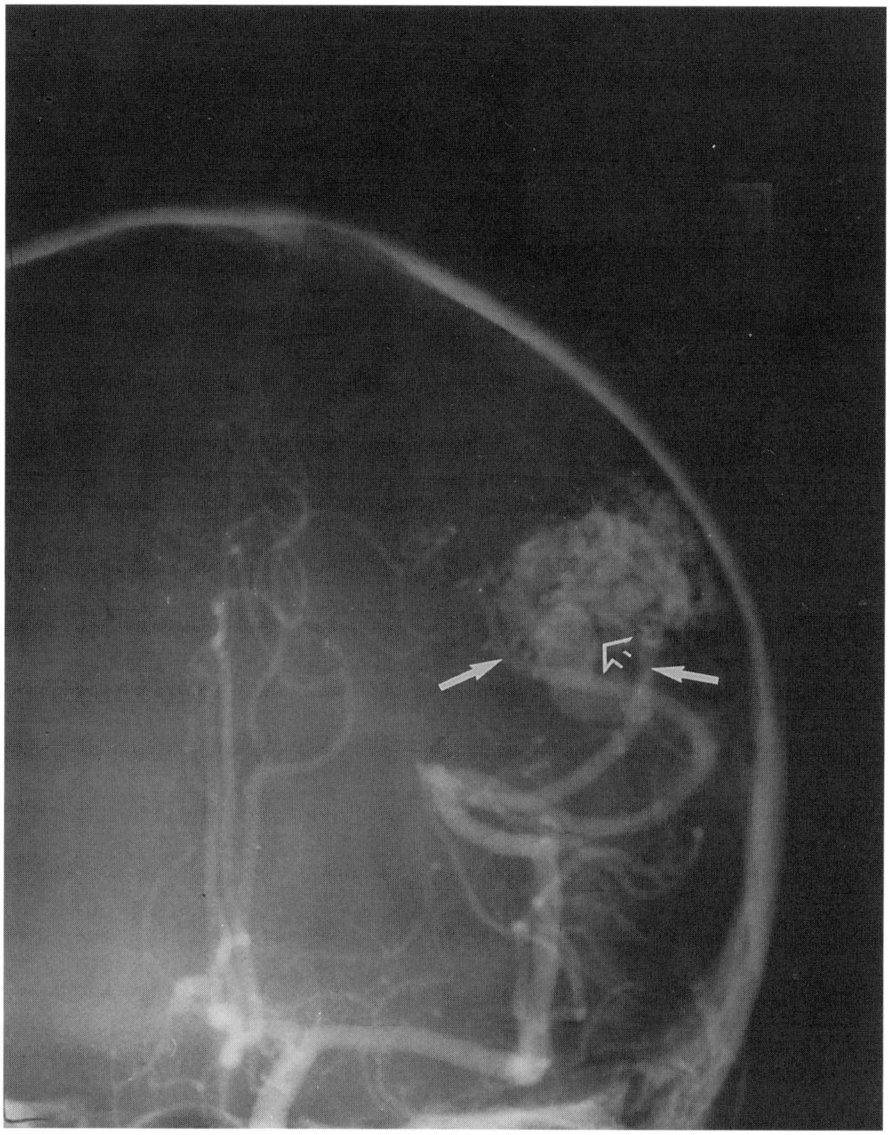

Figure 41C. The AP view shows two feeding arteries (arrows) and the major draining vein (arrowhead) originating from the deep posteromedial aspect of the core (see illustrative case 1).

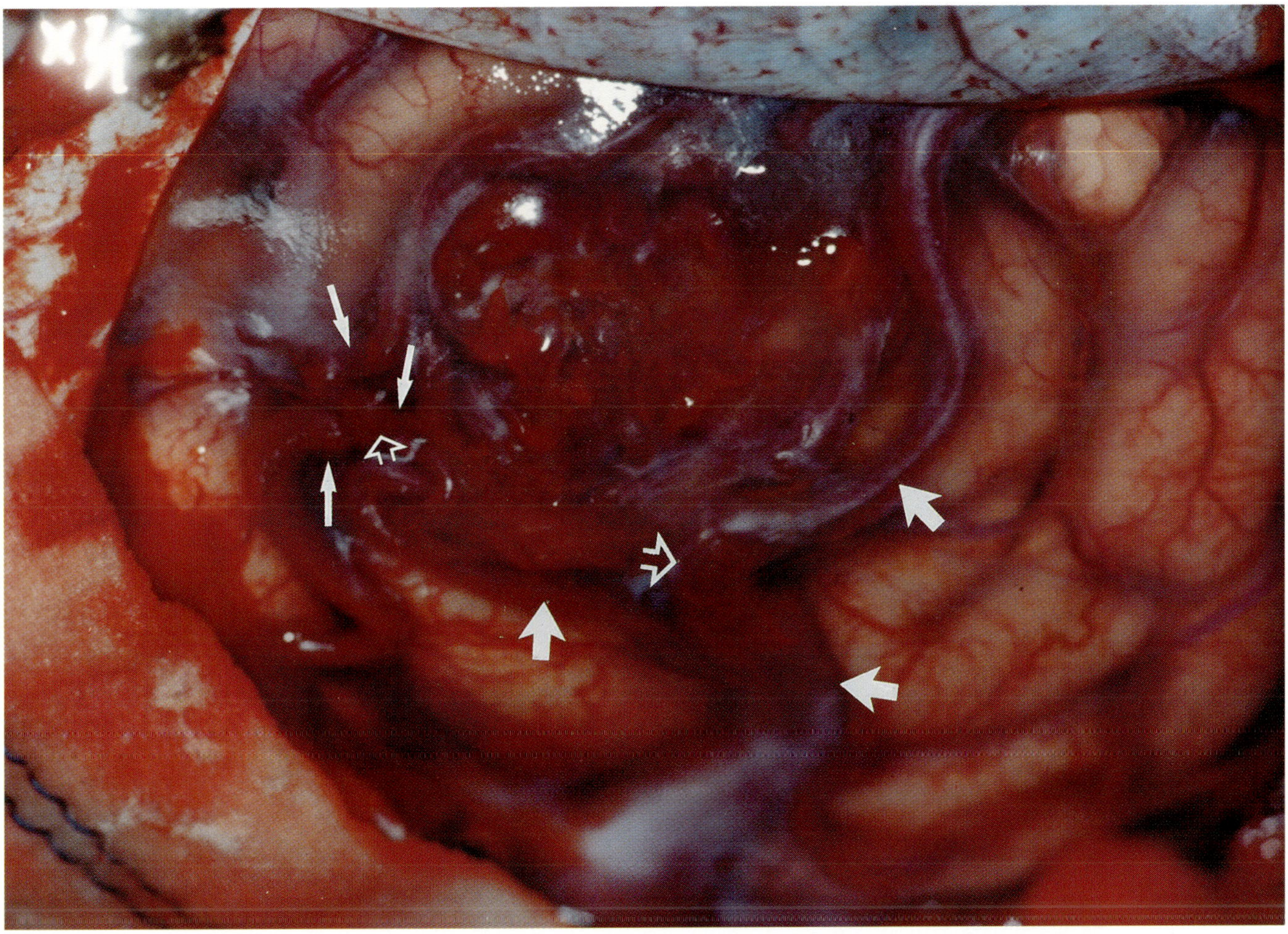

Figure 42A. A photograph of an AVM with a portion extending into the rolandic fissure flush with the hemispheric surface. The external end of the major draining vein (large open arrow) was connected to three cortical veins (arrows) posteriorly (right side of photo). Three small cortical veins (small arrows) were connected to the external end of the smaller draining vein (small open arrow) arising from the anterior portion of the AVM core (left side of photo) (see illustrative case 1). *Continued*

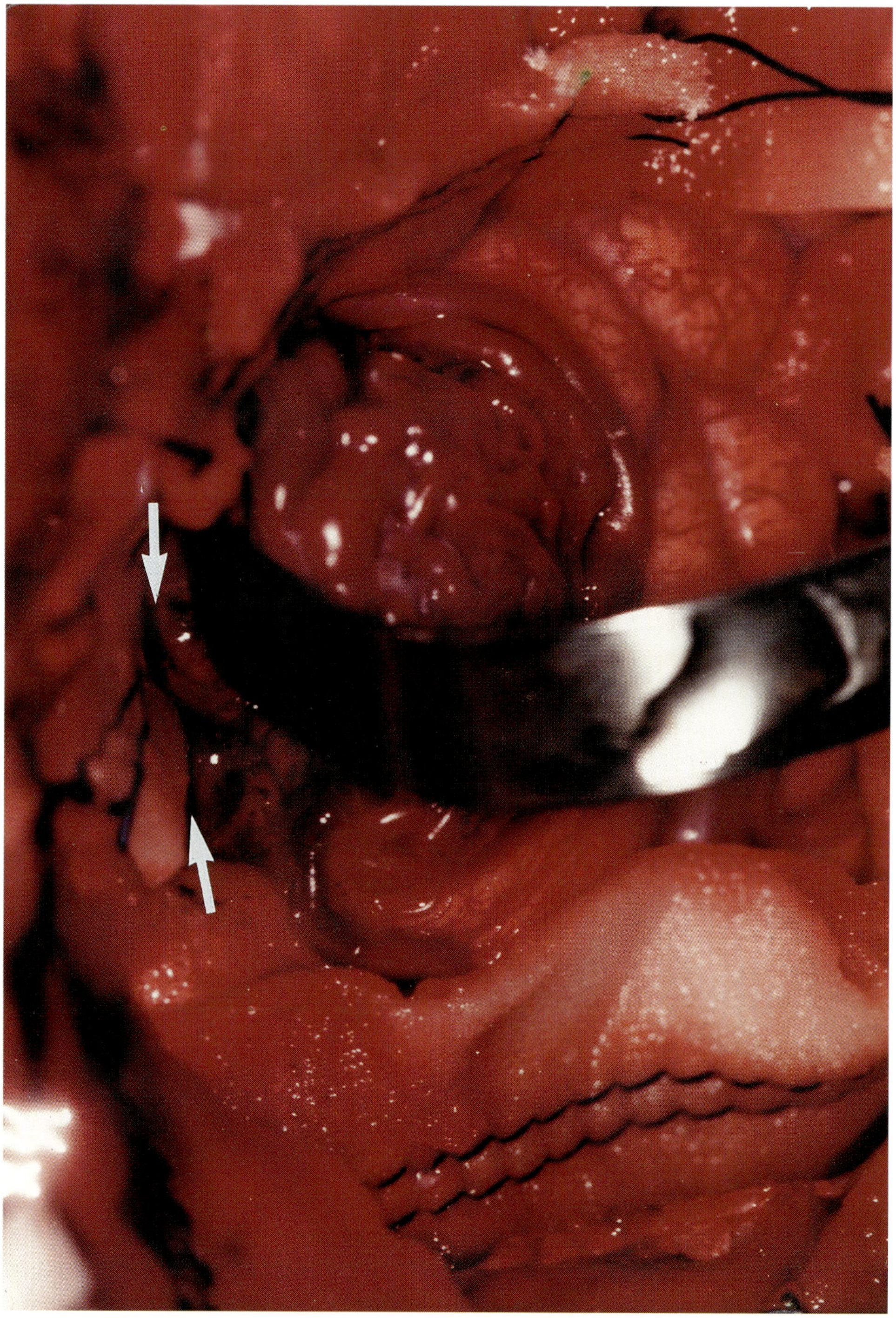

Figure 42B. A photograph of the AVM core retracted posteriorly on its anterior aspect while being dissected using the author's technique. A cleavage (arrows) was formed between the core and the sulcal cortex, which remained totally intact covered by a cottonoid patty (see illustrative case 1).

were interrupted circumferentially around the AVM. The AVM was totally resected after cauterizing and sectioning the major draining vein in the sulcus.

A cicatrix that formed in the sensory cortex (1.5 cm diameter, 0.5 cm thick) was removed away from the underlying normal brain tissue. Histologically it was found to be glial tissue.

Postoperative Course

The patient recovered without any neurological deficit except subjective numbness lateral to the thenar muscle bulk, which disappeared within 6 months. She continued to work as an escrow officer until age 65 years and now enjoys retirement.

Case 2: Three-Compartment Sensorimotor AVM

On January 8, 1978, this 54-year-old woman was admitted with the chief complaint of progressive weakness of her right leg associated with frequent seizures affecting that leg. About 20 years before admission, she began to have seizures, only occasionally involving the right extremities. Two months prior to admission, these seizures became frequent (>5 times a day). Leg weakness progressed and she began to use a short leg brace and a cane. She was placed on phenytoin and phenobarbital, which had no effect on the seizures. Examination showed mild right leg weakness with foot-drop (1/5 strength of the anterior tibial and peroneus longus muscles), hyperactive tendon reflexes, and Babinski's sign on the right.

Imaging Findings

An AVM with the lateral compartment supplied mainly by the middle cerebral artery branches, the medial compartment supplied primarily by the anterior cerebral artery (see Figures 4B, 14A and B), and the posterior compartment by the posterior branch of the middle cerebral artery (arrowhead in Figure 4C) was demonstrated by angiography and CT. The size of the AVM was 6.0 cm (lateral) × 5.5 cm (vertical) × 4.5 cm (AP) (77.5 cm^3 in volume). There were three major draining veins, one from the lateral compartment connected to the vein of Trolard and the other two arising from the medial compartment, verified at staged operations performed 6 months apart (as described in the previous section).

Operative Procedure

The major draining vein was followed in the central sulcus until the lateral compartment of the AVM core was reached. As the sensorimotor cortex was retracted outward, the lateral aspect of the core was isolated laterally and inferiorly. The junction of the draining vein to the core was found quite inferiorly. Numerous shunting arterioles were interrupted at the connections to the core vessels. Isolation of the core extended anteriorly, inferiorly, and posteriorly. When dissection extended farther posteromedially, a thin posterior compartment was identified separate from the lateral and medial (anteriorly located) compartments. The lateral compartment was cauterized loop by loop until it became a small mass of shrunken vessels. Another major draining vein came into view arising from the lateral aspect of the medial compartment. This vein passed between the medial and lateral compartments upward to connect to the cortical veins on the hemispheric convexity. On opening the central sulcus toward the midline and splitting part of the white matter, the mesial central sulcus was reached. A third major draining vein was located in this sulcus emerging in the mesial hemispheric surface to join the superior sagittal sinus. The superior of the two feeding arteries originating from the anterior cerebral artery was type 1, and traveled along the mesial surface of the hemisphere and then disappeared subcortically to join one of the large core vessels next to its junction to the draining vein (Figure 43A–C). This artery had a large diameter but a thin wall. It was doubly clipped and sectioned, and each sectioned end was cauterized to minimize the chance of later bleeding from this artery. The AVM core was resected after all three major draining veins were cauterized and sectioned (Figures 44 and 45).

Postoperative Course

The patient did well except for several transient episodes of difficulty moving her right hand with each lasting 30–60 minutes after the first stage operation. This seemed to correspond to propagation of the thrombosis in the AVM and probably spasms in the surrounding cerebral vessels. The patient was able to walk without a brace or a cane within 3 months, and returned to the management of her jewelry store. She lives well in retirement at the age of 74 years and is seizure-free without medication. Postoperative angiograms showed normalization of dilated feeding arteries, as described by Norlén.[74]

Case 3: Giant Sensorimotor AVM Extending to Surrounding Areas

On July 28, 1992, this 41-year-old woman was admitted with a history of excellent health until De-

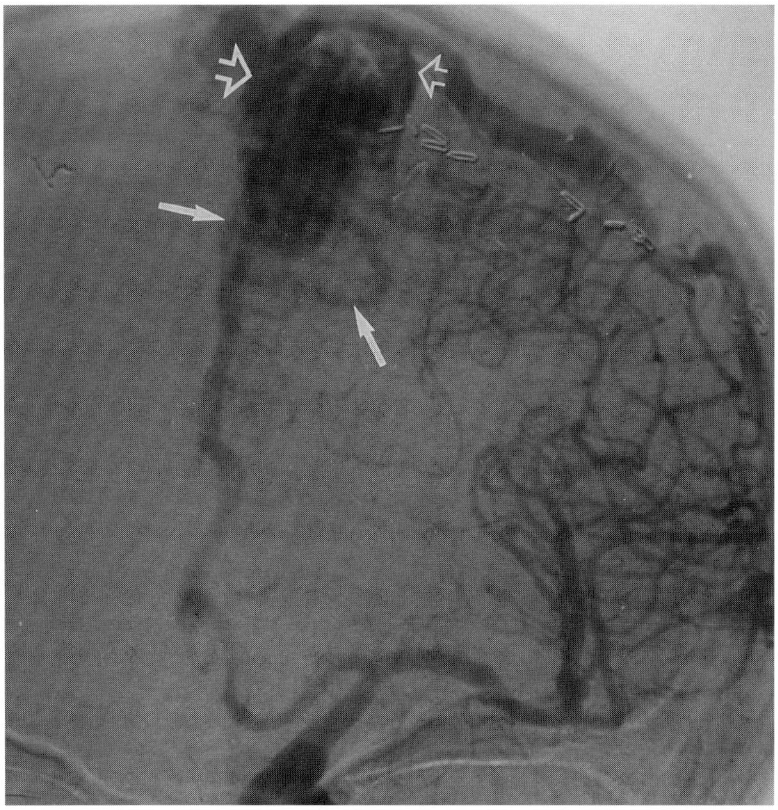

Figure 43A. The AP view of an angiogram after the obliteration of the lateral compartment showed two feeding arteries originating from the anterior cerebral artery (arrows) and two major draining veins (open arrows), one originating from the lateral aspect, and the other from the medial aspect of the medial compartment. Both connect to the enlarged vein of Trolard, which drains to the superior sagittal sinus as well as to the lateral sinus (see illustrative case 2). Figure used with permission of Neurological Research. *Continued*

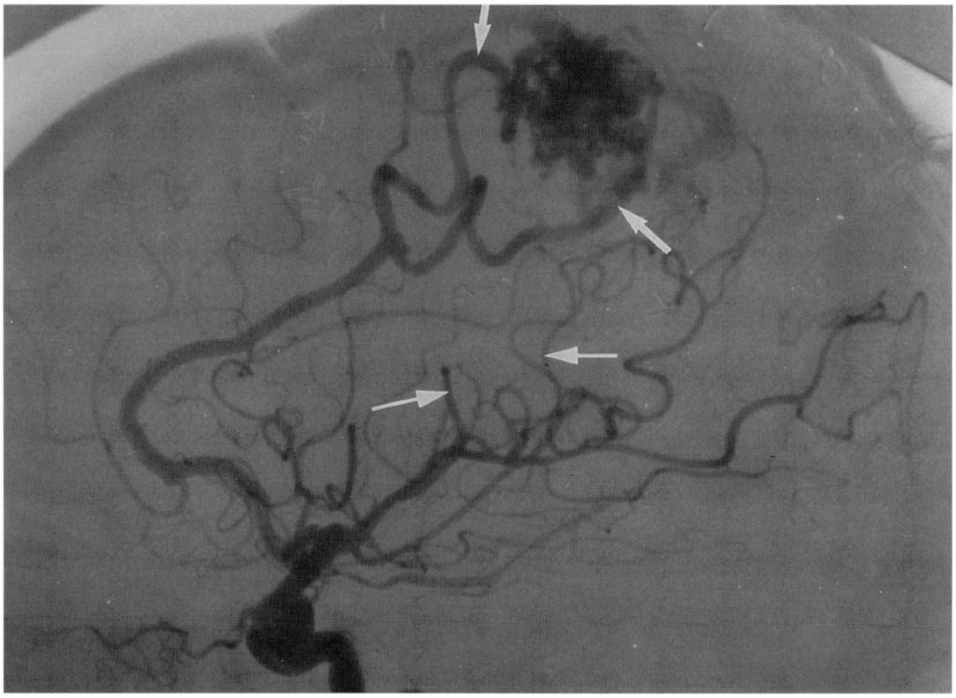

Figure 43B. The medial compartment is seen clearly in the lateral film, not superimposed by the lateral compartment. Of the two feeding arteries arising from the anterior cerebral artery, one approaches the compartment from anteriorly (top large arrow), and the other from posteriorly (lower large arrow). The arteries to the lateral compartment which were enlarged prior to the first stage operation returned to normal size (thin arrows) within 2 weeks after superselective interruption of arterioles and venules and obliteration of the lateral compartment (see illustrative case 2). Figure used with permission of Neurological Research. *Continued*

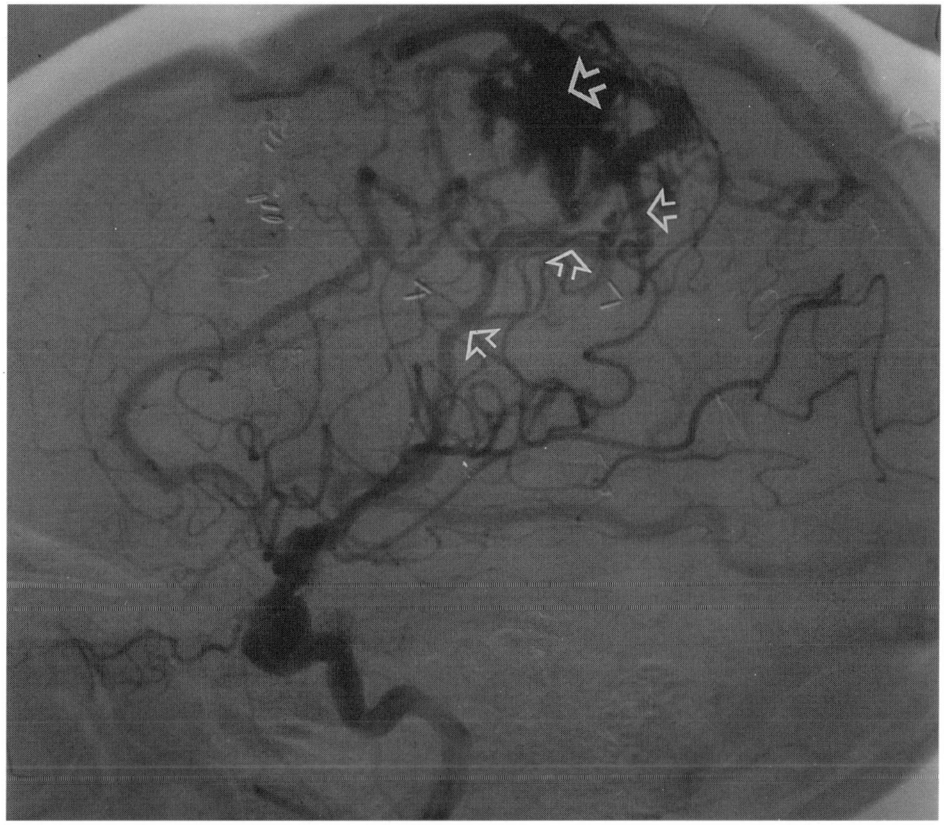

Figure 43C. Later phase of lateral angiogram showing two draining veins from the medial compartment superimposed on each other (large arrows). They are connected to the vein of Trolard (small arrows) (see illustrative case 2). Figure used with permission of Neurological Research.

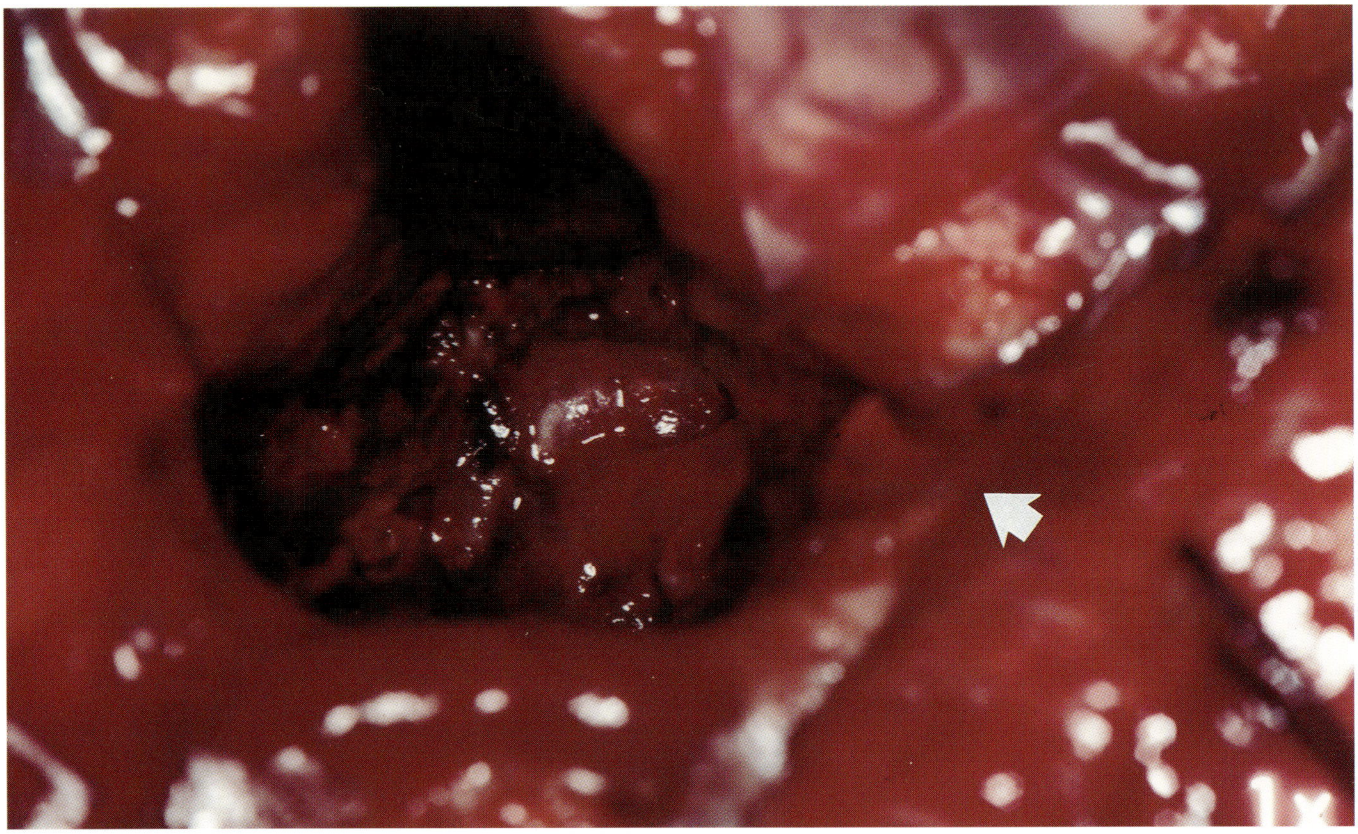

Figure 44. The AVM is shown in the widened rolandic fissure 2.5 cm in diameter. Further cauterization and shrinking of the core allows the removal of the shrunken core undermining the sensorimotor cortex through the sulcus (see illustrative case 2).

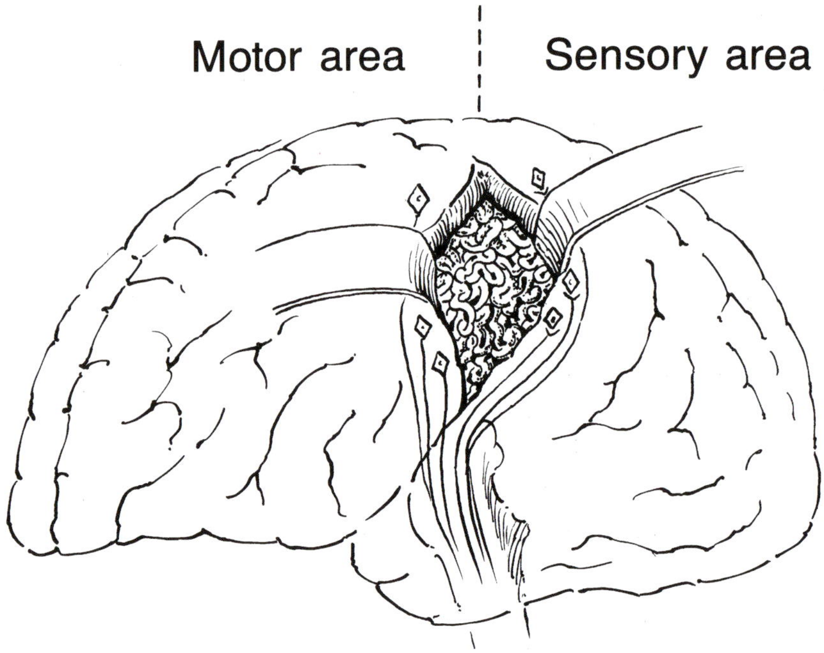

Figure 45. Schematic drawing of a large AVM surrounded by motor and sensory neurons. One of its major draining veins passes through the central sulcus (omitted in the drawing) (see illustrative case 2).

cember 8, 1990, when she experienced a Jacksonian seizure starting in her left upper extremity. She subsequently lost consciousness and developed a generalized seizure. She then began to have episodes of numbness of and inability to move the left arm, and also frequent paroxysmal severe throbbing headache every day. For 3 months the episodes of left arm numbness became increasingly frequent, to more than six times a day. Neurological findings were all within normal limits except for the inability to hop on either foot. She attributed it to "born clumsiness."

Imaging Findings

Angiography showed a giant AVM extending from the right premotor area to the posterior parietal area undermining the sensorimotor cortex, measuring 9.5 cm (AP) × 6 cm (coronal), × 6 cm (vertical), 180 cm^3 in volume (equivalent to 7 cm^3 sphere) (Figures 46A-D). MSI demonstrated left lower lip and second digit sensory area covering the AVM (Figure 47) and the left sensory forearm area in direct contact with the posterior aspect of the AVM (see Chapter 10, section 2). Similarly, the sensory foot area was in contact with the inferomedial aspect of the AVM core (not shown in Figure 47).

Operative Procedure

The subcortical AVM core was exposed compartment by compartment, and was resected in three stages. At the first stage, a part of the draining vein was found to be dilated, forming a venous aneurysm. This aneurysm was isolated by cauterizing and sectioning the communicating venules. Then the aneurysm was cauterized anteriorly, laterally, and posteriorly to shrink it to a smaller size. This procedure enabled the surgeon to visualize the AVM core. Adequate circulation was maintained in the draining vein. The anterior portion of the medial compartment (which was connected to the draining vein) was isolated first and the core vessels were cauterized. Then it became possible to isolate the lateral compartment located underneath the sensorimotor cortex, and the entire compartment was shrunken by cauterization. During the last stage, the posterior portion of the medial compartment was isolated through the routine technique. The posterior compartment was also isolated through the premotor sulcus opening. One retractor was inserted underneath the sensorimotor cortex (see Figures 33A and C) and another over the AVM core to isolate the communicating venules that connect the core and the cortical veins (Figure 48). Each of the shrunken AVM compartments was removed through a 2.5-cm opening of the precentral sulcus (Figure 49A).

The intact cerebral surface is seen with the arachnoid membrane covering the precentral sulcus at the beginning of the third stage (Figure 49B). This appearance would be expected after total resection.

Postoperative Course

The postoperative course was uneventful except for temporary foot-drop on the left after the last stage. However, the dorsiflexion of the foot began to return during the third postoperative week, and she walked without steppage gait in 2 months. She began to jump on both feet 5 years after surgery. She returned to part-time work as a grocery cashier and takes care of her children.

Case 4: Giant Dominant Frontotemporoparietal AVM

In July 1990, this 47-year-old right-handed man presented with a 20-year history of tonic and clonic seizures and severe headaches. The history dated back to his teenage years when he had the first generalized seizure. In 1970 he presented with subarachnoid hemorrhage, and angiography showed a giant AVM in the left frontotemporoparietal area. At another medical center in 1981, he underwent bead embolization, which was complicated with high fever and vomiting lasting 2–4 weeks. The patient simultaneously developed right arm and leg weakness and speech difficulty. These symptoms subsided within 2 months; however, he still had difficulty coordinating the left extremities, stuttered, and constantly complained of right occipital pain. He was taking Darvoset (propoxyphene napsylate and acetaminophen), Doxepin, and flurazepam. He experienced intermittent numbness and weakness of the right side of the body that required immediate sitting. The patient had been unable to work since 1971. The family noted his intermittent confusion and amnesia, suggestive of automatism. There was a history of depression associated with suicidal tendency dating to 1982.

On examination, he showed speech perseveration, repeating "occipital pain" with staccato rhythm to any question. Mild weakness of the right extremities was noted after repeated exertion of strength and tiptoe walking. No visual field defect was detected. Deep tendon reflexes were hyperactive, in general on the right, and associated with Babinski's sign. No sensory deficit was found except mild hypalgesia in the distal part of the right extremities.

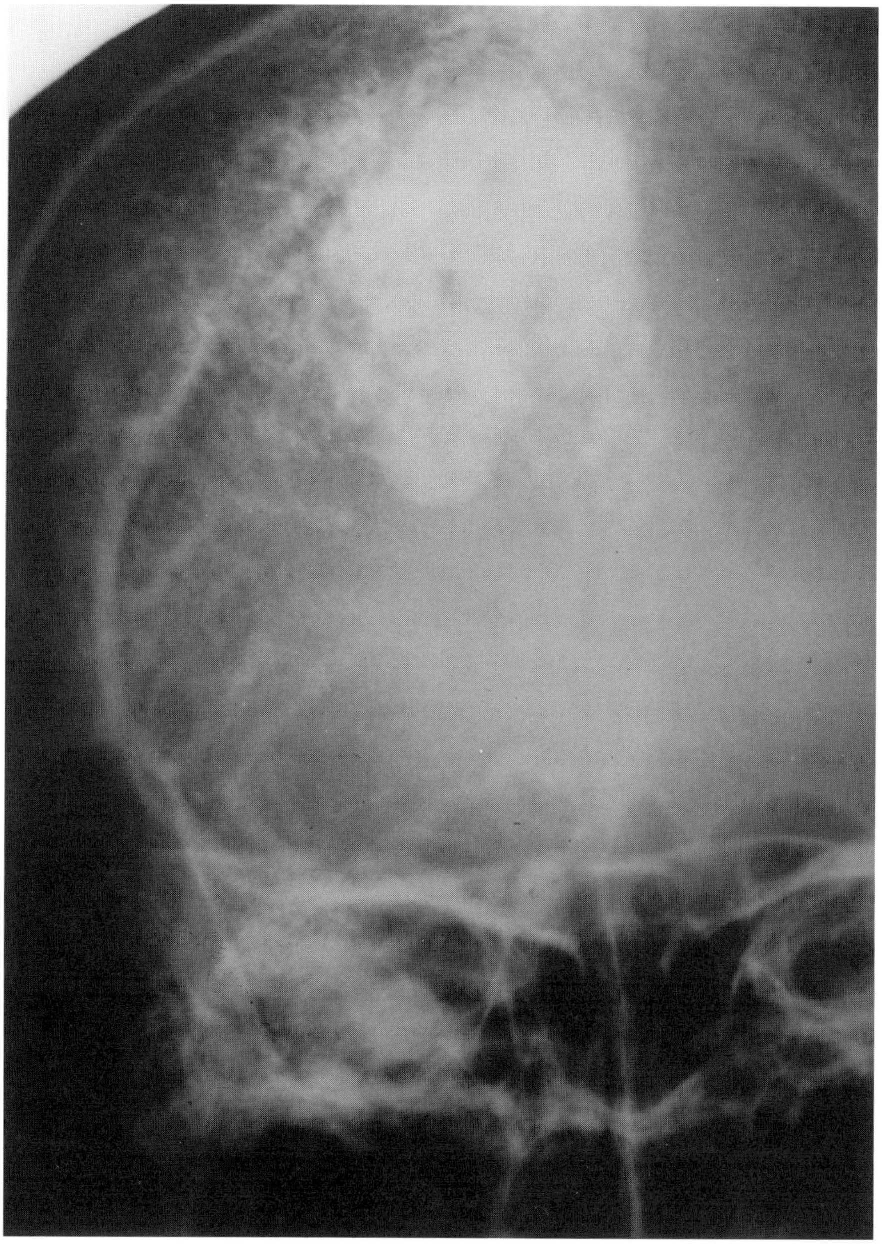

Figure 46A. An AP angiogram showing a 6 cm × 6 cm (coronal and vertical dimensions) AVM (see illustrative case 3).
Continued

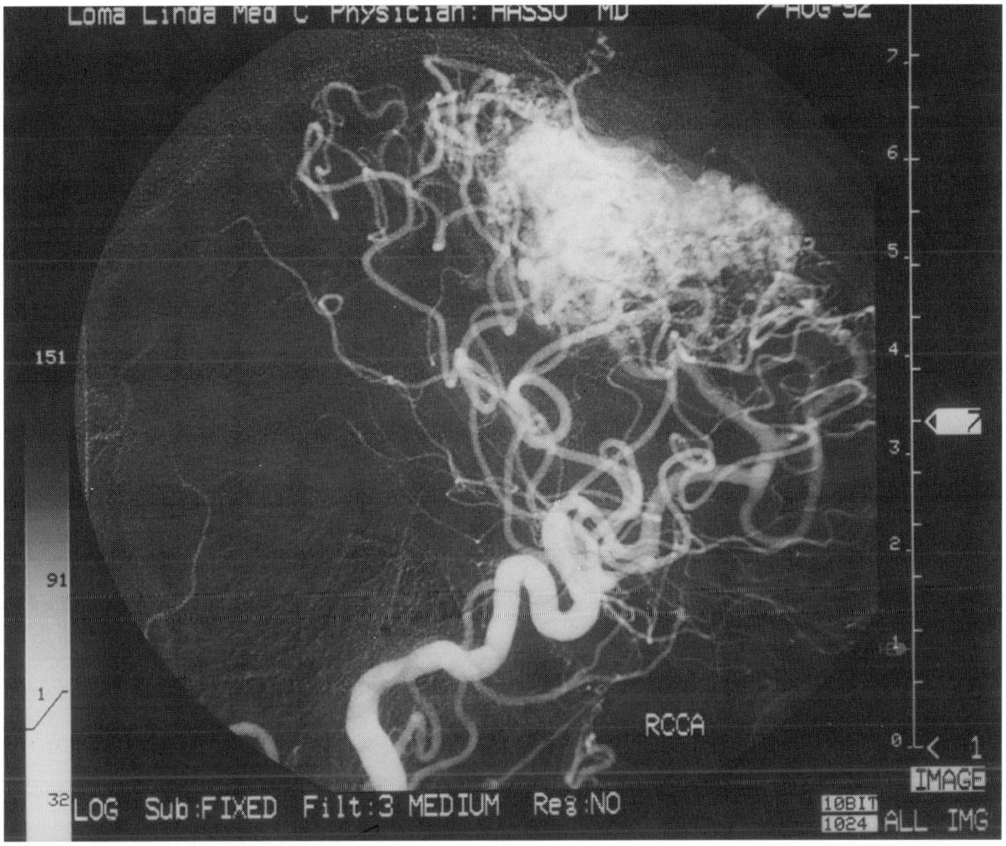

Figure 46B. An angiographic lateral film of early phase showing the contrast material filling the anterior portion of the AVM better than the later phase of filling (see illustrative case 3). *Continued*

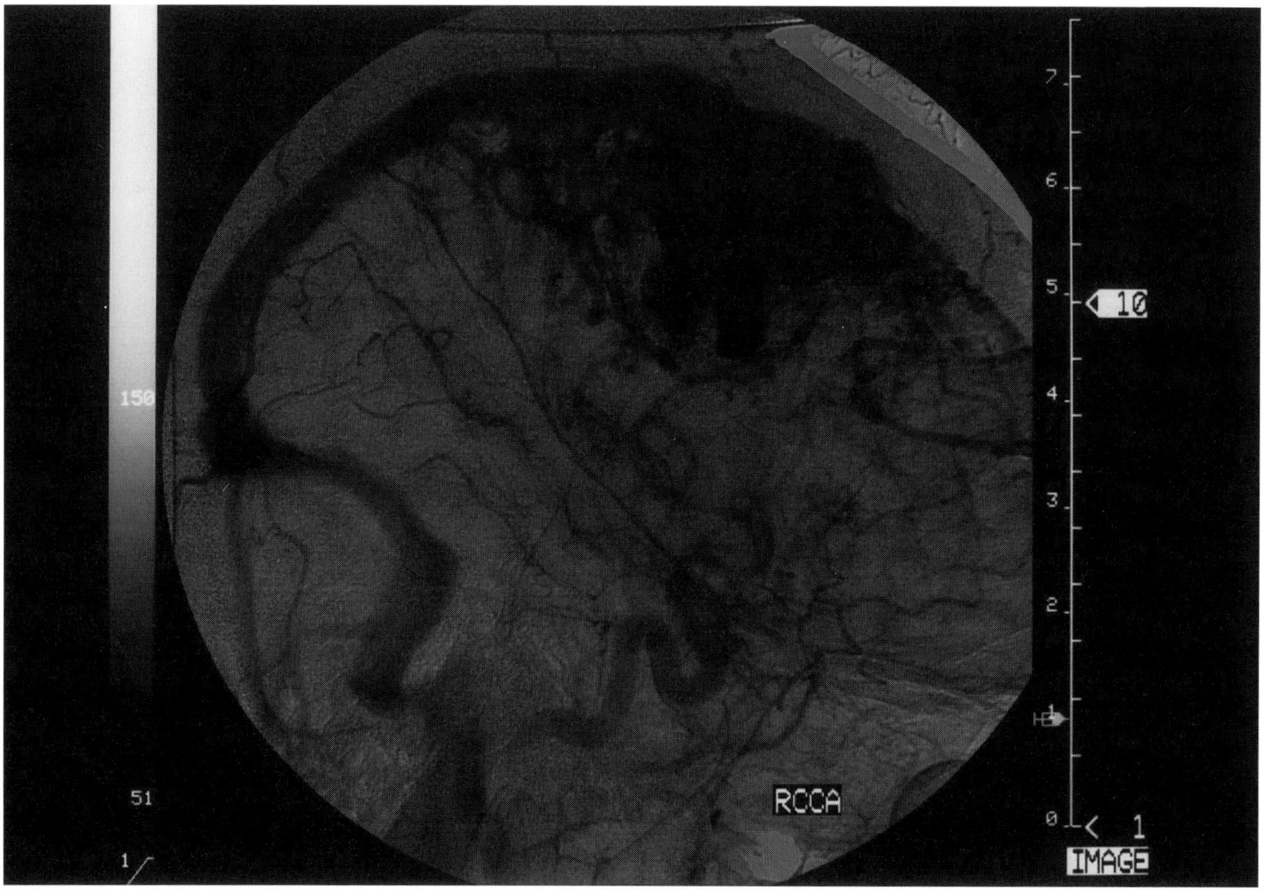

Figure 46C. A later angiographic film showing the posterior portion better than the earlier phase. By adding the two phases, the AP diameter of the AVM was calculated as 9.5 cm (see illustrative case 3). *Continued*

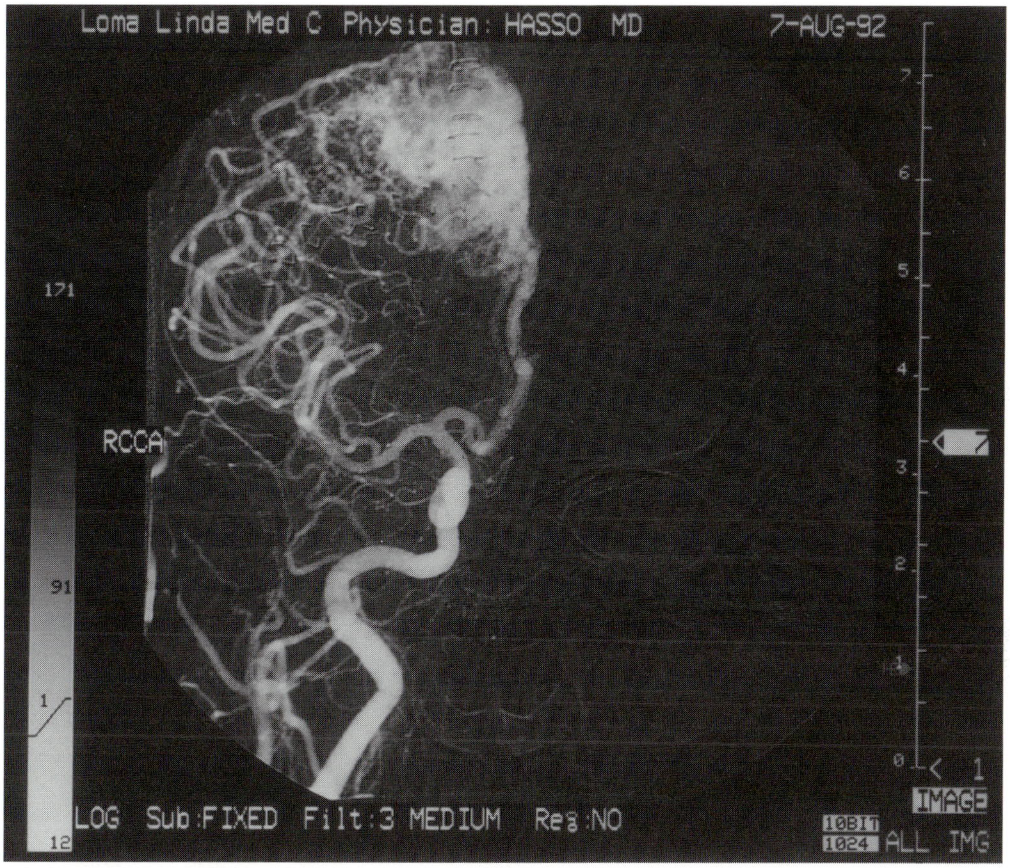

Figure 46D. AP view, showing the medial compartment better than the lateral compartment at this phase (see illustrative case 3).

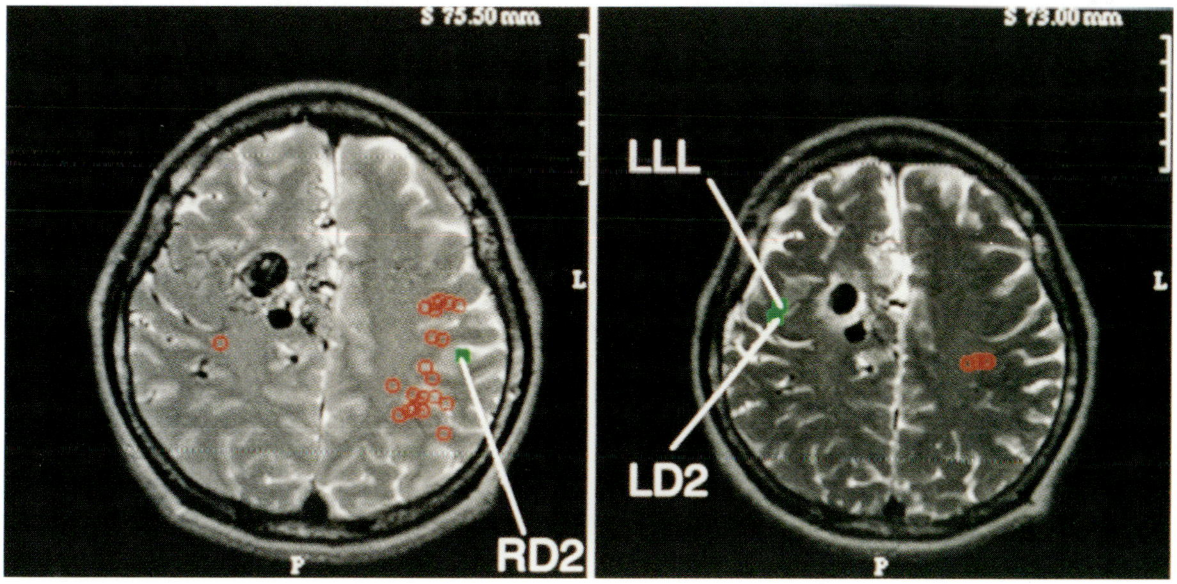

Figure 47. Axial view of MSI depicts the left lower lip (LLL) and the left second digit (LD 2) (indicated by green squares) overlying the AVM. Red circles indicate slow waves (see illustrative case 3).

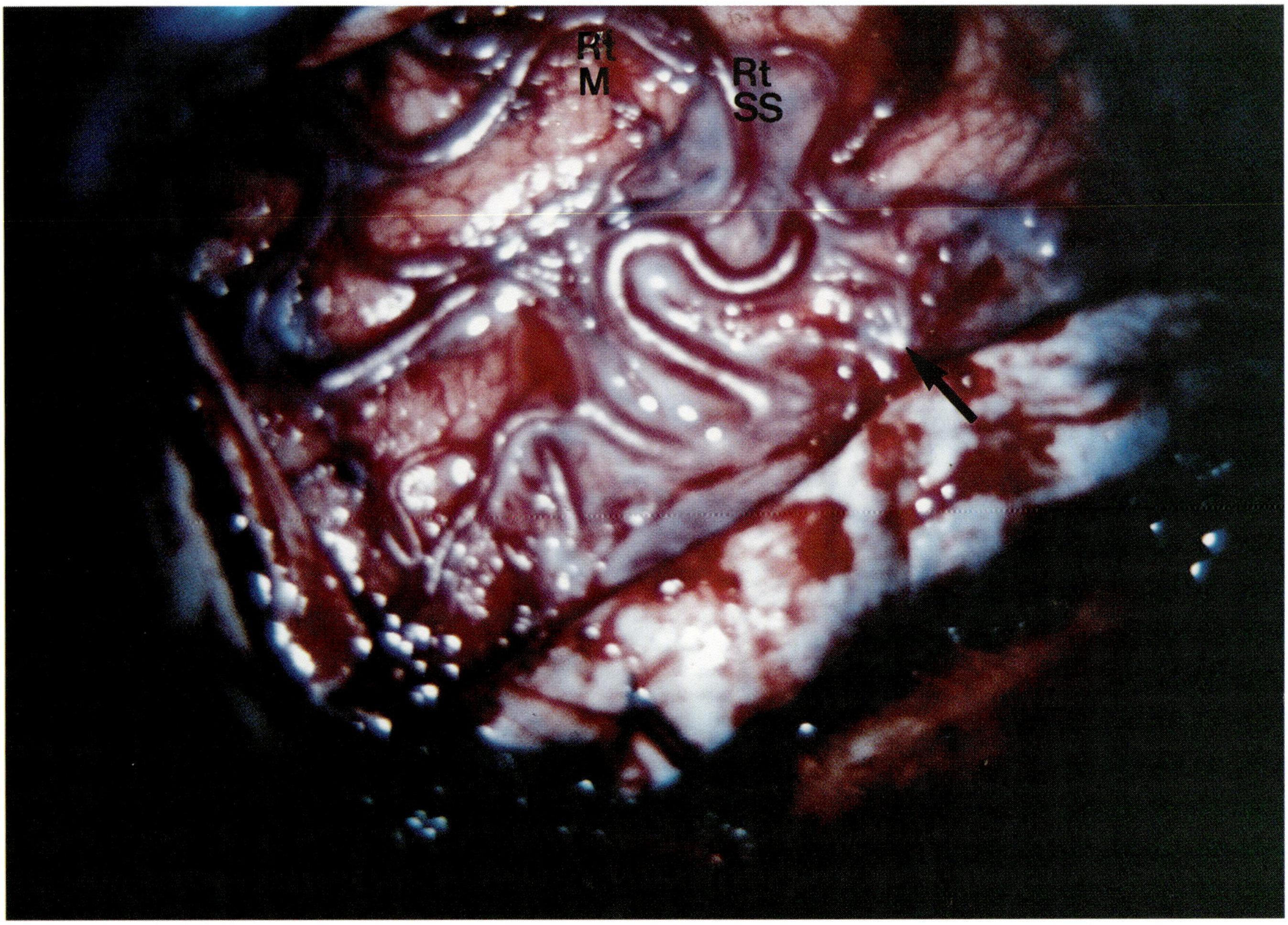

Figure 48. Cortical veins, passively dilated with arterial blood, were not a part of the AVM located underneath the sensorimotor cortex. The right sensory cortex (Rt SS) was determined by somatosensory evoked potentials elicited by stimulation of the left median nerve. The motor area (Rt M) was determined by phase reversal from the sensory cortex potentials with the same stimulation (see illustrative case 3).

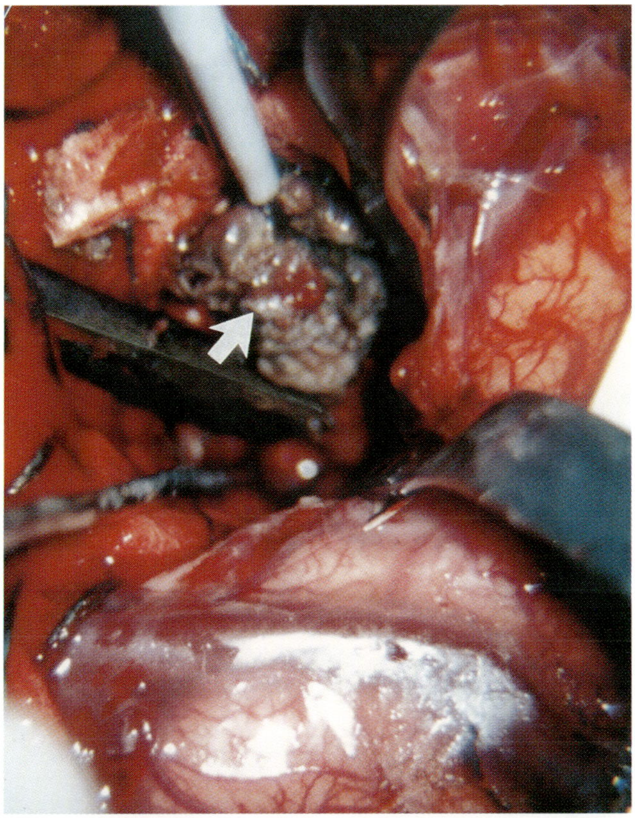

Figure 49A. The posterior compartment which has been cauterized and shrunken (arrows), is being removed through the open precentral sulcus (see illustrative case 3). *Continued*

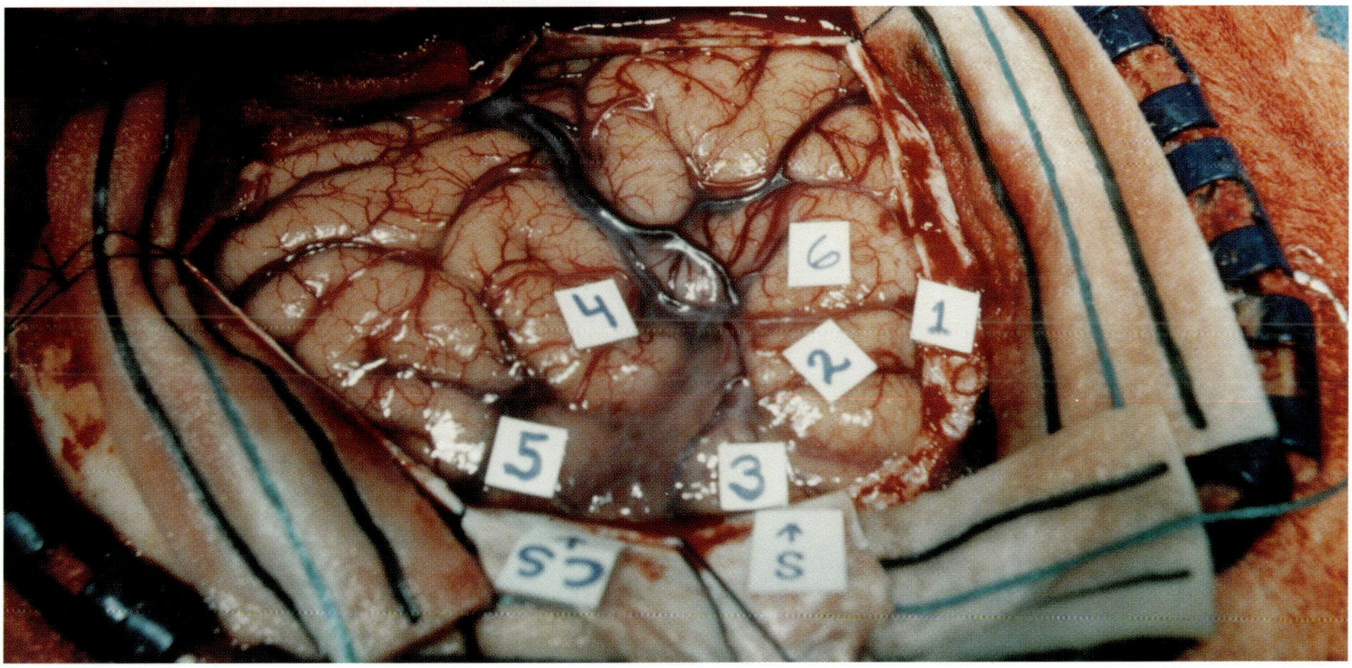

Figure 49B. The cortical surface of the same patient after two staged operations where the lateral and medial compartments were isolated and coagulated to two small shrunken masses. Cortical veins have gained normal size, color, and circulation (no arterial blood). No. 2 and no. 6 indicate the sensory cortex, no. 3 and no. 4 signify the motor cortex. No. 5 is the precentral sulcus, where the entry to the sulcus was made while following the major draining vein. The regenerated arachnoid membrane covers the entry zone and surrounding area. After total AVM resection at the third staged operation, the arachnoid is expected to heal as seen in this photograph (see illustrative case 3).

Imaging Findings

MRI findings supported the presence of the giant AVM extending from the area underneath the sylvian fissure to the temporal lobes, sensorimotor area, and posterior parietal area (Figure 50). Angiography showed the AVM core to be in the frontotemporoparietal area with only one draining vein, its connection being to the sylvian vein and then to the vein of Trolard, both of which were extremely dilated (Figures 51A and B). The external end of the draining vein was extremely narrow (similar to a bottleneck as seen between the two arrows in Figure 51B), and slowed AVM blood flow to the sylvian vein.

Operative Procedures

The AVM core was approached from the posterior end of the sylvian vein, following the small vein parallel and inferior to the sylvian vein (Figure 52). The AVM was circumscribed posteriorly, superiorly, inferiorly, and then inferomedially to the enlarged sylvian vein and the lower part of the vein of Trolard. As shunting arterioles were cauterized and the core pulsation diminished, the core vessels were cauterized. Finally, feeding arteries and the major draining vein, which were crowded at the bottleneck, and part of the AVM core were clipped together, cauterized, and sectioned next to the clip but away from the junction of the draining vein and sylvian vein. Thus, the AVM was totally resected.

Postoperative Course

After AVM resection, the patient was relieved of his severe throbbing headaches and stopped stuttering. His persevering "pain" complaint was replaced by natural conversation on various subjects. He gradually regained coordinated movements and cares for the household while his wife works.

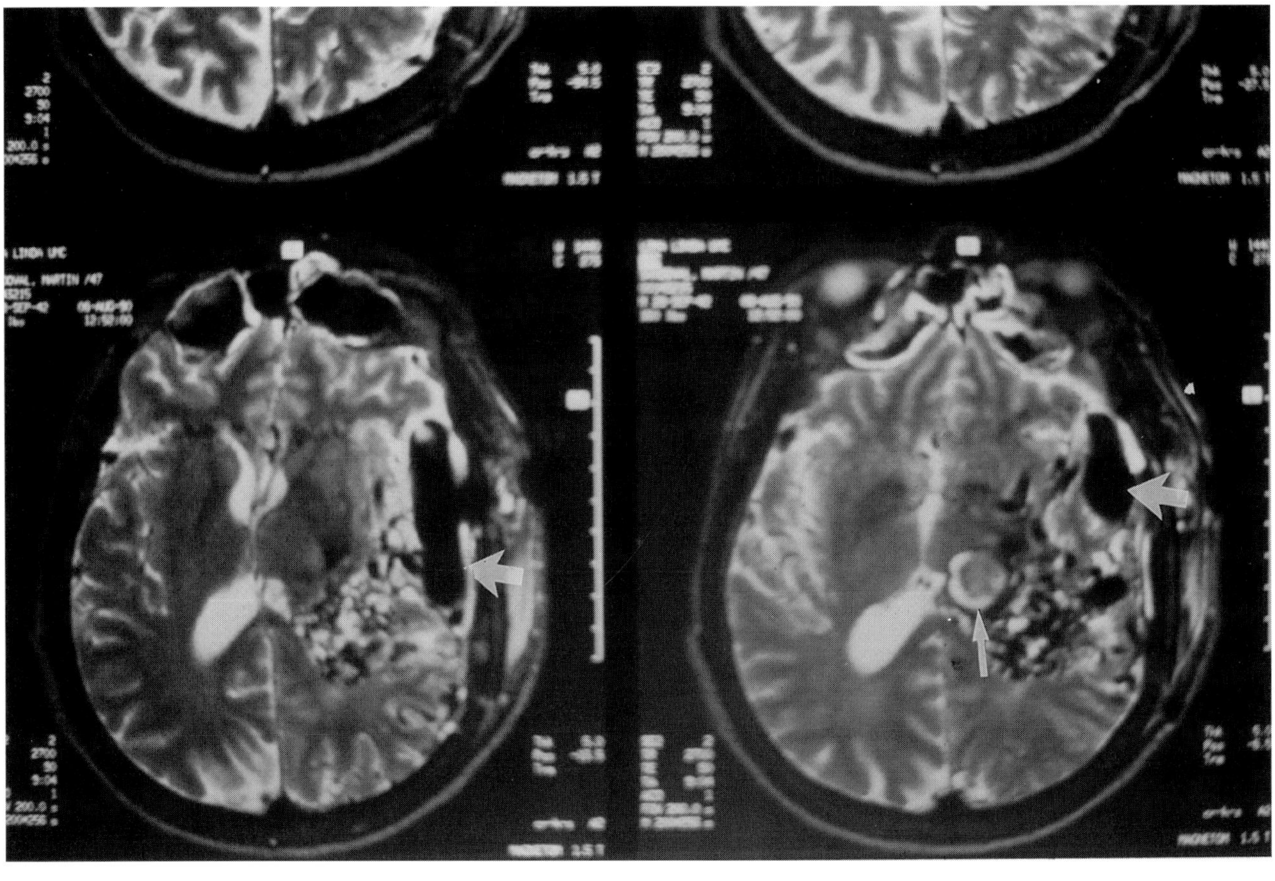

Figure 50. MRI axial view showing a giant AVM 9 cm (AP) × 7 cm (coronal) × 6 cm (vertical) dimension that includes the left parietal, temporal, and lower sensorimotor areas. A large draining vein is located in the sylvian fissure area (large arrows), and another along the vein of Galen forming aneurysmal dilation which appears thrombosed (small arrow) (see illustrative case 4).

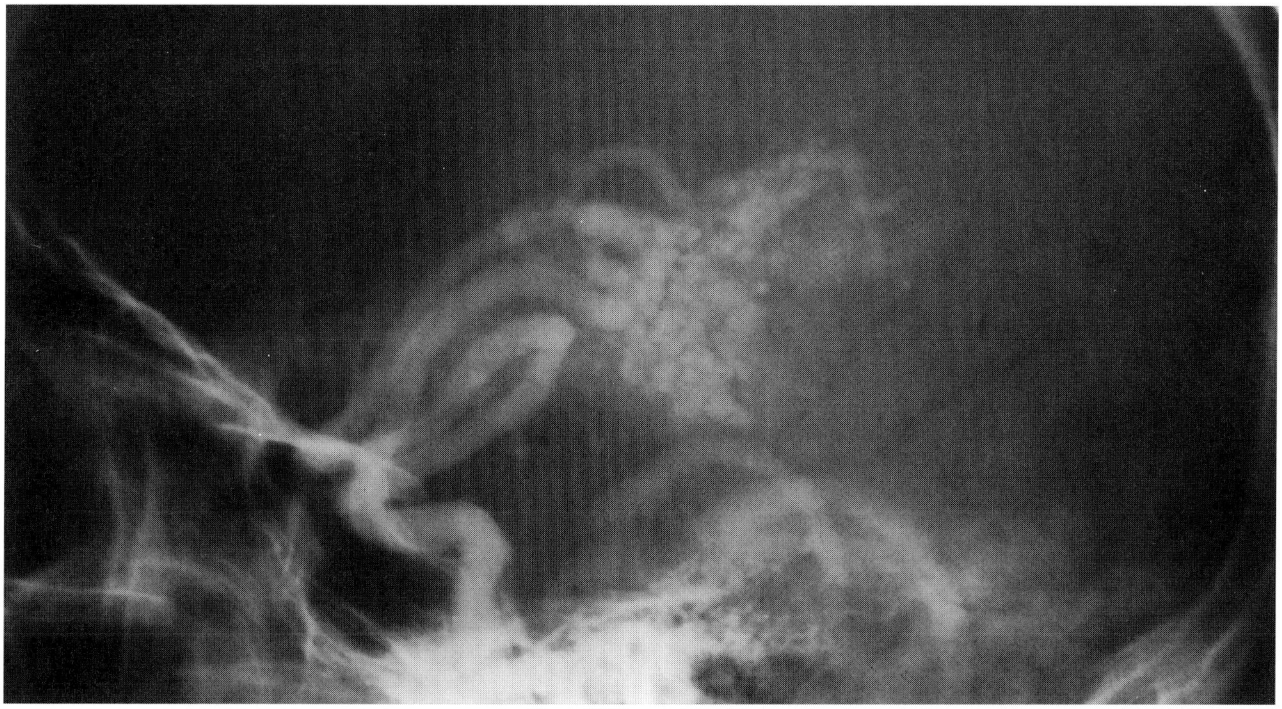

Figure 51A. The AVM core is filled by the middle cerebral artery and its branches, all of which are dilated. No immediate draining to the venous system is noted (see illustrative case 4). *Continued*

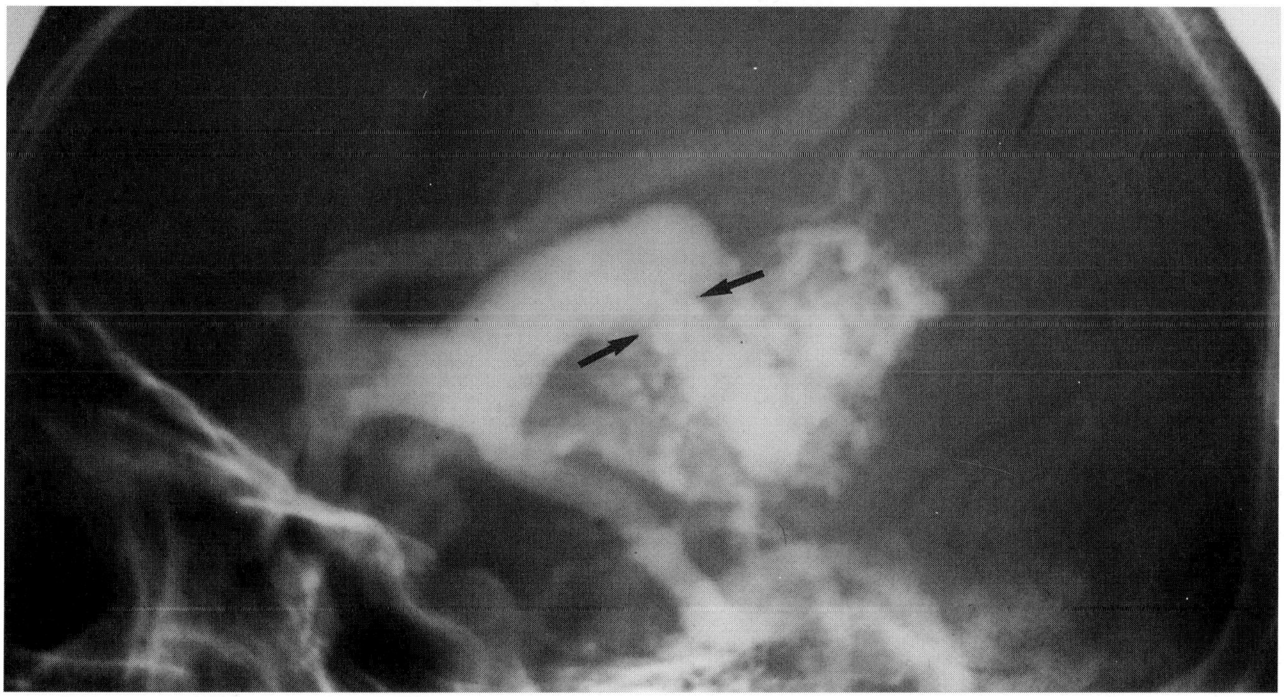

Figure 51B. Immediately after the major draining vein (arrows), an extremely enlarged sylvian vein, was filled, the vein of Trolard and vein of Labbé began to fill with the contrast material. The posterosuperior aspect of the AVM core is also connected to cortical veins through two small draining veins (see illustrative case 4).

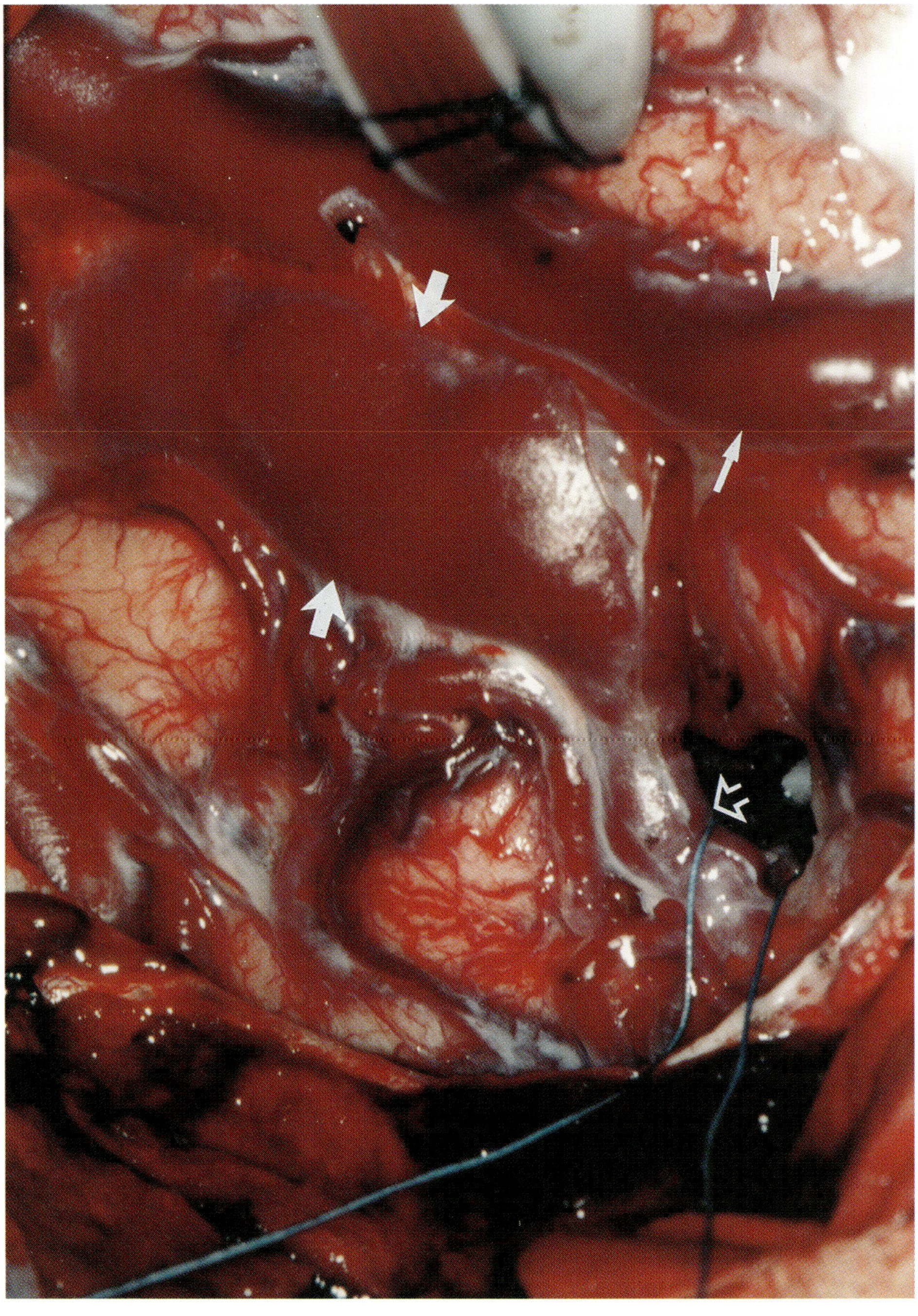

Figure 52. Operative photograph with the anterior on the left and the superior at the top. Anteriorly (left of the field shown in this photograph), the sylvian vein (large arrows) is connected to the vein of Trolard (thin arrows). Anteriorly (left superior to the field), there is a junction of the sylvian vein and the major draining vein where two cottonoid patties attached to strings were placed for hemostasis. The external end of this partially obliterated draining vein (open arrow) forms a bottleneck. Post-stenotic dilatation of the sylvian vein must have occurred after partial embolization of the AVM, which caused obstruction of other major draining veins (see illustrative case 4).

Case 5: Large Dominant Superior Temporal AVM

In May 1982, this 60-year-old man was admitted with a 6-year history of seizures consisting of: (1) staring followed by automatic behavior, (2) visual sensation (blinking light in the right visual field), (3) feeling as if being in a dream, often associated with twitching of the right upper extremity, and (4) postictal aphasia. These seizure patterns occurred separately or in combination, and increased in frequency to several times a week during the 6 months prior to admission. Anticonvulsants provided no significant benefit. No loss of consciousness, convulsions, or incontinence was experienced.

Imaging Findings

Angiography showed a large superior temporal AVM (see Figures 10B and C in the section on surgical procedure for AVMs in the superior temporal gyrus), including the frontal and temporal opercula, with supply from the left middle cerebral artery, posterior cerebral artery, and middle meningeal artery branches (including medial dura along the sphenoidal ridge). The draining veins were connected to the inferior anastomotic vein (Labbé), superficial middle cerebral vein (sylvian), sphenoparietal sinus, basilar vein (Rosenthal), and vein of Galen. The middle meningeal artery supply was obliterated with Gelfoam embolization.

Operative Procedure

The AVM was approached by following the draining vein of the anterior compartment (first stage operation), then following the second draining vein to the lateral compartment (second stage), and finally to the medioposterior compartment (third stage), as described in the surgical technique section for a large superior temporal gyrus AVM.

Postoperative Course

The patient recovered from each staged operation without developing neurological deficits and returned to work as an auto mechanic. Ten years after surgery, he reported that he is enjoying a healthy life in retirement.

Case 6: Large Dominant Inferior Frontal AVM Extending to the Capsulocaudatothalamic Area

In December 1986, this 33-year-old man was admitted with a history of generalized seizures, some of which were of an adversive type, since 25 years of age, for which he was taking phenytoin and phenobarbital. The frequency of seizures increased to several times daily during a spree of alcohol consumption (12 cans of beer a day), which he started to ease paroxysmal severe throbbing headaches. He had difficulty in speaking after each seizure, and difficulty with memory and comprehension gradually progressed.

Imaging Findings

Angiography showed a large AVM, 6 cm (AP) × 4 cm (coronal) × 5.5 cm (vertical), 70 cm^3 in volume in the left inferior frontal area; 3 cm × 3 cm × 3 cm, 15 cm^3 in volume, in the capsulocaudatothalamic area (Figures 53A and B).

Operative Procedure

A transcoronal skin incision and a frontotemporal craniotomy hinged over the temporal area and dural opening revealed convexity cortical veins dilated with half arterial (bluish-red) blood. The frontal lobe was retracted anterolaterally, and small arteries and veins coming through the cribriform plate were interrupted. The compact AVM was dissected circumferentially first anteriorly, then superolaterally, and finally inferiorly. As the medial aspect of the AVM was exposed, a feeding artery arising from the frontopolar artery was cauterized, but arterial pulsation did not diminish until the posterior frontal portion of the AVM was isolated. The portion of the AVM that extended to the capsulocaudatothalamic area was left untouched.

At the second stage, a stereotactic probe was inserted through a frontal area 2.5 cm lateral to the midline and 12 cm posterior to the glabella. A thin layer of brain tissue was removed and the AVM was exposed at the superoanterior surface. This portion of the compact AVM was resected using the author's technique, without removing any surrounding brain tissue. The draining vein of the AVM connected to the sylvian vein was the last to be interrupted.

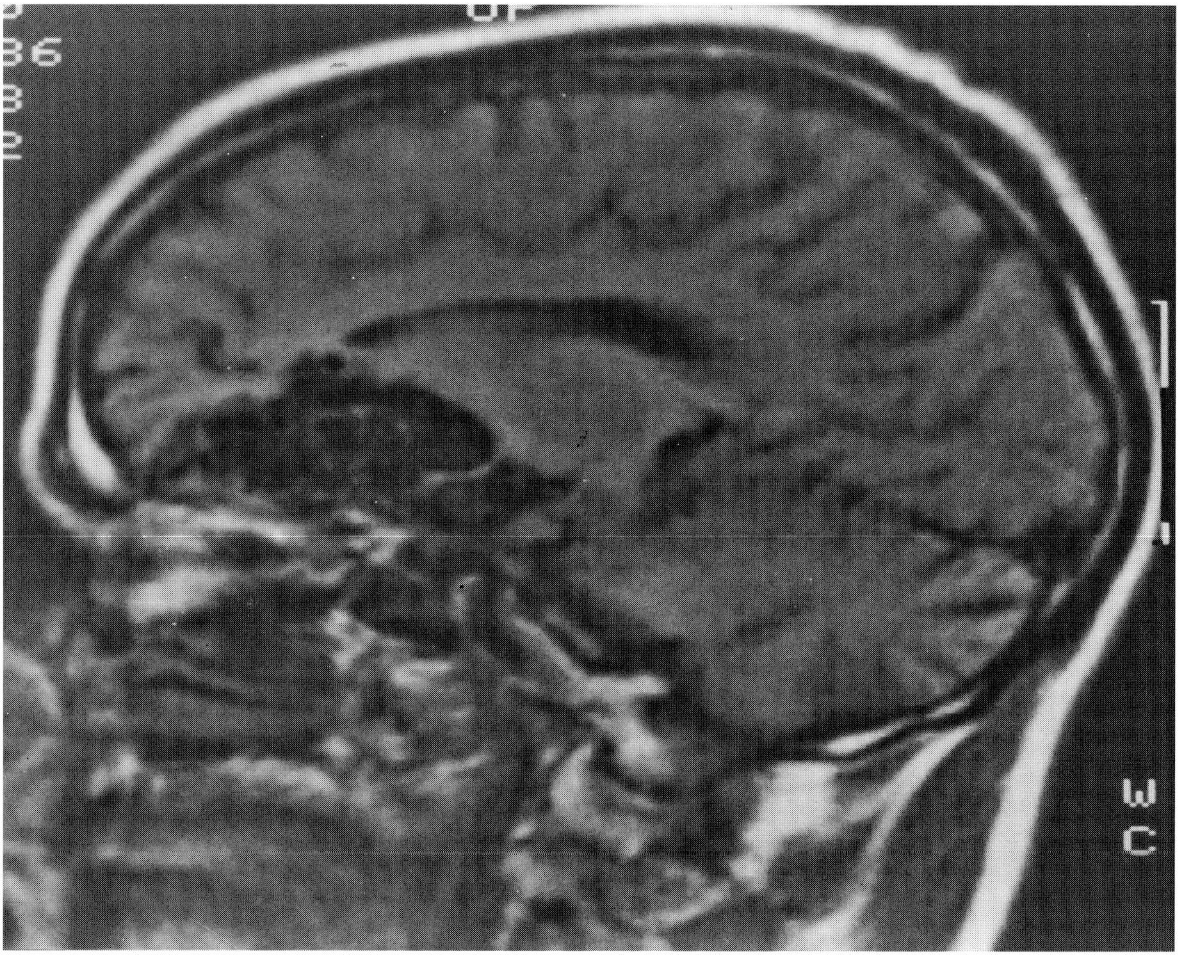

Figure 53A. Lateral MRI showing an inferior frontal area AVM extending to the basal ganglia and the internal capsule (see illustrative case 6). *Continued*

Postoperative Course

The patient recovered from the two-staged surgery without developing neurological deficit and regained a satisfactory lifestyle, refraining from constant drinking and having only an occasional social drink. He was referred for occupational rehabilitation, and now does voluntary work.

Case 7: Giant AVM Extending from the Frontal to the Subcortical Sensorimotor Area

This 43-year-old right-handed man presented with severe occipital headache, which began 8 months before admission. He later developed intermittent left hand numbness, dizziness, and difficulty with balance. Eight years before the consultation, he was involved in a head-on motor collision and was told that he underwent evacuation of right subdural hematoma and ventriculoperitoneal shunt. Soon afterward, he developed seizures, which became intractable to phenytoin, phenobarbital, and other anticonvulsant agents. Some of the seizures were noted to be focal in the left arm with elbow flexion, and occasionally associated with facial numbness. He drank a six-pack of beer and smoked two packs of cigarettes every day, hopefully to ease severe paroxysmal throbbing headache.

Imaging Findings

Angiography demonstrated a giant AVM extending from the right anterior frontal lobe to the sensorimotor area, 12.6 cm (AP) × 6 cm (coronal) × 8 cm (vertical) (Figures 54A-D).

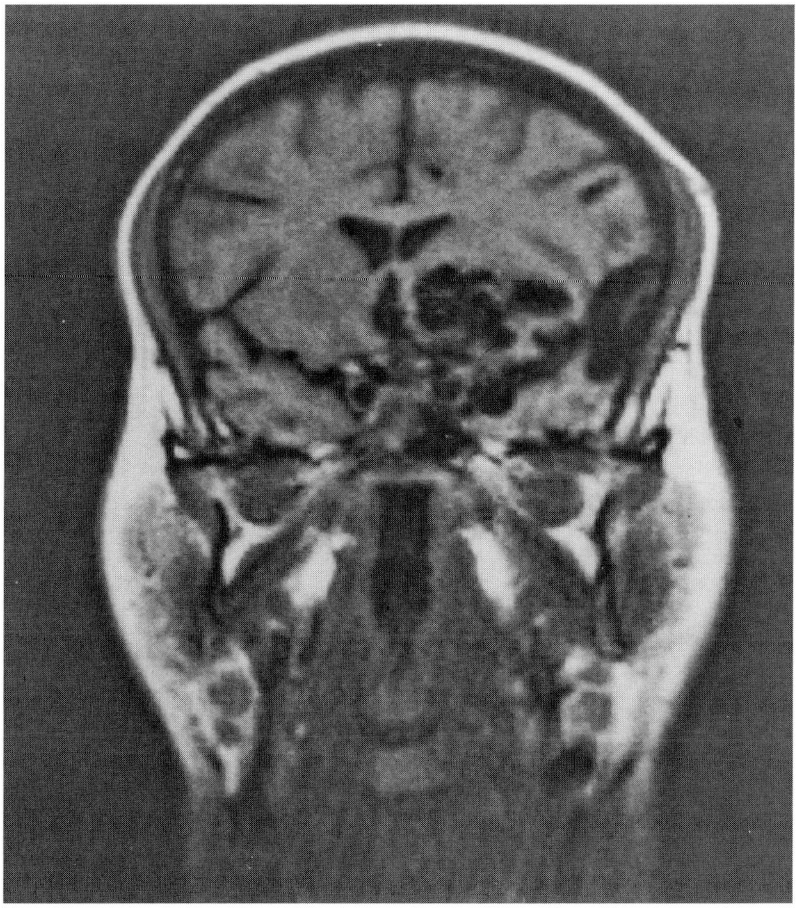

Figure 53B. An MRI AP view showing the AVM, including the basal ganglia, the internal capsule, and the draining vein in the sylvian fissure (see illustrative case 6).

Operative Procedure

The operative plan was to eliminate the giant AVM, elliptical on AP views, in three steps: isolation of the anterior one-third, the medial one-third, and finally the posterior one-third. The first two-thirds consisted of a medial compartment (supplied by the anterior cerebral artery and the posterior cerebral artery) and a lateral compartment (supplied by the middle cerebral artery and its perforating branches). The last one-third consisted of the posterior and lateral compartments. After a 12 cm (sagittal) × 7 cm (corneal) craniotomy, the dura was opened in a rectangular flap. First the draining vein was followed in the sulcus 4 cm lateral to the midline. One gyrus was removed to provide adequate exposure to the AVM. The anterior one-third of the AVM was isolated by interrupting shunting arterioles and communicating venules, and occasionally removing a thin layer of brain tissue around the AVM.

The second step included removal of part of the anterior one-third, which was thrombosed after the first step, followed by meticulous isolation of the middle one-third of the AVM without removing brain tissue laterally, medially, and inferiorly. Additionally, a small area (2 cm) of the cingulate gyrus was resected, allowing exposure of the right anterior cerebral artery for a short distance and of a large tortuous draining vein (1 cm in diameter) arising from the posterior portion of the medial compartment and traveling toward the superior sagittal sinus (indicated by the open arrow in Figure 54D). Dissection of this vein resulted in profuse bleeding, requiring tamponade. Another draining vein (4 mm in diameter) was noted arising from the posterior compartment and draining into the superior sagittal sinus.

The third step was to isolate the posterior one-third of the AVM, which consisted of the posterior compartment and the posterior part of the lateral compartment. Resection began superiorly and laterally underneath the sensorimotor cortex (Figure 55) which was displaced more posteriorly than expected from anatomical localization (confirmed by somatosensory evoked potentials); and continued, anteriorly and anteroinferiorly, and finally, posteroinferiorly (where a pair of pericallosal arteries were identified).

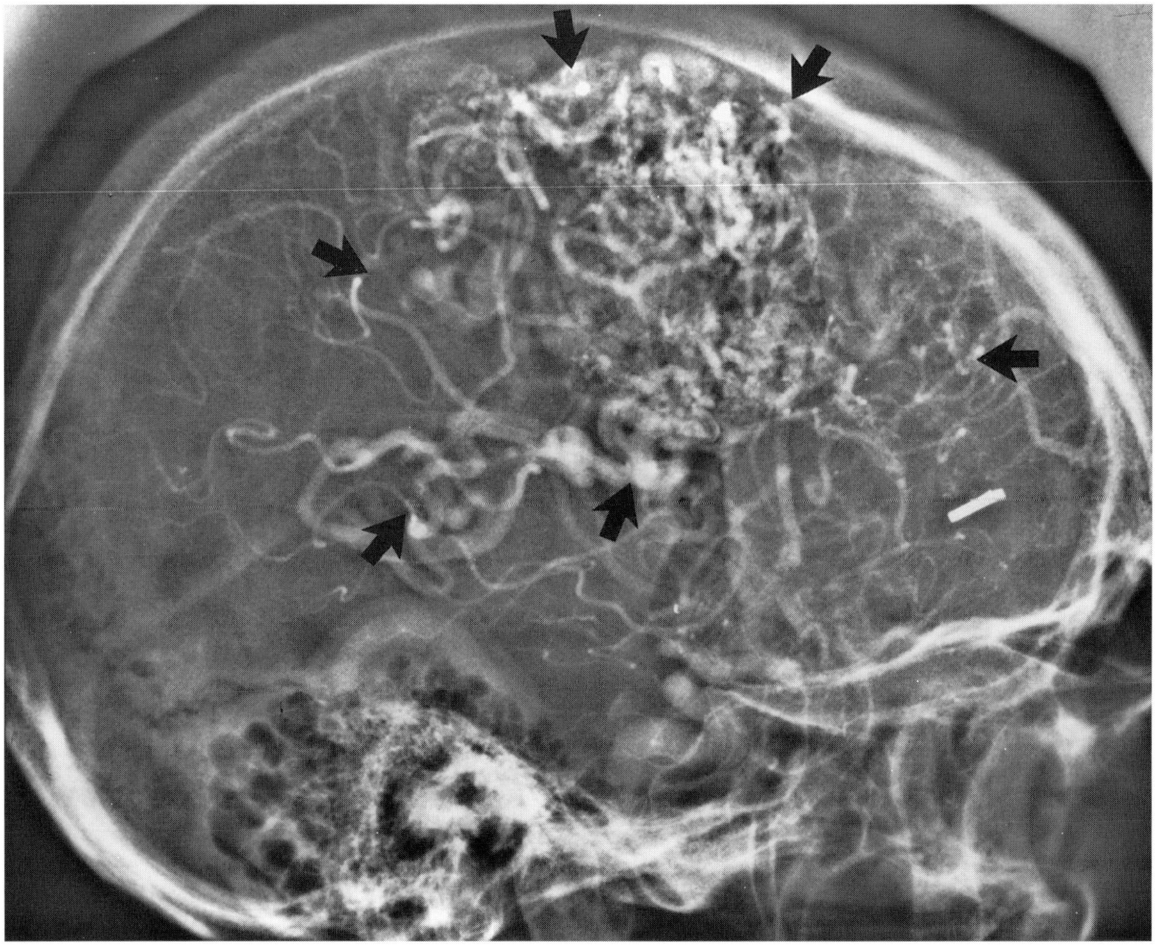

Figure 54A. The lateral view of the carotid angiogram showing a giant AVM extending from the right frontal area to the posterior parietal area. The posterior compartment, which was filled only by vertebral angiogram, is outlined by three posteriorly placed arrows. *Continued*

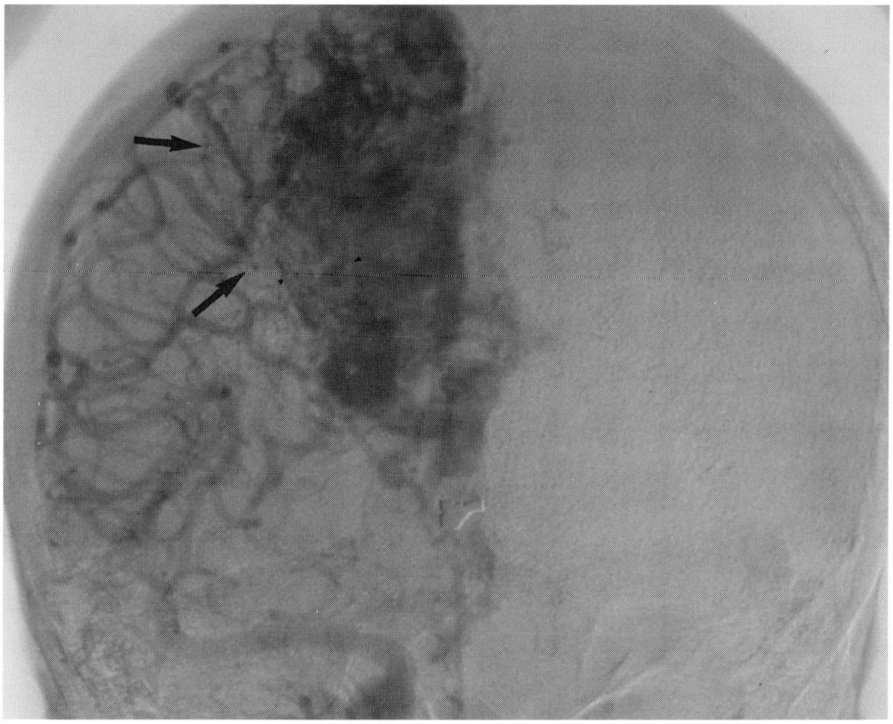

Figure 54B. The AP view of the medial compartment showing the contrast material in the lateral compartment, which had almost been washed out by dilution effect. *Continued*

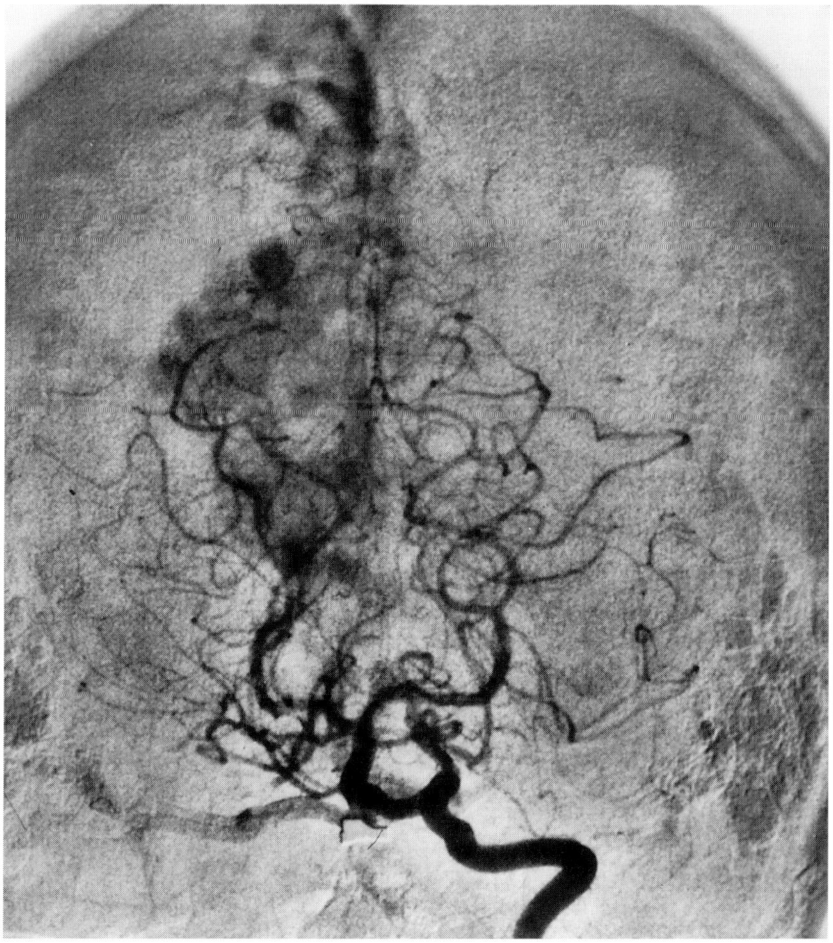

Figure 54C. The AP view of the posterior compartment supplied by the right posterior cerebral artery. *Continued*

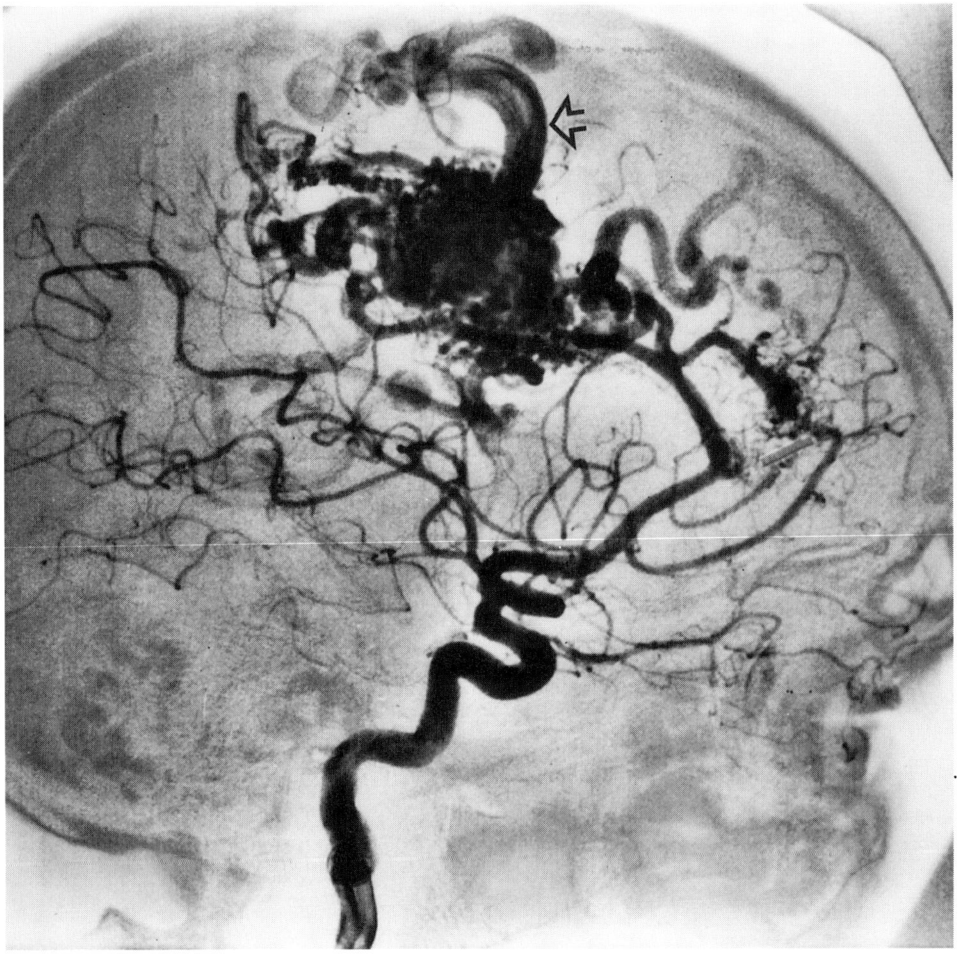

Figure 54D. Lateral view of the medial compartment of the middle third of the AVM (between the anterior and posterior two-thirds) is the last to be dissected (see illustrative case 7). The arrow indicates the major draining vein.

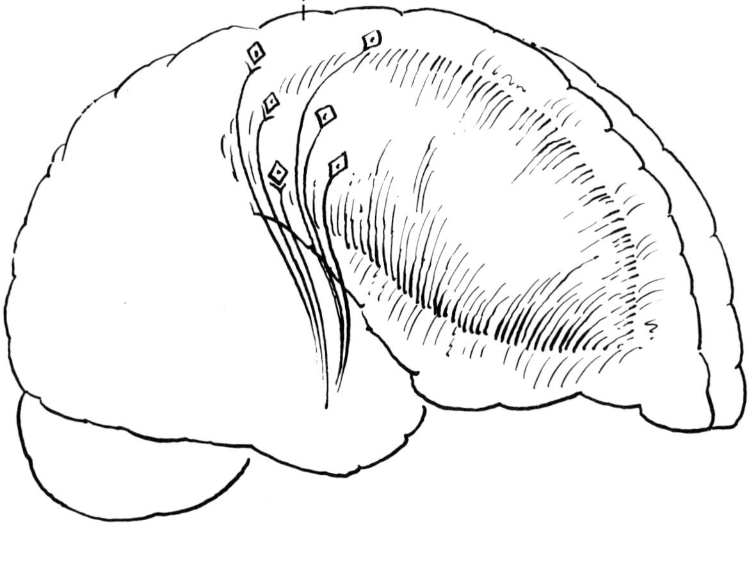

Figure 55. A schematic drawing of an AVM extending from the frontal area to the sensorimotor area underlying the sensorimotor cortex, more posterior than the usual anatomical location (see illustrative case 7).

The fourth step was to dissect the medial compartment of the middle one-third. This required: (1) isolation of small draining veins medioinferiorly to disrupt the connection to the internal cerebral vein, and cauterization of the AVM that extruded to the ventricular wall; (2) isolation and interruption of the huge major draining vein connected to the superior sagittal sinus; and (3) interruption of another draining vein from the posterior side of the AVM. After cauterization of the entire AVM, the operation was concluded.

Postoperative Course

Angiography showed total elimination of the AVM anteriorly with resection and posteriorly with thrombosis. The patient did well except for temporary weakness on the left, which lasted for several weeks. He returned to an independent lifestyle helping with various odd jobs. He stopped drinking and smoking, and his attitude changed from an argumentative to a more amicable disposition.

Case 8: Large Mesial Occipital AVM

In September 1988, a 23-year-old right-handed woman was admitted with a history of visual seizures. The history dated back to age 14 years when she had the first seizure, seeing flashing lights in the left visual field, followed by a severe throbbing headache. Similar episodes occasionally occurred and she had to lie down and sleep for 2–3 hours to relieve the headache. At the age of 17 years, she began to experience nausea and vomiting in addition to sudden onset of flashing light and headache. At age 20, similar attacks occurred 3–4 times per week. Inderal (propranolol) was prescribed to control episodes of palpitation. These symptoms were thought to be associated with a gallbladder infection for which she underwent a cholecystectomy (at age 21 years). She then began to have weakness and numbness of the left arm, which was relieved with phenobarbital medications. For 2 years before admission, attacks of headaches, nausea, and flashing light increased to daily occurrence.

Imaging Findings

Angiography demonstrated a large AVM in the occipital lobe partly extending subcortically into the striate cortex. The size of the irregular spherical AVM was 5 cm in diameter (Figures 56A and B).

Operative Procedure

The AVM was approached through the occipital convexity surface, following the major draining vein. The AVM core was circumscribed laterally and superiorly. The medioinferior portion was then dissected and the core was totally circumscribed. However, another small satellite AVM (0.5 cm) was found mediosuperiorly. This cluster of vessels was isolated and cauterized to total obliteration (rather than resection) and the draining vein from the satellite AVM was also obliterated. The major portion of the AVM was removed without removal of surrounding brain tissue.

Postoperative Course

The patient recovered from surgery with only left lower quadrantanopia, which subsided within 2 months. She is now 32 years old, free of seizures without medication, and takes care of her two young children, who were born after surgery.

Case 9: Dominant Posterior Parietal Area (Superior and Inferior Lobules) AVM

During pregnancy in 1982, this 24-year-old left-handed ballet dancer had an episode of subarachnoid hemorrhage manifested by a sudden onset of severe headache, mild nuchal rigidity, difficulty with left visual fields, and mental obtundation. Following the recovery from these symptoms, she underwent an elective cesarean section on January 30, 1983, at 21 weeks' gestation. She had several Jacksonian seizures, starting with left arm numbness followed by aphasia. She recalled that as a child she had sudden attacks of throbbing headaches on the right side of the head. On admission on February 21, 1983, she was neurologically intact and the left homonymous hemianopia was already resolved.

Imaging Findings

Cerebral angiography showed a large AVM 7.2 cm × 4.6 cm × 7.2 cm (125 cm^3, equivalent to a 6.2-cm sphere) in three dimensions with three compartments supplied by the middle (Figures 57A and B), anterior (Figure 57C), and posterior cerebral arteries (Figure 57D).

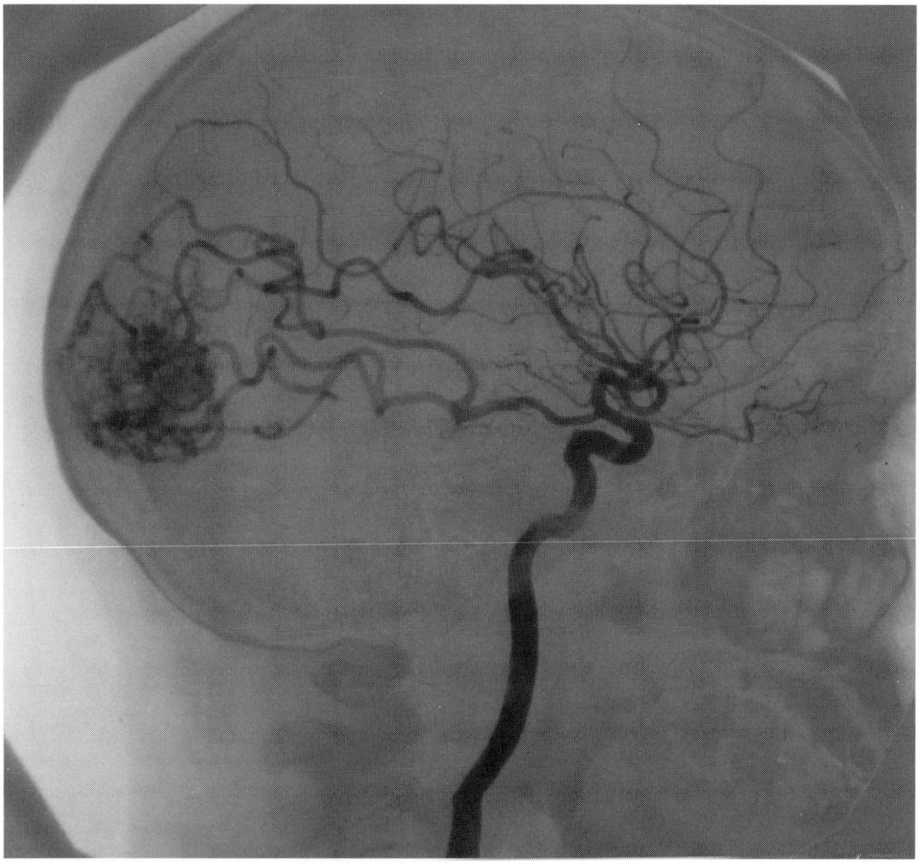

Figure 56A. Lateral view of the angiogram of an occipital AVM supplied by both posterior cerebral and middle cerebral arteries (see illustrative case 8). *Continued*

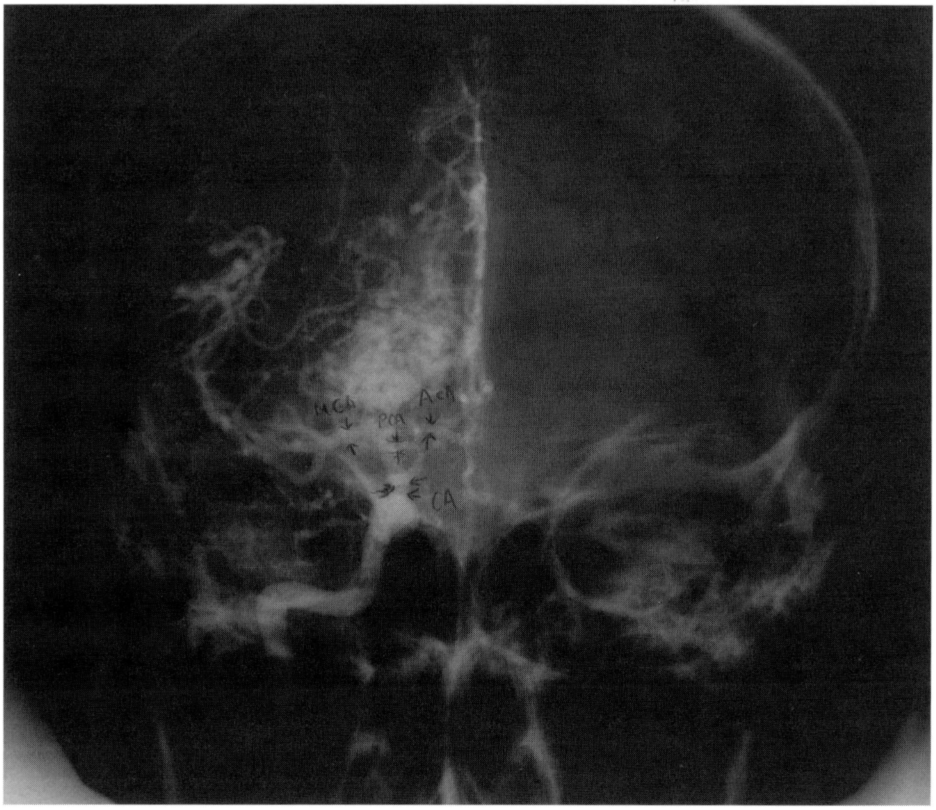

Figure 56B. AP view of the same AVM (see illustrative case 8).

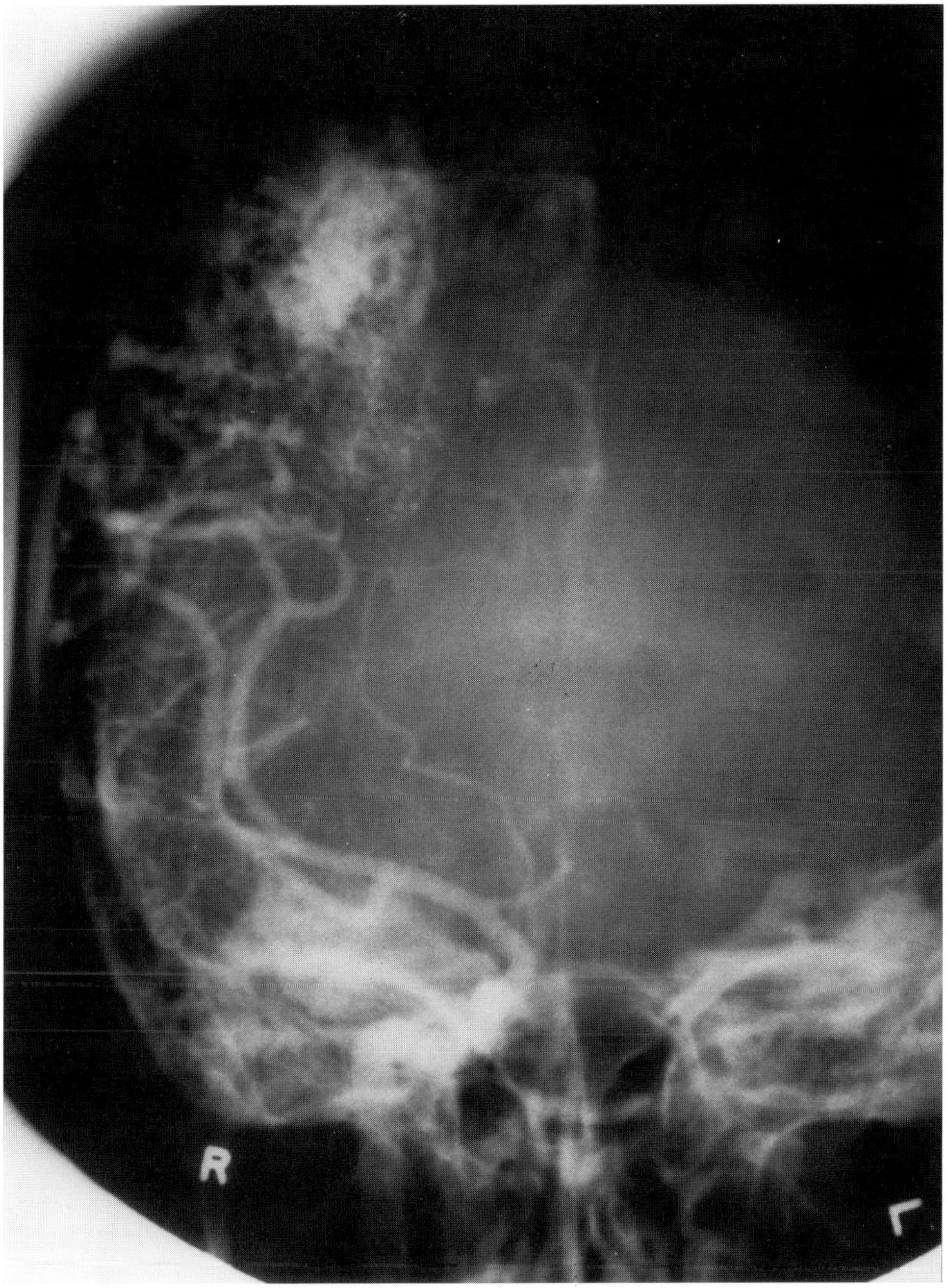

Figure 57A. An AP view of the right carotid angiogram showing the lateral compartment of the right dominant posterior parietal AVM (a left-handed patient), supplied by the middle cerebral artery branches and the faintly filled medial compartment supplied by the anterior cerebral artery (see illustrative case 9). *Continued*

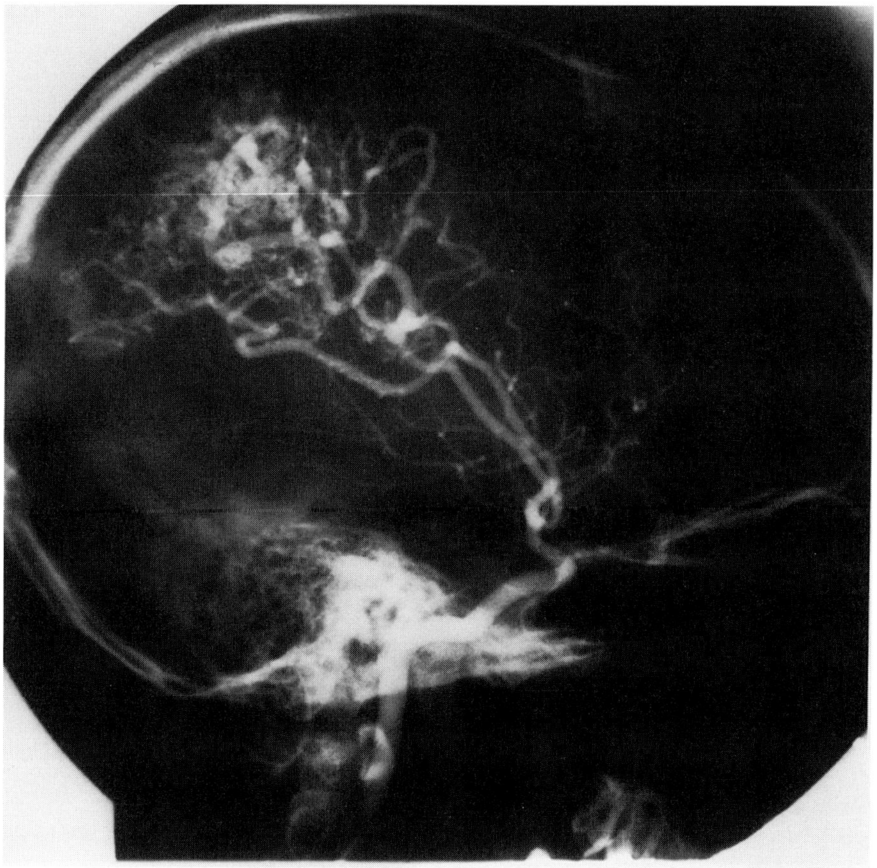

Figure 57B. The right lateral carotid angiogram clearly showing the lateral compartment (see illustrative case 9). *Continued*

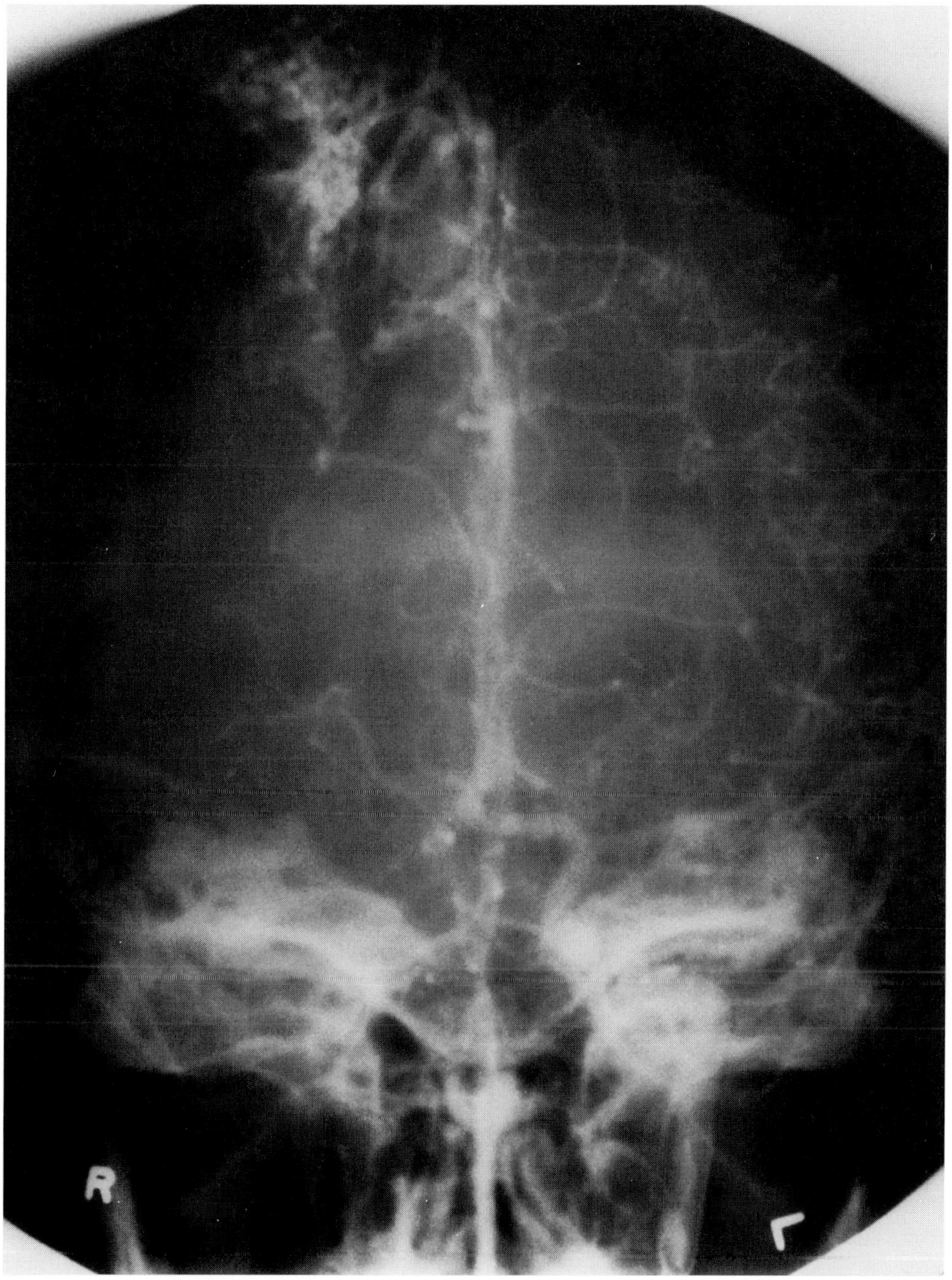

Figure 57C. The left AP carotid angiogram filling the medial compartment of the right posterior parietal AVM by cross filling through the anterior communicating artery (see illustrative case 9). *Continued*

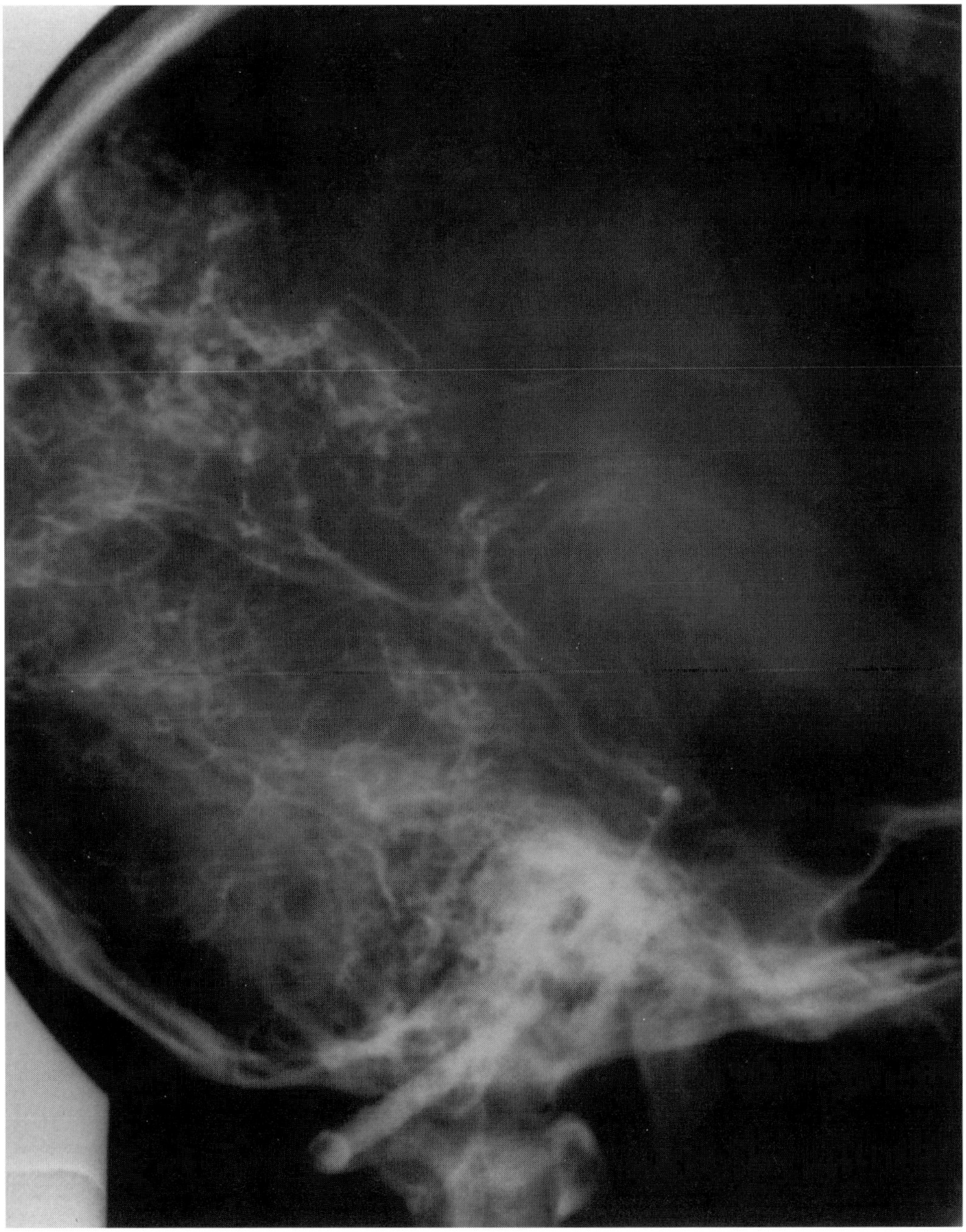

Figure 57D. The right vertebral angiogram showing the posterior compartment supplied by the right posterior cerebral artery (see illustrative case 9).

Operative Procedure

The AVM was approached through the intraparietal sulcus, which passed one of the major draining veins, and was totally resected in four stages.

Postoperative Course

The patient recovered without neurological deficit. Three months after the last stage, she was able to perform a pirouette.

Case 10: Capsulostriatothalamic and Hypothalamic AVM

For 3 years, this 6-year-old girl had a progressive course of left-sided weakness, difficulty with mentation, and speech dysfunction. The first symptom the parents noticed was blindness of the left eye. On evaluation, she perceived objects only with the nasal field of the right eye and was able to walk approximately 10 yards dragging her left leg. She was unable to write or draw and her speech was limited to simple expressions.

Imaging Findings

MRI and angiography demonstrated a left capsulostriatothalamic and hypothalamic AVM, which grew larger over 2 years (from 3 cm × 3 cm × 3.5 cm to 4 cm × 6 cm × 5 cm), with an intraorbital extension (2 cm × 2 cm × 3 cm) (Figures 58A-C).

Operative Procedure

The AVM was approached through the occipitoparietal cortex, which allowed entry to the posterior lateral ventricle. The first step was to cauterize the AVM in the dorsal portion of the thalamus followed

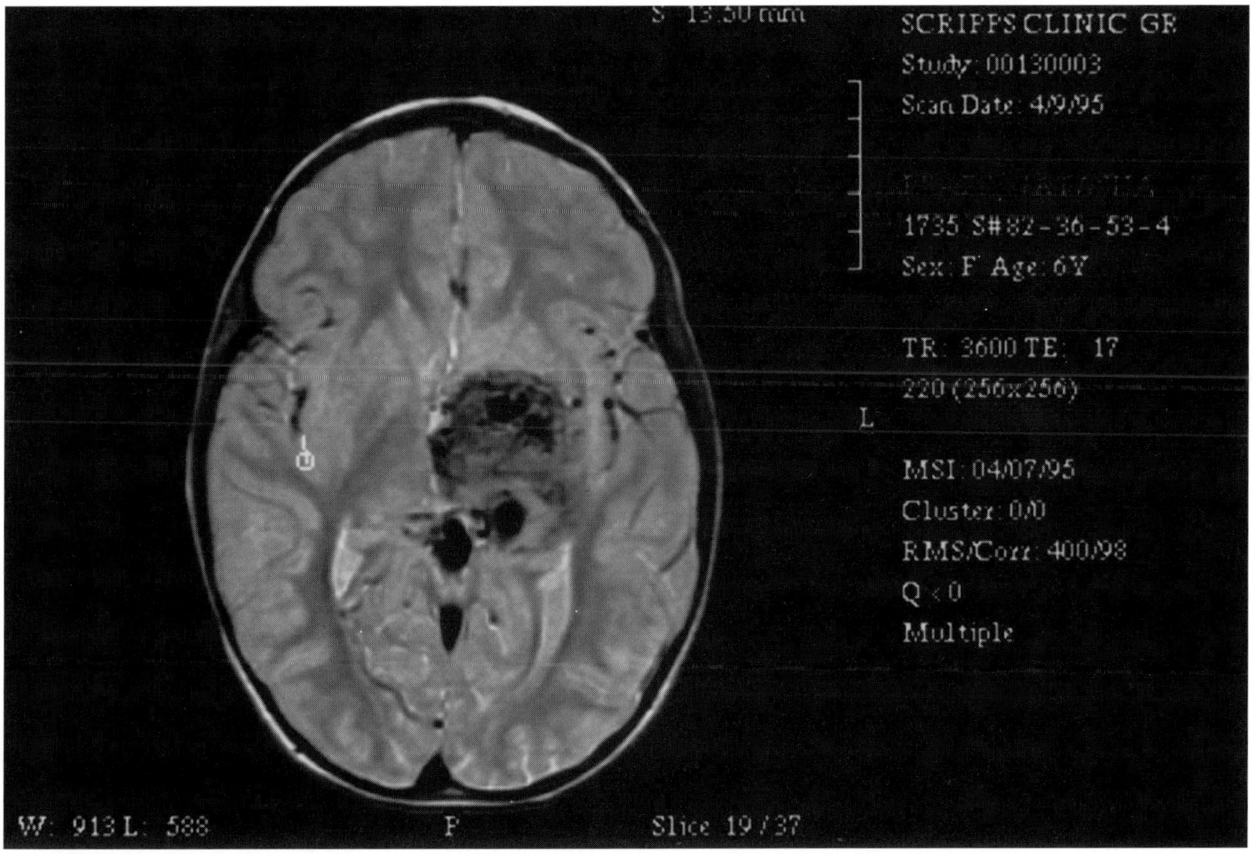

Figure 58A. A larger AVM is located by an axial MRI film in the left thalamus, internal capsule (mainly posterior limb), and basal ganglia (putamen and caudate nucleus) (see illustrative case 10). *Continued*

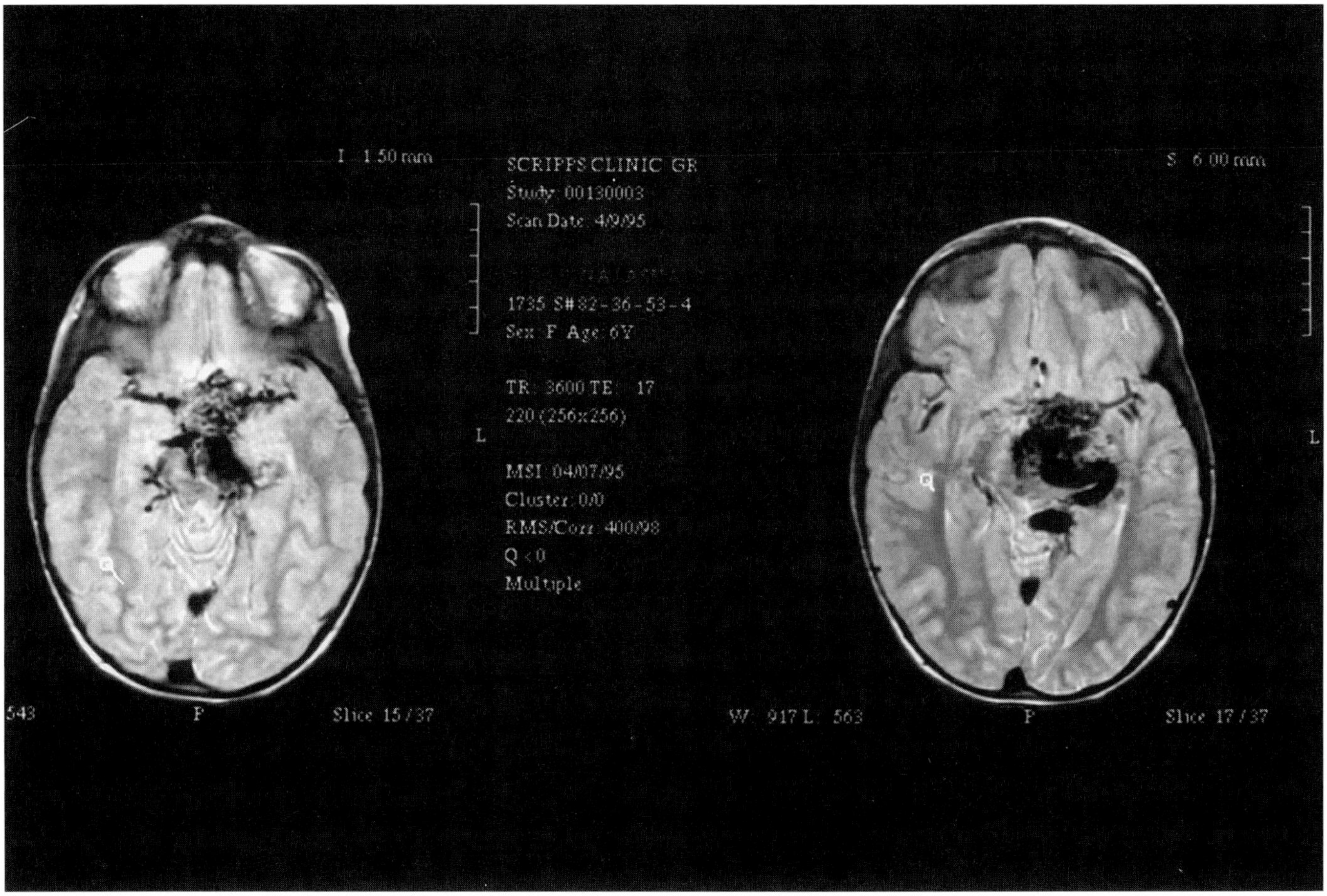

Figure 58B. The lower cuts of the axial view, demonstrating AVM involvement of the globus pallidus, internal capsule, and hypothalamus (see illustrative case 10). *Continued*

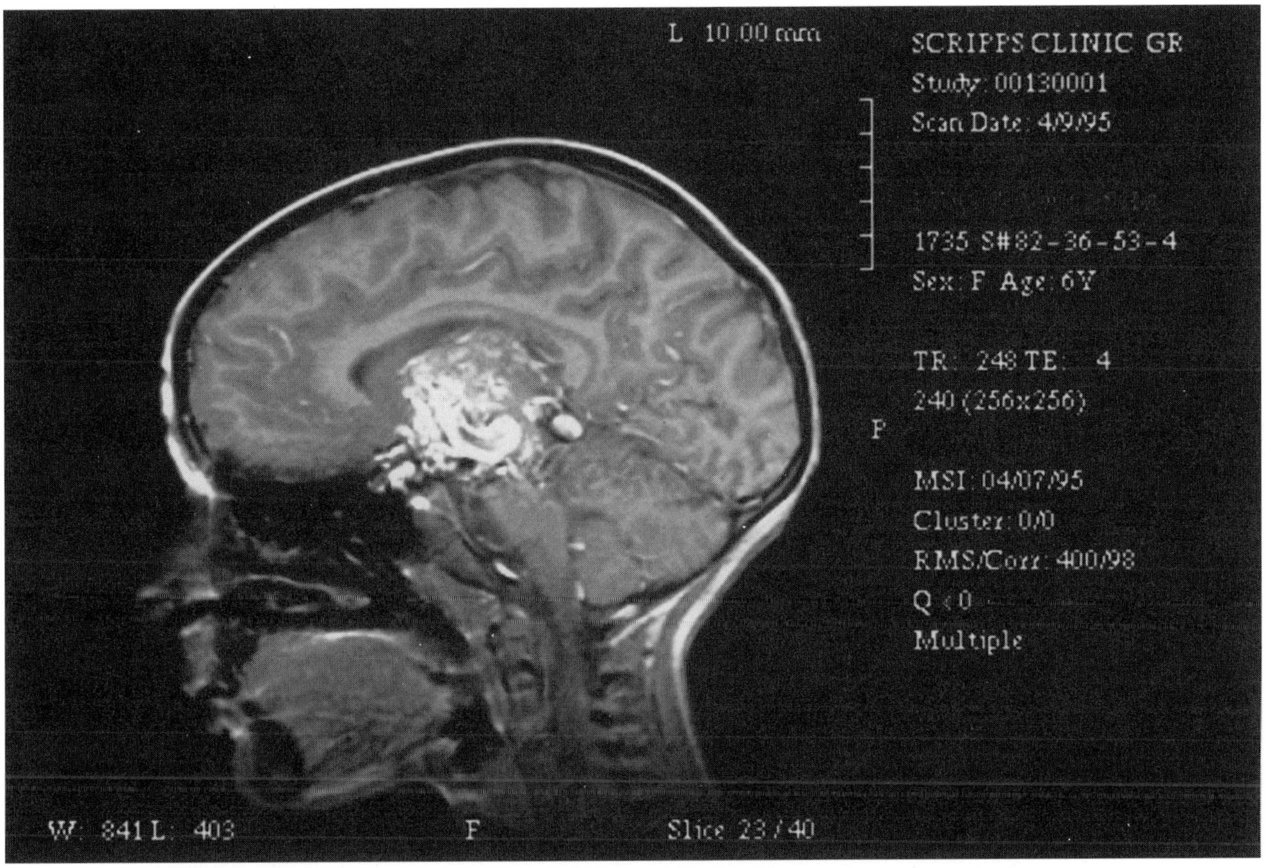

Figure 58C. The lateral MRI film confirming the involvement of the previously mentioned structures and the extension into the left orbit (see illustrative case 10).

by (the second step) cauterization of the AVM in the caudate nucleus and the putamen.

The third step was to eliminate the extension of the AVM into the left orbit. This was accomplished by means of the left pterional approach and additional bone removal of the roof and posterior wall of the orbit, including the sphenoid ridge and anterior clinoid. The intraorbital AVM was exposed posterior to the globe, and its intracranial extension through the superior and inferior orbital fissure and optic foramen. The intraorbital AVM was eliminated totally by cauterization.

Postoperative Course

The patient improved in strength and coordination after surgery. The first improvement noted by the parents included "beginning to color the drawing with the right hand," and "swimming on her own without any training." After surgery, she received gamma knife irradiation to the remaining AVM by Ladislau Steiner, MD, PhD, at University of Virginia Gamma-Knife Institute. She attends school with ordinary students, although she is still slower mentally and physically than the average student. About $2\frac{1}{2}$years later, the thalamic portion of the AVM was obliterated and only the hypothalamic portion remains open (Figures 59A and B). She had two episodes of lethargy, speech difficulty, and weakness of the right arm and leg that lasted for 2 weeks, probably related to progression of intraluminal closure of the AVM.

Case 11: Cerebellar and Brain Stem AVM

This 25-year-old woman was admitted to Loma Linda University Medical Center in 1994 with a chief complaint of double vision, incoordination, and gait disturbance. The history dated back to June 1986 when at the age of 17 she experienced a sudden onset

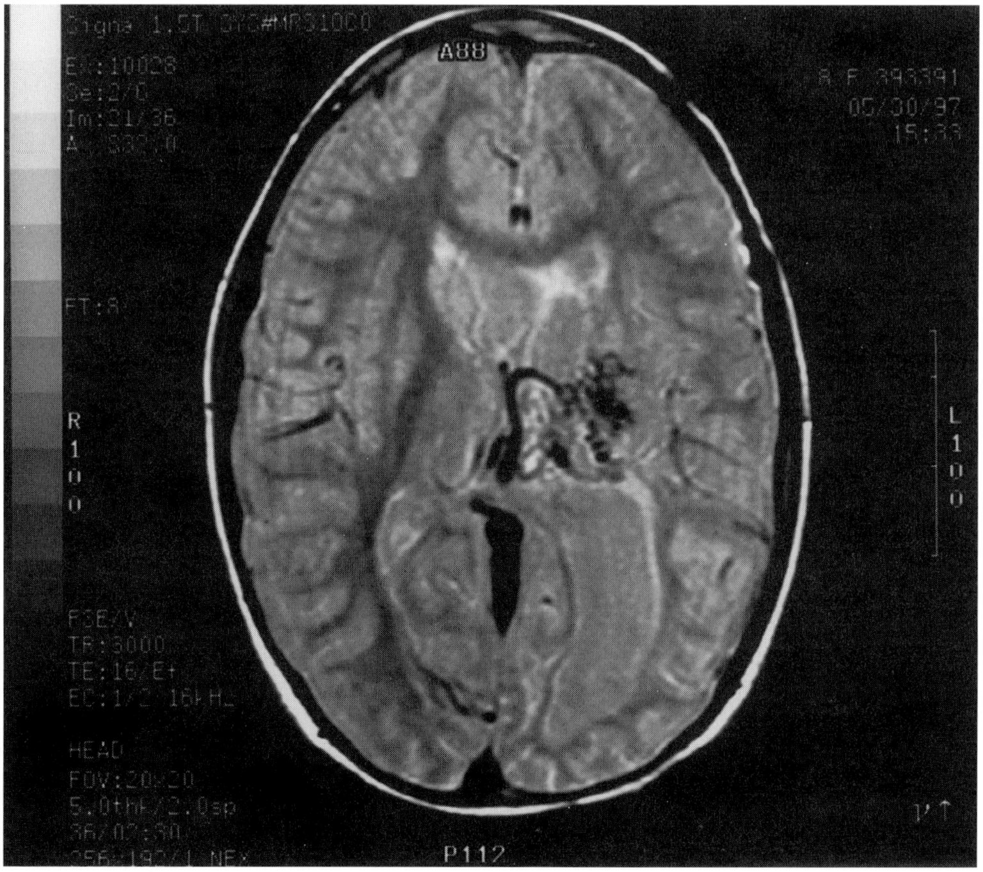

Figure 59. A, B. One month after the last staged surgery, this patient underwent gamma knife treatment. About $2\frac{1}{2}$ years after irradiation, extensive obliteration of the thalamic portion of the AVM was noted in MRI, but the hypothalamic portion was still patent. *Continued*

of headache associated with meningismus. The CT scan showed subarachnoid hemorrhage primarily in the cistern ambiens, and the angiogram revealed a large AVM in the brain stem and cerebellum supplied by the three major cerebellar arteries. She had two additional episodes of hemorrhage. In July 1986, she underwent embolization which reportedly decreased the size of the AVM by 70%. After the embolization, she was noted to have right upper quadrant anopia, double vision, memory loss, gait difficulties, some right-sided weakness, and bilateral dysmetria. However, all of these symptoms almost completely subsided to the point that she was able to drive and to work as a sales clerk in her parent's pet shop. About 1 year later she again began to have worsening of her symptoms. In January 1991, 5 years after the onset of the symptoms, she fell and began to note worsening of her double vision, which required prism glasses. Otherwise, there was only the drooping of one side of the face (not clear as to which side). In October 1991, she experienced excruciating headaches, confusion, ataxia, occasional incontinence and intermittent facial weakness. The MRI at that time showed persistent AVM in the same area and marked hydrocephalus. Partly because of financial difficulty, she did not have medical treatment other than dexamethasone, which caused some improvement in her neurological conditions. The patient's own neurologist described mild impairment of adduction of each eye on lateral gaze, mild (4±5) left hemiparesis, tendency to tilt her body toward the right while walking, inability to perform tandem walking, and finger-to-nose dysmetria. In December 1991, she underwent a VP shunt which was followed by reduction of the ventriculomegaly. Her mother felt that all of her symptoms were worse following the VP shunt and she was unable to walk because she had "floppy legs." When she arrived at Loma Linda, she had diplopia with skew deviation of the eyes, marked spasticity, and ataxic gait using walker, and was able to walk only a few steps unassisted. She had severe dysmetria in the upper and lower extremities, the left being worse than the right. Coordinating movements were severely impaired, more so on the left than the

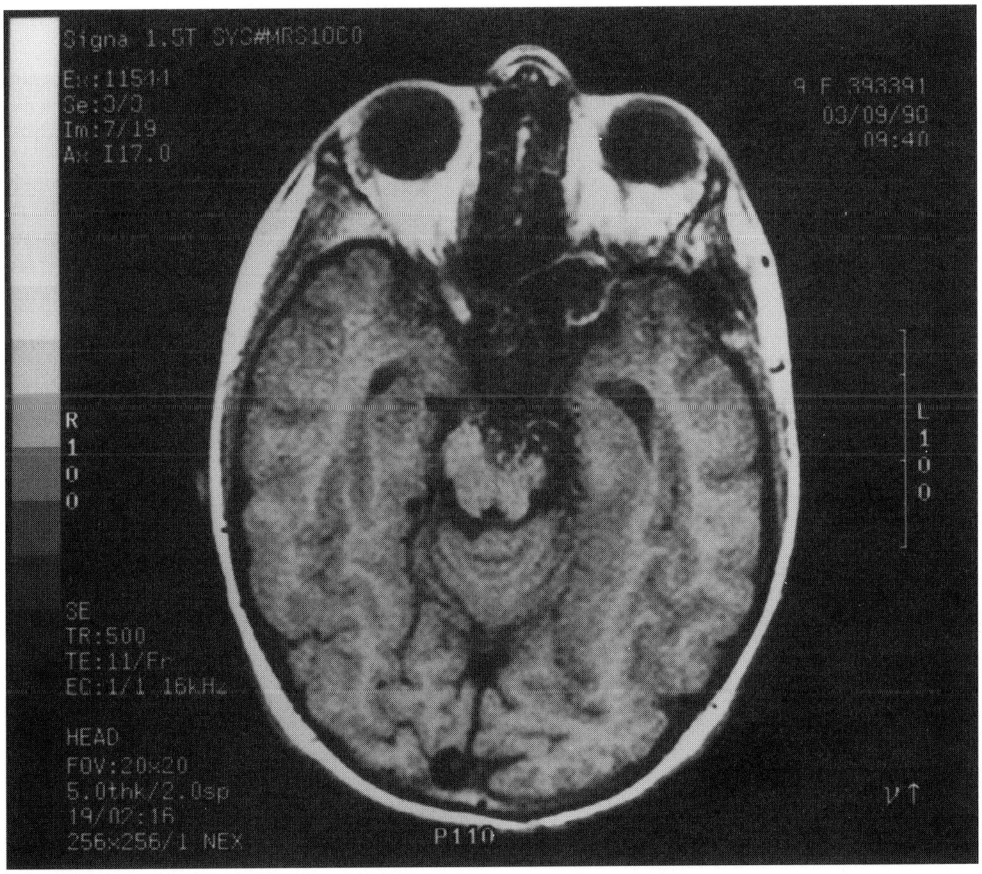

Figuure 59B. Same patient as in **A.**

right. No sensory changes were noted in any of the modalities. She showed marked emotional lability, crying almost constantly with anger.

Imaging Findings

CT scan, MRI and conventional angiogram were compatible with a large AVM 6 cm vertical, 5.5 cm axial, and 3.5 cm lateral in dimension in the cerebellar and brain stem (Figures 60A and B). A large draining vein connected to the straight sinus near the vein of Galen. The AVM was indenting into the brain stem, splitting the midbrain almost in half.

Operative Procedure

The first stage operation consisted of lateral isolation of the AVM. A large occipital craniotomy was performed including above and below the transverse sinus. The S-shaped large draining vein was followed from the surface of the vermis to 1 cm depth, and the AVM core was exposed and then dissected along its lateral aspect, first on the right and then on the left, by interrupting shunting arterioles, which were the terminal branches of the superior cerebellar, the anterior inferior cerebellar and the posterior inferior cerebellar arteries. The AVM was shrunk to 4 cm × 3 cm × 2.5 cm (Figures 61A and B).

At the second stage surgery, the AVM was isolated along the medulla oblongata inferiorly to expose the fourth ventricle upward underneath the vermian cortex to the quadrigeminal plates. The AVM was extending into the upper brain stem including the midbrain. After circumferential isolation of shunting arterioles and communicating venules, the AVM was shrunken to about 2.5 cm in diameter, the size considered to be appropriate for gamma knife radiation. Four months later she was treated by gamma knife at the University of Virginia.

Postoperative Course

Core vessels have been almost eliminated and only the major draining vein of decreased size still

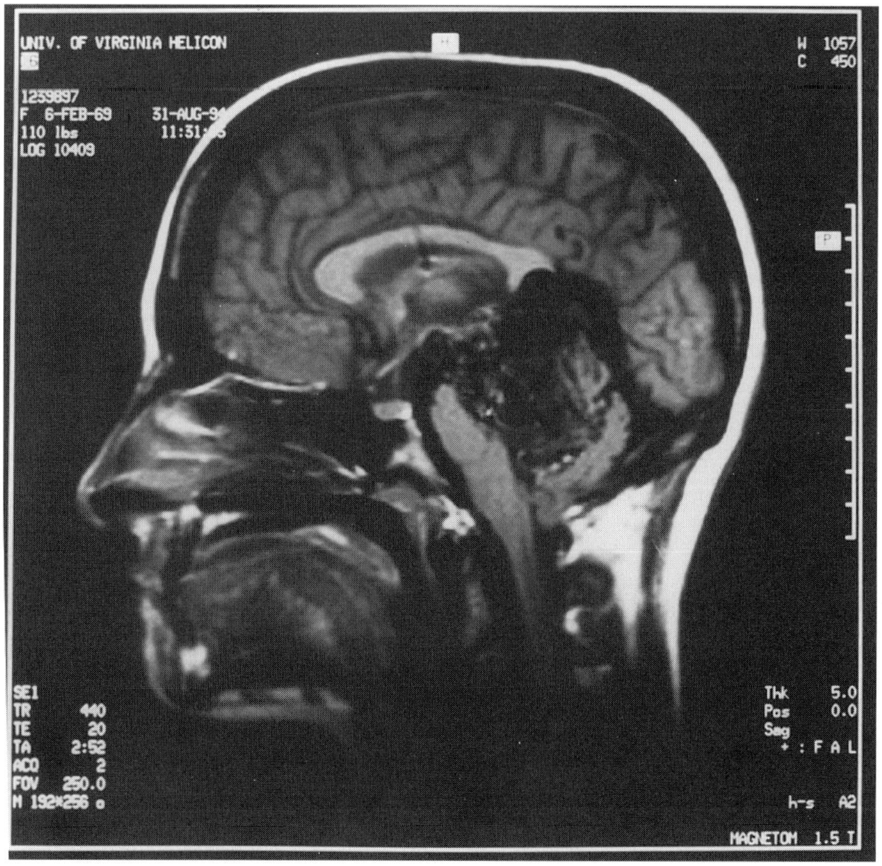

Figure 60. A, B. A large AVM 6 cm (vertical) × 5.5 cm (horizontal) × 3.5 cm (lateral) included the cerebellar vermis and midbrain, pons, and medulla oblongata. *Continued*

persists by MRI and angiogram. The patient was relieved from the attacks of severe throbbing headaches, and she gradually improved in speaking, swallowing, and thinking, although she still forgets recent happenings when she is under pressure. She has been in a stable pleasant emotional state, and the constant crying has ceased. She now lives in her own apartment and is able to walk alone for approximately 10 feet without a walker, 3 years following surgery and radiation.

Discussion and Conclusion

As illustrated in this section, patients with AVMs in functional areas often present with seizures and progressive neurological deficits, and are candidates for surgical treatment. Smaller AVMs (less than 4 cm in diameter) in sensorimotor, speech, visual (occipital), and dominant parietotemporal areas can be surgically treated in one stage. Safer resection of AVMs greater than 4–5 cm in diameter may be accomplished by using two or more staged surgical procedures. Embolization and irradiation may have a place for treatment of small AVMs in those areas, but no data are available.

Moderate or severe neurological deficit caused by AVM hemorrhage may require urgent surgery. However, it is best to wait until surgical procedures are less harmful to surrounding vital but severely edematous and fragile brain tissue, unless the signs of increased intracranial pressure dominate the other signs and symptoms.

Neurological improvement usually parallels the capacity of the patient to return to his/her occupation. However, even mild speech difficulty is detrimental to intellectually oriented professionals, whereas manual workers may function well. Mild weakness of arms or legs may be a threat to the occupational capacity of athletic professionals, although the same degree of weakness may not interfere with other professionals. Homonymous hemianopia can be compensated well by a housewife and many professionals, but professional drivers or pilots may be severely handicapped.

The patients in the cases described in this chapter were able to return to work or undergo occupational rehabilitation. Better control of seizures, neurological improvement, relief of severe throbbing headaches, alleviation of anxiety associated with

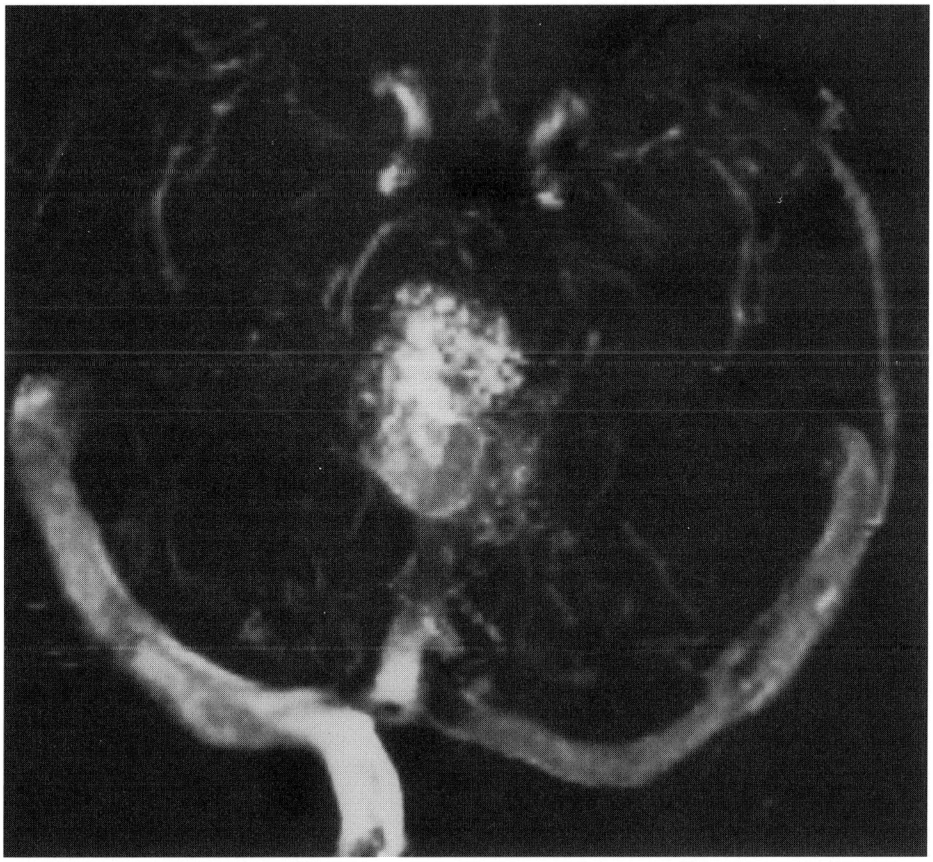

Figure 60B. The same AVM as shown in **A.**

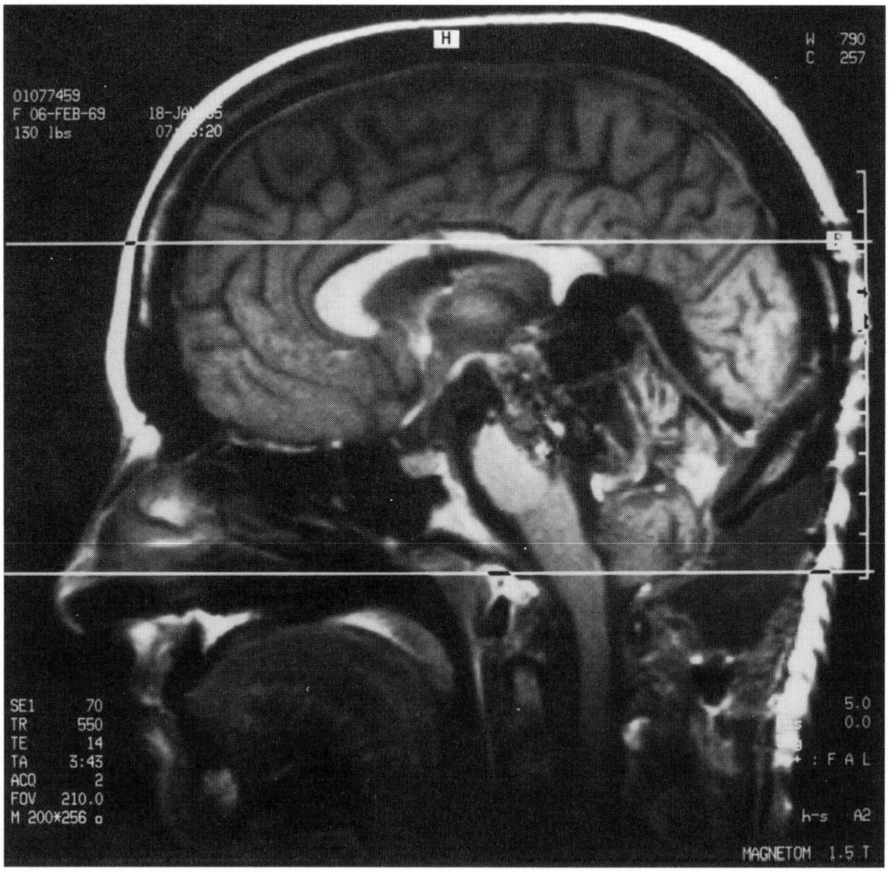

Figure 61. A, B. After the first staged operation, the size of the AVM reduced to 4 cm × 4 cm × 2.5 cm as shown in the MRI. After the second staged surgery, the size was 3 cm × 2 cm × 2 cm, and the AVM was irradiated by gamma knife. *Continued*

postictal paralysis, aphasia, increasing transient ischemia, or of the fear of the risks from the natural history led the patients to the quality of life that they desired before surgery. Although the risks involved in surgical treatment of AVMs in functional areas must be evaluated, carefully planned surgical intervention reduces the risks to patients. Medical professionals, as well as laymen, must be fully acquainted with the balance between the surgical risks and the dangers of this disorder without surgical intervention.

Summary

Arteriovenous malformations in functional areas of the brain have been considered unapproachable. It is through the efforts of a limited number of neurosurgeons that these AVMs became operable without serious complications. For safe AVM resection in functional areas, it is necessary to adhere to the following principles: (1) the surgeon must thoroughly understand the hemodynamic anatomy of the AVM so he/she can identify its type and location; (2) meticulous techniques are required to avoid removing essential brain tissue and to maintain microcirculation in the functional areas; (3) different approaches are applicable for different types and locations of AVMs in the functional areas; (4) the compartmental isolation of large AVMs is an enormous advantage in minimizing the insult to the surrounding brain tissue and in maintaining circulation of the cerebral vasculature around the AVM core; and (5) good outcomes are possible after surgical treatment, as demonstrated by the case reports.

In conclusion, the surgical risks involved in resection of small, medium, large, and even giant AVMs have reached an acceptable level when applied to sensorimotor, speech, and visual areas. However, from the author's experience, diffuse AVMs in the capsulocaudatothalamic area and brain stem re-

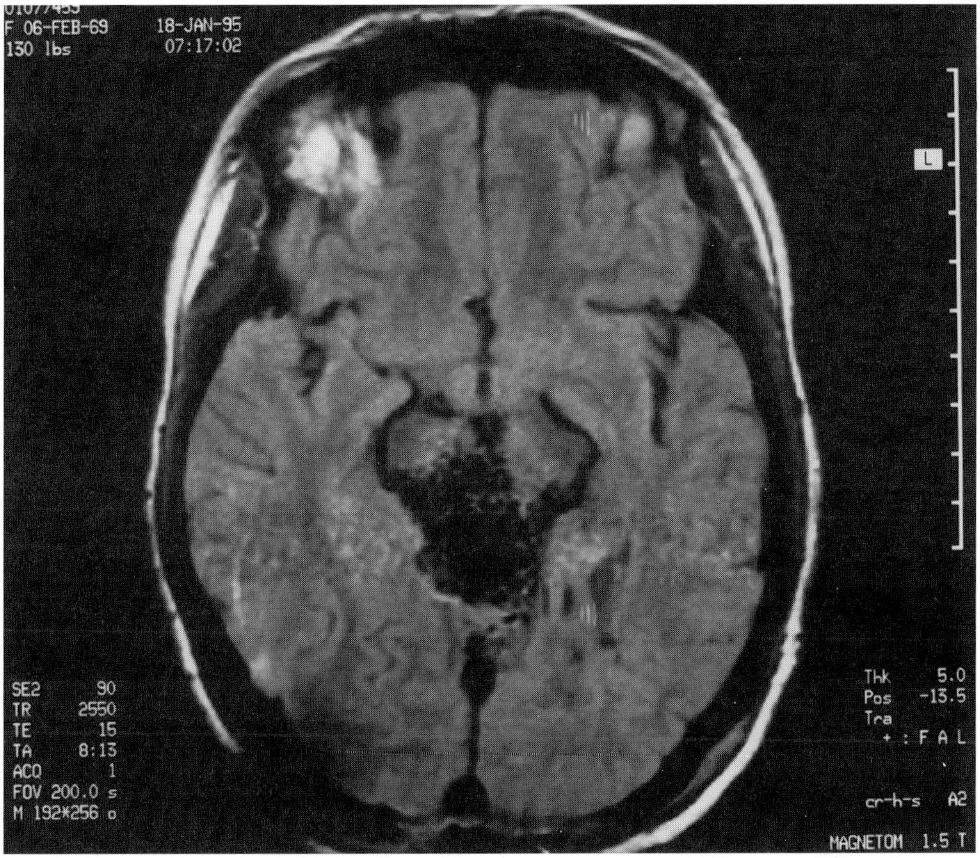

Figure 61B. Same AVM as shown in **A.**

quire radiosurgery. Large diffuse AVMs in these areas must first be surgically treated until reduced to a size suitable for radiosurgery. Embolization is a supportive measure for enhancing surgical resection or radiosurgery of large AVMs by reducing the part of the AVM that extends into the silent area of the brain.

References

1. Albin MS, Bunegin L, Helsel P, et al. Intracranial pressure and regional blood flow responses to experimental brain retraction pressure. In Shulman K, Marmarou A, Miller JD, et al (eds): Intracranial Pressure IV. Berlin: Springer, 1980, pp 131–134.
2. Allen MB Jr, Doetsch GS, Gindin RA, et al. A Manual of Neurosurgery. Baltimore: University Park Press, 1978.
3. Aronson SM. Vascular malformations. In Minckler J (ed): Pathology of the Nervous System. New York: McGraw-Hill, 1972.
4. Benzel EC, Lewine JD, Bucholz RD, et al. Magnetic source imaging: a review of the Magnes System of Biomagnetic Technologies Incorporated. Neurosurgery 33:252–259, 1993.
5. Benzel EC, Rupp FW, McCormack BM, et al. A comparison of fluoroscopy and computed tomography-derived volumetric multiple exposure transmission holography for the guidance of lumbar pedicle screw insertion. Neurosurgery 37:711–716, 1995.
6. Berenstein A, Kricheff II. Catheter and material selection for transarterial embolization: technical considerations, Part I. Catheters. Radiology 132:619–630, 1979a.
7. Berenstein A, Kricheff II. Catheter and material selection for transarterial embolization: technical considerations, Part II. Materials. Radiology 132:631–639, 1979b.
8. Berger MS, Cohen WA, Ojemann GA. Correlation of motor cortex brain mapping data with magnetic resonance imaging. J Neurosurg 72:383–387, 1990.
9. Bergstrand H, Olivecrona H, Tönnis W. Gefässmissbildungen und Gefässgeschwüste des Gehirns. Leipzig: Thieme, 1936.
10. Black KL, Rubin JM, Chandler WF, et al. Intraoperative color-flow Doppler imaging of AVMs and aneurysms. J Neurosurg 68:635–639, 1988.

11. Brown RD Jr, Wiebers DO, Forbes G, et al. The natural history of unruptured intracranial arteriovenous malformations. J Neurosurg 68:352–357, 1988.
12. Burchiel KJ, Clarke H, Ojemann GA, et al. Use of stimulation mapping and corticography in the excision of arteriovenous malformations in sensorimotor and language-related neocortex. Neurosurgery 24: 322–327, 1989.
13. Bushe KA, Bockhorn J, Schaefer ER, et al. Macro- and microsurgery of central angiomas. In Pia HW, Gleave JRW, Grote E, et al (eds): Cerebral Angiomas: Advances in Diagnosis and Therapy. Berlin: Springer, 1975, pp 123–128.
14. Carter LP, White WL, Atkinson JR. Regional cortical blood flow at craniotomy. Neurosurgery 2:223–229, 1978.
15. Colombo F, Benedetti A, Pozza F, et al. Linear accelerator radiosurgery of cerebral arteriovenous malformations. Neurosurgery 24:833–840, 1989.
16. Crawford PM, West CR, Chadwick DW, et al. Arteriovenous malformations of the brain: natural history in unoperated patients. J Neurol Neurosurg Psychiat 49: 1–10, 1986.
17. Cushing H, Bailey P. Tumors Arising from the Blood Vessels of the Brain: Angiomatous Malformations and Hemangioblastomas. Springfield, IL: Charles C Thomas, 1928.
18. Dandy WE. Arteriovenous aneurysms of the brain. Arch Surg 17:190–243, 1928.
19. Dandy WE. Venous abnormalities and angiomas of the brain. Arch Surg 17:715–793, 1928.
20. DaPian R, Pasqualin A, Scienza R, et al. Microsurgical treatment of ten arteriovenous malformations in critical areas of the cerebrum. J Microsurg 1:305–320, 1980.
21. Davis C, Symon L. The management of cerebral arteriovenous malformations. Acta Neurochir 74:4–11, 1985.
22. Debrun G, Vinuela F, Fox A, et al. Emobilization of cerebral arteriovenous malformations with bucrylate: experience in 46 cases. J Neurosurg 56:615–627, 1982.
23. Doppman JL, DiChiro G, Ommaya AK. Obliteration of spinal-cord arteriovenous malformation by percutaneous embolization. Lancet 1:477, 1968.
24. Drake CG. Cerebral arteriovenous malformations: considerations for and experience with surgical treatment in 166 cases. Clin Neurosurg 26:145–208, 1979.
25. Duma CM, Lundsford LD, Kondziolka D, et al. Radiosurgery for vascular malformations of the brain stem. Acta Neurochir 58:92–97, 1993.
26. Fabrikant JI, Lyman JT, Hosobuchi Y. Stereotactic heavy-ion Bragg-peak radiosurgery for intra-cranial vascular disorders: method for treatment of deep arteriovenous malformations. Br J Radiol 57:479–490, 1984.
27. Feindel W, Yamamoto YL, Hodge CP. Cerebral microcirculation. Red cerebral veins and the cerebral steal syndrome: evidence from fluorescein angiography and microregional blood flow by radioisotopes during excision of an angioma. J Neurosurg 35:167–179, 1971.
28. Filatov YM, Konavolov AM, Serbinenko FA. Surgical treatment of poorly accessible arteriovenous malformations. In Carrea R (ed): Neurological Surgery with Emphasis on Noninvasive Methods of Diagnosis and Treatment, Proc. 6th International Congress of Neurological Surgery. Amsterdam: Excerpta Medica, 1978, pp 157–161.
29. Forster DMC, Steiner L, Håkanson S. Arteriovenous malformations of the brain: a long-term clinical study. J Neurosurg 37:562–570, 1972.
30. French LA, Seljeskog EL. Arteriovenous malformations of the brain. In Youmans JR (ed): Neurological Surgery Vol 2. Philadelphia: WB Saunders, 1973, pp 827–836.
31. Friedman WA, Bova FJ. Linear accelerator radiosurgery for arteriovenous malformations. J Neurosurg 77: 832–841, 1992.
32. Fults D, Kelly DL Jr. Natural history of arteriovenous malformations of the brain: a clinical study. Neurosurgery 15:658–662, 1984.
33. Gallen CC, Schwartz BJ, Bucholz RD, et al. Presurgical localization of functional cortex using magnetic source imaging. J Neurosurg 82:988–994, 1995.
34. Gallen CC, Sobel DF, Waltz T, et al. Noninvasive presurgical neuromagnetic mapping of somatosensory cortex. Neurosurgery 33:260–268, 1993.
35. Garretson HD. Arteriovenous malformation. In Rosenberg RN, Grossman RG (eds): The Clinical Neurosciences, Vol 2. New York: Churchill Livingstone, 1983, pp 1089–1100.
36. Girvin JP, Fox AJ, Viñuela F, et al. Intraoperative embolization of cerebral arteriovenous malformations in the awake patient. Clin Neurosurg 31:188–247, 1983.
37. Gjindjian R, Merland JJ. Superselective Arteriography of the External Carotid Artery. New York: Springer, 1978.
38. Graf CJ, Perret GE, Torner JC. Bleeding from cerebral arteriovenous malformations as part of their natural history. J Neurosurg 58:331–337, 1983.
39. Guglielmi G, Viñuela F, Sepetka I, et al. Electrothrombosis of saccular aneurysms via endovascular approach: Part 1: Electrochemical basis, technique, and experimental results. J Neurosurg 75:1–7, 1991.
40. Guidetti B, Delitala A. Intracranial arteriovenous malformations: conservative and surgical treatment. J Neurosurg 53:149–152, 1980.
41. Hamby WB. The pathology of supratentorial angiomas. J Neurosurg 15:65–75, 1958.
42. Henderson WR, Gomez RD. Natural history of cerebral angiomas. Br Med J 4:571–574, 1967.
43. Heros RC. Arteriovenous malformations of the medial temporal lobe: surgical approach and neuroradiological characterization. J Neurosurg 56:44–52, 1982.
44. Heros RC, Tu Y. Unruptured arteriovenous malformations: a dilemma in surgical decision making. Clin Neurosurg 33:187–236, 1985.
45. Hieshima GB, Mehringer CM, Grinnell VS, et al. Preoperative balloon occlusion: The intravascular ligature. Surg Neurol 17:191–196, 1982.
46. Hilal SK, Michelsen JW. Therapeutic percutaneous embolization for extra-axial vascular lesions of the head, neck, and spine. J Neurosurg 43:275–287, 1975.
47. Hoang TA, Hasso AN. Intracranial vascular formations. Neuroimaging Clin N Am 4:823–847, 1994.
48. Houdart R. Problèmes thérapeutiques des anévrismes artérioveineux. Rev Prat (Paris) 17:4147–4167, 1967.

49. Hunter J, Ogilvy R, Schulz R, et al. Holograph versus maximum-intensity projection display of neurovascular anatomy and pathology. In Takahashi M, Korogi Y, Mosely I (eds): Proceedings of the XV Symposium Neuroradiologicum. Berlin: Springer, 1994, pp 69–71.
50. Kelly DL Jr, Alexander E Jr, Davis CH, et al. Intracranial arteriovenous malformations: clinical review and evaluation of brain scans. J Neurosurg 31:422–428, 1969.
51. Kerber CW, Bank WO, Cromwell LD. Calibrated leak balloon microcatheter: a device for arterial exploration and occlusive therapy. Am J Roentgenol 132: 207–212, 1979.
52. Kjellberg RN, Davis KR, Lyons S, et al. Bragg-peak proton beam treatment of arteriovenous malformation of the brain. Clin Neurosurg 31:248–290, 1983.
53. Kunc Z. Surgery of arteriovenous malformations in the speech and motor-sensory regions. J Neurosurg 40:293–303, 1974.
54. Kunicki A. Discussion of arteriovenous anomalies. 3rd Europ Congr Neurosurg, Madrid. Amsterdam: Excerpta Medica, 1967, p 33.
55. Kusske JA, Kelly WA. Embolization and reduction of the "steal" syndrome in cerebral arteriovenous malformations. J Neurosurg 40:313–321, 1974.
56. Lewis AI, Tew JM Jr. Management of thalamic-basal ganglia and brain-stem vascular malformations. Clin Neurosurg 41:83–111, 1993.
57. Lonser R, Yamada S, Liwnicz B, et al. Scanning EM demonstration of shunting arterioles in arteriovenous malformations (AVMs). Annual meeting Congress of Neurological Surgeons: Oral Poster # 66. September 22 - October 2, 1997 pp 282–283.
58. Luessenhop AJ. Natural history of cerebral arteriovenous malformations. In Wilson CB, Stein BM (eds): Intracranial Arteriovenous Malformations. Baltimore: Williams & Wilkins, 1984, pp 12–23.
59. Luessenhop AJ, Kachmann R Jr, Shevlin W, et al. Clinical evaluation of artificial embolization in the management of large cerebral arteriovenous malformations. J Neurosurg 23:400–417, 1965.
60. Lunsford LD, Kondziolka D, Flickinger JC, et al. Stereotactic radiosurgery for arteriovenous malformations of the brain. J Neurosurg 75:512–524, 1991.
61. Malik GM, Seyfried DM, Morgan JK. Temporal lobe arteriovenous malformations: surgical management and outcome. Surg Neurol 46:106–115, 1996.
62. Malis LI. Bipolar coagulation in microsurgery. In Donaghy RMP, Yasargil MG (eds): Microvascular Surgery. Stuttgart: Theime, 1967, pp 126–130.
63. Malis LI. Arteriovenous malformations of the brain. In Youmans JR (ed): Neurological Surgery, Vol 3. Philadelphia: WB Saunders, 1982, pp 1786–1806.
64. Martin N, Jordan S, Viñuela F, et al. Preoperative and intraoperative localization of eloquent cortex adjacent to arteriovenous malformation. Neurosurgery 24: 633, 1989 (abstract).
65. Martin NA, Wilson CB. Medial occipital arteriovenous malformations: surgical treatment. J Neurosurg 56:798–802, 1982.
66. McCormick WF. The pathology of vascular ("arteriovenous") malformations. J Neurosurg 24:807–816, 1966.
67. McCormick WF. Pathology of vascular malformations of the brain. In Wilson CB, Stein BM (eds): Intracranial Arteriovenous Malformations. Baltimore: Williams & Wilkins, 1984, pp 44–63.
68. Michelsen WJ. Natural history and pathophysiology of arteriovenous malformations. Clin Neurosurg 26: 307–313, 1979.
69. Mingrino S. Supratentorial arteriovenous malformations of the brain. In Krayenbühl H (ed): Advances and Technical Standards in Neurosurgery, Vol 5. New York: Springer, 1978, pp 93–123.
70. Moniz E. L'encéphalographie artérielle, son importance dans la localisation des tumeurs cérébrales. Rev Neurol 2:72–90, 1927.
71. Moody RA, Poppen JL. Arteriovenous malformations. J Neurosurg 32:503–511, 1970.
72. Mullan S, Brown FD, Patronas NJ. Hyperemic and ischemic problems of surgical treatment of arteriovenous malformations. J Neurosurg 51:757–764, 1979.
73. Newton TH, Troost BT, Mosely I. Angiography of arteriovenous malformations and fistula. In Wilson CB, Stein BM (eds): Intracranial Arteriovenous Malformations. Baltimore: Williams & Wilkins, 1984, pp 64–104.
74. Norlén G. Arteriovenous aneurysms of the brain: report of ten cases of total removal of the lesion. J Neurosurg 6:475–494, 1949.
75. Nornes H, Lundar T, Wikeby P: Cerebral arteriovenous malformations: results of microsurgical management. Acta Neurochir 50:243–257, 1979.
76. Okazaki H, Scheitauer BW: Atlas of Neuropathology. New York: Gower, 1988.
77. Olivecrona H, Ladenheim J: Congenital Arteriovenous Aneurysms of the Carotid and Vertebral Arterial Systems. Berlin: Springer, 1957.
78. Parkinson D. Cerebral arteriovenous aneurysms: surgical management. Can J Surg 1:313–325, 1958.
79. Parkinson D. Arteriovenous malformations. Neurol Res 4:163–175, 1982.
80. Paterson JH, McKissock W. A clinical survey of intracranial angiomas with special reference to their mode of progression and surgical treatment: a report of 110 cases. Brain 79:223–266, 1956.
81. Patterson RH, Voorhies RM. Surgical approaches to intracranial and intraspinal arteriovenous malformations. Clin Neurosurg 25:412–424, 1978.
82. Pellettieri L, Carlsson CA, Grevsten S, et al. Surgical versus conservative treatment of intracranial arteriovenous malformations: A study in surgical decision-making. Acta Neurochir Suppl 29:1–86, 1980.
83. Penfield W, Erickson TC. Epilepsy and Cerebral Localization. Springfield: Charles C Thomas, 1941, pp 52–154.
84. Perret G, Nishioka H. Arteriovenous malformations: an analysis of 545 cases of cranio-cerebral arteriovenous malformations and fistulae reported to the cooperative study. J Neurosurg 25:467–490, 1966.
85. Pertuiset B, Ancri D, Goutorbe G. Variation de volume sanguin cérébral local en fonction de la pression artérielle moyenne chez l'homme. Rev Neurol (Paris) 132: 213–218, 1976.
86. Pertuiset B, Ancri D, Sichez JP, et al. Radical surgery in cerebral AVM: tactical procedures based upon hemodynamic factors. In Krayenbühl H: Advances and

Technical Standards in Neurosurgery, Vol 10. Wien: Springer, 1983, pp 83–143.
87. Pertuiset B, Posada T, Metzger J, et al. L'exérèse rétrograde des malformations artério-veineuses des hémisphères cérébraux sans hématome: technique, indications et résultats. Ann Chir 22:803–809, 1968.
88. Pertuiset B, Sichez JP. The backward technique in the total resection of cerebral arteriovenous malformations: experience with 86 cases. Adv Neurosurg 6: 148–153, 1978.
89. Pertuiset B, Sichez JP, Philippon J, et al. Mortalité après et morbidité après exérèse chirurgicale totale de 162 malformations artérioveineuses intrâcraniennes (1958–1978). Rev Neurol (Paris) 135(4):319–327, 1979.
90. Pia HW. The indications and contraindications for treatment or assessment. In Pia HW, Gleave JRW, Grote E, et al (eds): Cerebral Angiomas: Advances in Diagnosis and Therapy. New York: Springer, 1975, pp 1–8.
91. Pilcher C. Angiomatous malformations of the brain: sucessful extirpation in three cases. Ann Surg 123: 766–784, 1946.
92. Pool JL. Treatment of arteriovenous malformations of the cerebral hemispheres. J Neurosurg 19:136–141, 1962.
93. Pool JL. Excision of cerebral arteriovenous malformations. J Neurosurg 29:312–321, 1968.
94. Riechert T, Mundinger F. Combined stereotactic operation for treatment of deep-seated angiomas and aneurysms. J Neurosurg 21:358–363, 1964.
95. Sano S, Aiba T, Jimbo M. Surgical treatment of cerebral aneurysms and arteriovenous malformations. Neurologia Med Chir 7:128–131, 1965.
96. Schatz S, Botterell EH. The natural history of arteriovenous malformations. In Milliken C (ed): Cerebrovascular Disease. Vol XLI, Chapter X. Baltimore: Williams & Wilkins, 1966, pp 180–187.
97. Seifert V, Stolke D, Mehdorn HM, et al. Clinical and radiological evaluation of long-term results of stereotactic proton beam radiosurgery in patients with cerebral arteriovenous malformations. J Neurosurg 81: 683–689, 1994.
98. Serbinenko FA. Balloon catheterization and occlusion of major cerebral vessels. J Neurosurg 41: 125–145, 1974.
99. Shi Y, Chen X. A proposed scheme for grading intracranial arteriovenous malformations. J Neurosurg 65: 484–489, 1986.
100. Shi Y, Chen X. Surgical treatment of arteriovenous malformations of the striatothalamocapsular region. J Neurosurg 66:352–356, 1987.
101. Solomon RA, Stein BM. Interhemispheric approach for the surgical removal of thalamocaudate arteriovenous malformations. J Neurosurg 66:345–351, 1987.
102. Spetzler RF, Martin NA. A proposed grading system for arteriovenous malformations. J Neurosurg 65: 476–483, 1986.
103. Spetzler RF, Wilson CB, Weinstein P, et al. Normal perfusion pressure breakthrough theory. Clin Neurosurg 25:651–672, 1978.
104. Stein BM, Wolpert SM. Arteriovenous malformations of the brain, II: current concepts and treatment. Arch Neurol 37:69–75, 1980.
105. Steiner L. Treatment of arteriovenous malformations by radiosurgery. In Wilson CB, Stein BM (eds): Intracranial Arteriovenous Malformations. Baltimore: Williams & Wilkins, 1984, pp 295–314.
106. Sundt TM. Surgical Techniques for Saccular and Giant Intracranial Aneurysms. Baltimore: Williams & Wilkins, 1990.
107. Suzuki J, Onuma T, Kayama T. Surgical treatment of intracranial arteriovenous malformations. Neurol Res 4:191–207, 1982.
108. Svien HJ, McRae JA. Arteriovenous anomalies of the brain: fate of patients not having definitive surgery. J Neurosurg 23:23–28, 1965.
109. Taveras JM, Wood EH (eds). Diagnostic Neuroradiology. Baltimore: Williams & Wilkins, 1964.
110. Tönnis W. Die chirurgische therapie der cerebralen Durchblutungsstörungen infolge Gefässmissbildungen. Acta Neurochir Suppl 7:268–282, 1961.
111. Tönnis W, Schiefer W, Walter W. Signs and symptoms of supratentorial arteriovenous aneurysms. J Neurosurg 15:471–480, 1958.
112. Wilson CB, Martin NA. Deep supratentorial arteriovenous malformations. In Wilson CB, Stein BM (eds): Intracranial Arteriovenous Malformations. Baltimore: Williams & Wilkins, 1984, pp 184–208.
113. Wilson CB, U HS, Domingue J. Microsurgical treatment of intracranial vascular malformations. J Neurosurg 51:446–454, 1979.
114. Wilson CB, Yorke C. Intracranial arteriovenous malformations. In Wilson CB, Hoff JT (eds): Current Surgical Management of Neurologic Disease. New York: Churchill Livingstone, 1980, pp 182–190.
115. Yamada S. Arteriovenous malformations in the functional area: surgical treatment and regional cerebral blood flow. Neurol Res 4:283–322, 1982.
116. Yamada S, Brauer F. Surgical approach to arteriovenous malformations (AVMs) of the superior temporal gyrus, including the speech area. Neurosurgery 20: 990, 1987 (abstract).
117. Yamada S, Brauer F, Dayes L, et al. Surgical techniques for arteriovenous malformations in functional areas focused on superior temporal gyrus. Neurologia Med Chir (Suppl) 38:122–126, 1998.
118. Yamada S, Brauer F, Iacono RP. Surgical importance of venous channels in arteriovenous malformations. In Hakuba A (ed): Surgery of the Intracranial Venous System. Tokyo: Springer, 1995, pp 499–505.
119. Yamada S, Brauer FS, Knierim DS. Direct approach to arteriovenous malformations in functional areas of the cerebral hemisphere. J Neurosurg 72:418–425, 1990.
120. Yamada S, Brauer F, Knierim D, et al. Safety limits of controlled hypotension in humans. Acta Neurochir (Suppl) 42:14–17, 1988.
121. Yamada S, Brauer F, Knierim D, et al. Can somatosensory evoked potential monitoring predict energy dynamics during controlled hypotension? Neurol Res 14:325–329, 1992.
122. Yamada S, Cojocaru T. Arteriovenous malformations. In Wood JH (ed): Cerebral Blood Flow. New York: McGraw-Hill, 1987, pp 580–590.
123. Yamada S, Gallen CC. Biomagnetic Technologies: Magnetic source imaging (MSI). Magnes Biomagnetometer. Neurosurgery 33:166–168, 1993.

124. Yamada S, Iacono RP, Mandybur GT. Endoscopic procedures for AVMs resection in functional areas of the brain. 65th Annual Meeting The American Association of Neurological Surgeons, Poster 1102. Denver: April 12–17, 1997, p 72.
125. Yamada S, Knierim D, Brauer F, et al. Direct surgical attack on AVMs located in functional area: intraoperative recording of evoked potentials and oxidative metabolism. In Brihave J, Vigouroux R, Achslogh J, et al (eds): Advances in the Management of Intracranial AVMs. 7th European Congress of Neurosurgery. Brussels: August 28-September 3, 1982, p 8.
126. Yamada S, Ritland S, Knierim D. Stereotactic localization of deep-seated arteriovenous malformations in the functional area. Appl Neurophysiol 46:231–235, 1983.
127. Yamada S, Rouse G, Iacono RP, et al. Color Doppler ultrasonography during arteriovenous malformation (AVM). surgery. Annual Meeting, Section on Cerebrovascular surgery of AANS and CNS, Poster # 51. Anaheim: February 4–6, 1997, p 96.
128. Yamada S, Thio S, Iacono RP, et al. Total blood flow to arteriovenous malformations. Neurol Res 15: 379–383, 1993.
129. Yasargil MG. Operations on intracranial arteriovenous malformations. In Yarsargil MG (ed): Microsurgery Applied to Neurosurgery. Stuttgart: Thieme, 1969, pp 143–148.
130. Yasargil MG. Microneurosurgery, Vol IIIA. AVM of the Brain, History, Embryology, Pathological Considerations, Hemodynamics, Diagnostic Studies, Microsurgical Anatomy. New York: Thieme, 1987.
131. Yasargil MG. Microneurosurgery, Vol IIIB. AVM of the Brain, Clinical Considerations, General and Specific Operative Techniques, Surgical Results, Nonoperated Cases, Cavernous and Venous Angiomas, Neuroanesthesia. New York: Thieme, 1988.
132. Yeh H, Tew JM. Management of arteriovenous malformations of the brain. Contemp Neurosurg 9:1–6, 1987.
133. Zoltan L. Some remarks to the operability of the centrally located arteriovenous angiomas. 3rd European Congr Neurosurg, Madrid. Amsterdam: Excerpta Medica, 1967, p 34.

Chapter 2

Postoperative Care for Arteriovenous Malformations in Functional Areas of the Brain

Shokei Yamada, MD, PhD, Daniel J. Cole, MD, and Sigmund Teichman, MD

Introduction

Postoperative care must be managed as meticulously as surgical procedures, particularly in the case of intraoperative bleeding that requires blood transfusion and fluid supplementation. Each of the following factors must be evaluated carefully and treatment must be practiced appropriately.

Prevention of Postoperative Bleeding

Postoperative bleeding may occur from several sources: (1) shunting arterioles; (2) type 1 and type 2 final feeding arteries; (3) communicating venules; (4) juxtanidal veins; and (5) the arteriovenous malformation (AVM) residuum. The AVM cavity wall may bleed from these sources after complete surgical hemostasis if a coagulation defect occurs, if an increase in blood pressure occurs suddenly after the completion of surgery, particularly during the recovery process from controlled hypotension, or if venous congestion causes increases in venous pressure. A combination of these factors can cause bleeding from the final feeding arteries. Bleeding from the residual AVM after a staged operation or unrecognized residual AVM is likely due to venous congestion or a coagulation defect. The sources of bleeding are at either end of the coagulated and sectioned communicating venules or juxtanidal veins. Type 1 or type 2 final feeding arteries can be the source of a large amount of bleeding if blood pressure rises rapidly. Usually, sectioned arteries (or arterioles) on the brain side and venules that are left connected to the core venous loops are the most likely sources of bleeding in cases of staged operation, because the holes developed in the core venous loops enlarge more profoundly and more rapidly than the other sectioned ends of these vessels on the brain side. Postoperative bleeding from the AVM residuum after a staged operation can be prevented by intraoperative isolation, followed by coagulation and shrinking of the compartment venous loops. Partial resection should be avoided,[5] because the actively circulating compartment may rupture along the border between the resected and the unresected portions.

Methods of Prevention

The coagulation mechanism must be regulated properly. Prothrombin time (PT) and partial prothrombin time (PTT) must be tested immediately after surgery and every day thereafter, for at least 3 days. The authors have found that PT is often delayed (i.e., >14.1 seconds and international normalized ratio (INR) >1.2) during or after surgery if blood loss is >1000 mL requiring multiple blood transfusions, or if a large amount of crystalloid is given. Vitamin K (5 mg) may be given intramuscularly or intravenously over 15 minutes twice a day.

If PTT is prolonged, transfusion of fresh frozen plasma often corrects the coagulopathy. If platelets are lower than normal (<150,000/mL), several units

From Yamada S (ed): *Arteriovenous Malformations in Functional Areas of the Brain.* © Futura Publishing Co, Inc, Armonk, NY, 1999.

of platelets should be given. If the platelet count is normal but platelet function is impaired, as may be noted after a large amount of blood loss treated with blood transfusion, prior use of acetylsalicylic acid (ASA) or nonsteroidal anti-inflammatory drugs (e.g., ibuprofen), uremia, or crystalloid infusion, a transfusion of platelets reverses this coagulopathy as well.[2]

Low hematocrit (less than 28%) or hemoglobin (less than 9 g/dL) causes a bleeding tendency because cellular components do not stick together.[1] Transfusion of packed cells or whole blood facilitates coagulation in the opened vessels. An iatrogenic decrease in hematocrit should be avoided by limiting the amount of crystalloid that is given.

There are pros and cons for administration of hydroxyethyl starch (Hetastarch) as blood volume expanders during or immediately after AVM surgery. It is more effective to increase cardiac output than plasma, crystalloid, or blood.[2] However, it has several disadvantages that must be considered. Hetastarch affects coagulation: (1) by prolonging PTT, PT, and bleeding times by lowering clotting proteins such as fibrinogen via hemodilution; (2) by lowering clotting factor VIII to a greater degree than can be explained by hemodilution; and (3) by shortening thrombin, reptilase, and urokinase-activated clot lysis time.[6] Since AVMs have a propensity for hemorrhagic events by nature, the authors advise avoiding the use of Hetastarch during and immediately following AVM surgery.

Blood Pressure Control

Postoperative mean arterial pressure must be kept at 60 mm Hg, where pulsation of the residual AVM is negligible. After a 12- to 24-hour period, the mean pressure may be maintained at 60–80 mm Hg.

At the present time, nitroprusside (Nipride) is the most effective agent to maintain blood pressure at an optimal level.[3,8,9] The Nipride dose may be increased to 5 μg/kg/min, as necessary. A dose of 10 mg/kg/min is considered to be toxic. The serum thiocyanate level may be estimated periodically (e.g., every 3 days) if Nipride is administered at a rate of about 5 μg/kg/min continuously. It is preferable to supplement Nipride with labetalol (Normodyne), at a dose of 10 mg every 15 minutes as needed. Labetalol is a selective competitive alpha-1 adrenergic blocking and nonselective competitive beta adrenergic blocking agent that maintains the pulse rate at an optimal level. Sedative agents, such as pentobarbital (Nembutal), augment stable control of low blood pressure while using Nipride. Nembutal is known to suppress activity of interneurons and anterior horn cells,[4] and may interrupt reflex arcs for blood vessel constriction at the spinal cord level.

Management of Medications

Controlled hypotension may be done effectively with nitroprusside, labetalol, or esmolol. The half-life of esmolol is too short and titration of this hypotensive medicine, which requires frequent adjustment, may not be as practical on the ward as in the operating room, where the anesthesiologist can devote total attention to pressure monitoring. If the patient is hypertensive (essential or secondary), ordinary antihypertensive medicines may be administered to maintain the basic pressure control.

Prevention of Postoperative Cerebrovascular Thrombosis

Coagulation of the AVM is typically followed by propagation of a thrombus to the remaining AVM loops. Thrombosis that is produced by partial or subtotal isolation of the AVM core causes AVM stasis and a precoagulant environment. Transient neurological deficits have also been reported due to thrombosis after partial or subtotal isolation of the AVM.[8,9] These temporary deficits are similar to those related to transient ischemic attacks in occlusive disease and are thought to be due to vasospasms of cerebral arterioles that share blood flow with shunting arterioles. Excessive thrombosis propagation can be prevented by adequate fluid maintenance at a rate of at least 100 mL/hr.

Fluid Balance

Hypernatremia, hyponatremia, or hypomagnesemia cause impairment of consciousness or frank seizures. Hyperkalemia or hypokalemia can cause cardiac dysrhythmias and may interfere with the cerebral circulation, particularly when associated with low cardiac output or cardiac failure. Osmotic pressure is usually calculated using the formula: ($Na^+ + K^+$ (in mEq) $\times$ 2 (for both cation and anion), e.g. (140 Na^+ + 4 K^+) $\times$ 2 = 288 mEq. If laboratory values for osmolarity show a higher value than the value calculated above, high glucose or blood urea nitrogen must be suspected, and their values must be examined. Normal Na^+ and K^+ maintenance is 55–70 mEq (1 mEq/kg in children) per day. Normal saline, which contains 154 mEq/L, is more than adequate for maintenance if 2400 mL/day is provided. However, the intake must be adjusted when cerebral edema occurs.

Blood Volume Management

Blood volume should remain normal (4.5–5.0 liters in adults). Blood loss should be replaced by an amount equal to or slightly less than the blood loss. When controlled hypotension is induced intraoperatively, slight hypovolemia may augment the beneficial effect of less AVM pulsation observed at the operative site. Occasionally, phlebotomy may be done immediately before surgery to decrease blood volume if the hematocrit is 39 or greater (or the hemoglobin is 13 or higher). The drawn blood can be transfused when blood loss occurs. The hemoglobin or hematocrit level is basically a good indication of blood volume if crystalloid infusion is appropriately adjusted for fluid maintenance. Generally, if blood loss is less than 800 mL in adults, extracellular fluid is transferred to the intravascular space and infused crystalloid fills in the extravascular space and compensates the blood loss.[2] However, if crystalloid is overloaded beyond the blood loss without increases in urinary output, the hemoglobin is diluted and its value may be misleading. For example, if crystalloid is overloaded by 1 liter and remains intravascularly, hemoglobin decreases by 2.5 g/dL. Diuresis is usually delayed for 24–36 hours and further overloading with blood or blood substitutes may cause hypervolemia or extracellular water accumulation. Hypervolemia may accentuate the bleeding tendency.

Because the blood flow to the brain is 20% of the total cardiac output, it can be postulated that the extracellular space of the brain would imbibe more water than that of other parts of the body, if the blood-brain barrier is impaired. Therefore, overloading of crystalloid should be avoided to prevent cerebral edema. On the other hand, low blood volume and underhydration tend to cause vasoconstriction associated with low flow and can result in ischemia, which is detrimental to cerebral function, especially in the region surrounding cerebral vessels adjacent to where thrombosis is propagating in the AVM. Transient neurological deficit or even permanent deficit may ensue. Blood volume can be evaluated by hemoglobin or hematocrit level, intake and output calculation, electrolytes, specific gravity of urine (concentrated or diluted), central venous pressures, or pulmonary artery wedge pressure. These are indirect means to evaluate blood volume. Body weight measurements allow for estimation of water volume changes in the intravascular space if extravascular fluid remains constant. Isotope studies with tagged blood cells for blood volume may be more accurate than other methods, but the complexity and expense of such studies reserve them for patients with multiple complications.

Electrolyte Balance

Along with fluid balance and blood volume adjustment, electrolytes must be tested periodically, especially after a large amount of blood loss and supplementation with blood or crystalloid. The normal levels of sodium (135–145 mEq/L) and potassium (3.5–4.5 mEq/L) must be maintained to prevent lethargy or seizures, and cardiac arrhythmias, respectively, particularly for patients with expected cerebral edema or hemorrhage and for patients with cardiac failure or atrial fibrillation.

Both sodium and potassium intake must be maintained at 1 mEq/kg/day, i.e., 55–75 mEq/kg/day for average adults. When the sodium level approaches or exceeds 150 mEq/L, 5% dextrose in one-half normal saline solution should be given; a 5% dextrose in water solution must be avoided, otherwise pontine myelinolysis may develop.

Inappropriate antidiuretic hormone syndrome or cerebral salt-wasting syndrome[7] is treated with water restriction, although the possibility of blood volume depletion must be kept in mind. Surgery of AVMs in the hypothalamic area may be associated with diabetes insipidus. It is the authors' routine to test specific gravity every 4 hours for at least a few days postoperatively until homeostasis is established.

Respiratory Regulation

The patient must be well oxygenated during and after AVM surgery. Oxygen saturation must be kept at 98%–100%. If it is lower than this level, the oxygen content steeply decreases following the dissociation curve of blood oxygen. Patients with chronic pulmonary disease must, however, be kept at their highest level, which can be attained by hyperventilation. After partial obliteration of AVMs with staged operations, it is the authors' routine to keep the patients intubated and maintained on mechanical ventilation. When the patient begins to awaken, breathes spontaneously, and cooperates in performing a voluntary effort of respiration, a weaning method may be used, e.g., the ventilation rate is decreased from 10 per minute to 8 and then to 6. The mechanical ventilation may be changed to continuous positive airway pressure and then to pressure support of 5 mm H_2O before the patient breathes independently.

In complicated cases, such as those with cerebral edema or postoperative cerebrovenous congestion, or in the cases of pulmonary disorders, the weaning procedures may be delayed. Systemic and cerebral oxygenation must be kept at an optimal level. From the authors' experimental work on oxidative metabolism with cytochrome *a,a*$_3$ measured by noninvasive reflectance spectrophotometry, oxidation of this enzyme continues to increase as PaO_2 increases and plateaus at 145 mm Hg in the brain.[10] To maximize energy production in the brain, PaO_2 must be kept at 145 mm Hg for maintaining the ion pump and action potentials of neurons at their maximum.

Postoperative Patient Positioning

The patient may be placed in the recumbent, horizontal, or slightly head-elevated (up to 15°) positions. Excessive head and neck flexion caused by a thick pillow underneath the head must be avoided, to maintain a free airway and jugular circulation.

When the patient is fully awake, the head side of the bed may be gradually elevated to 30°, then to 45°, and then to 60° before he/she is allowed to sit up. Straining, which can result in increased intracranial pressure, must be avoided in patients after a staged operation.

Summary

Postoperative care of a smoothly performed resection of a small or medium-sized AVM can be managed in a routine manner with blood pressure control, adequate fluid supplementation, and a balance of intake and output and electrolytes. Patients with a large or giant AVM who had one or more staged operations or surgery that was complicated with large intraoperative blood loss associated with postoperative cerebral edema, venous congestion, or a small hemorrhage that does not require surgical evacuation must be carefully treated with a combination of the abovementioned modes of management.

References

1. Fukusaki M, Maekawa T, Miyako M, et al. Acute haemodilution and prostaglandin E1-induced hypotension: effects on the coagulation-fibrinolysis system. Eur Anaesthesiol 14(4):443–449, 1997.
2. Marino PL. ICU Book. Philadelphia: Lea & Febiger, 1991.
3. Martin NA, Wilson JB. Preoperative and postoperative care: management of intracranial hemorrhage. In Wilson CB, Stein BM (eds): Intracranial Arteriovenous Malformations. Baltimore: Williams & Wilkins, 1984, pp 121–129.
4. McCouch G. Physiology. In Austin GM (ed): The Spinal Cord. New York: Igaku-Shoin, 1983, pp 73–91.
5. Olivecrona H, Ladenheim J. Congenital Arteriovenous Aneurysms of the Carotid and Vertebral Arterial Systems. Berlin: Springer-Verlag, 1957.
6. Strauss RG, Stansfield C, Henriksen RA, et al. Pentastarch may cause fewer effects on coagulation than hetastarch. Transfusion 28 (3):257–260, 1988.
7. Taylor SL, Tyrell JB, Wilson CB. Delayed onset of hyponatremia after transsphenoidal surgery for pituitary adenomas. Neurosurgery 37:649–654, 1995.
8. Yamada S. Arteriovenous malformations in the functional area: surgical treatment and regional cerebral blood flow. Neurol Res 4:283–322, 1982.
9. Yamada S, Brauer FS, Knierim DS. Direct approach to arteriovenous malformations in functional areas of a cerebral hemisphere. J Neurosurg 72:418–425, 1990.
10. Yamada S, Sanders D, Haugen G. Functional and metabolic responses of the spinal cord to anoxia and asphyxia. In Austin GM (ed): Contemporary Aspects of Cerebrovascular Disease, 1976. Dallas: Professional Information Library, 1976, pp 239–246.

Chapter 3

Blood Flow to Arteriovenous Malformations and the Brain, and Cerebral Metabolism

Introduction

The intricacy of the balance between blood flow into the arteriovenous malformation (AVM) and that into the brain tissue adjacent to and remote from the AVM has been the interest of clinicians and basic scientists for decades. The difficulties with blood flow studies were partly due to the lack of knowledge about the hemodynamic anatomy of AVMs. Because of a direct connection between arteries and veins in AVMs, preferential blood flow into the AVM compromises the circulation to the surrounding cerebral tissue (the so-called "steal" phenomenon). This situation poses a number of questions in regard to the autoregulation of cerebral blood flow (CBF) in patients with AVMs. The influence of not only the arterial phase on AVM pressure and blood flow, but also the influence of the venous phase must be considered for autoregulation mechanisms. This review discusses the preoperative and postoperative regional cerebral blood flow (rCBF) status in patients who underwent removal of their AVMs.

Arterial blood passes through shunting arterioles (50–250 μm) into the AVM core (or nidus) and then to the draining vein. Although this flow pattern is unidirectional, there is another venous system that connects the core and cerebral veins through communicating venules (20–200 μm).[18] These venules likely function as a cushion for the AVM core. Blood flow may be directed either from the core to the cerebral vein or vice versa, depending on the gradient between the core pressure and the cerebral vein pressure.

There are at least three mechanisms acting against free or passive conduit: (1) communicating venules; (2) cortical veins or draining veins constricted at their junctions to the sinus;[5] and (3) constriction of shunting arterioles. Draining veins and cortical veins connected to them contain arterial blood and have blood pressures higher than that in normal veins. Junctions of draining veins or dilated cortical veins to the sinuses are relatively constricted because these junctions are surrounded by nonelastic dura mater and are resistant to dilation (unlike cortical veins). This relative constriction of the junctions suppresses passive blood flow from the AVM to the sinus. Thus, the AVM core draining vein and dilated cortical veins act as a reservoir rather than as a passive or free conduit. Rupture of the AVM, which is a high-pressure reservoir, immediately causes pulsatile bleeding. Shunting arterioles have elastica and muscularis and are capable of constricting against pressure to some degree, particularly during hypotension.

Diversion of a large amount of blood from the cerebral arteries is called "blood steal" or "vascular steal,"[6] although to Malis[8] the term "steal" should be used only when blood flow is reversed from normal vessels into an abnormal vascular system.

Subclavian steal occurs when the subclavian artery is occluded proximal to the origin of the vertebral artery. Blood flow into the brachial artery is compensated by flow from the vertebral artery contralateral to the lesion. Subclavian syndrome, syncopal episode, or other brain stem signs occur when flow of the basilar artery is reversed while the patient is exerting muscle activity in the ipsilateral arm.[21]

From Yamada S (ed): *Arteriovenous Malformations in Functional Areas of the Brain.* © Futura Publishing Co, Inc, Armonk, NY, 1999.

Section 1

Regional Cerebral Blood Flow in Arteriovenous Malformation Patients

Shokei Yamada, MD, PhD, Russell R. Lonser, MD, and David Knierim, MD

The brain is dependent on the cerebral vasculature to supply it with adequate amounts of oxygen and substrates for proper metabolic and physiological functions. CBF is controlled by autoregulatory mechanisms that maintain a perfect balance between the arterial and the venous systems, and between oxygen and substrate supply and consumption.

Techniques of Blood Flow Studies

The authors utilized the xenon intravenous method to study CBF. This method is based on the Fick equation, as follows:

$$C = \frac{dc}{dt} = f(A(t) - C/\lambda$$

where C = concentration of ^{133}xenon in brain (mL/g),
t = time (minutes),
f = perfusion flow (mL/100 g/min),
λ = partition coefficient for xenon
$A(t)$ = concentration of ^{133}xenon in arteries as a function of time.

The term "F_1" is used throughout this chapter to describe the mean regional blood flow in the gray matter.

Shielded sodium iodide scintillation detectors were placed in four areas on both sides of the brain (frontal, parietal, temporal, and occipital) to continuously record the gamma radiation. Twenty to 30 millicuries of xenon were dissolved in 0.5 mL of normal saline and then injected into an arm vein.

The intake from the air sinuses was excluded from recording. An additional scintillation detector recorded the gamma radiation in the exposed air. The analysis of the head curves was done by generating an envelope of the expired air curve, *A(t)*, on a function generator and feeding this into each integrator. The amplitude of *A(t)* was varied according to the portion of the head curve being fitted, as follows:

Fick equation:

$$C_i + f_i/\lambda_i C = f_i A(t)$$

Intracarotid method:

$$C_i(t) = C_{oie}{}^{-kit};\ k_i = f_i/\lambda_i$$

Intravenous method:

$$C_i(t) = f_i \int_0^t A(\tau)e^{-k_i(t-\tau)}\,dt$$

The intravenous method requires a specific digital computerization to solve the clearance curve, in contrast to the arterial injection method, which negates the consideration of the recirculation of ^{133}xenon.[2]

Clinical Data

The study included 16 patients (5 males and 11 females) with AVMs located in the functional areas: sensorimotor area, 12 patients; the speech area, 1 patient; and the occipital area, 3 patients. Patient ages ranged from 14 to 53 years (average 34.1 years). The size of the AVMs ranged from 14.0 cm^3 (3.0 cm in diameter of the spherical AVM with the same volume) to 81.0 cm^3 (5.3 cm in diameter). Functional area AVMs were selected versus silent area AVMs so that possible correlation between neurological signs and symptoms and blood flow could be made.

In all cases, blood flow, F_1, was measured by the technique outlined previously, at 1–4 weeks before surgery, and at 2–8 weeks after surgery. The data from the gamma counters were converted to percentages based on the ratio:

$$\frac{F1 \text{ of patient}}{F_1 \text{ of normal individual of corresponding age}}$$

The F_1 percentages were then calculated for three areas:

1. F_1 in the area adjacent to the AVM (AVM area).
2. F_1 as an average of the three areas ipsilateral to the AVM.
3. F_1 as an average of the four areas contralateral to the AVM.

Calculations and Results

These results were summarized from a previous publication.[21]

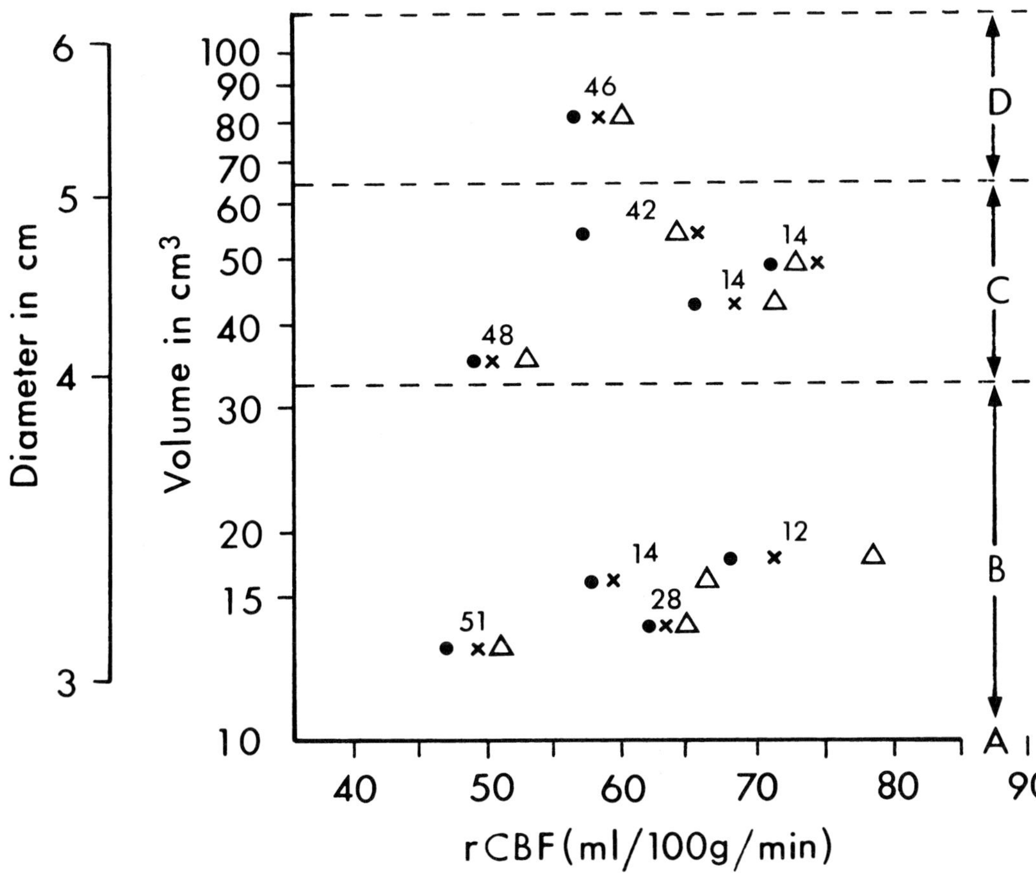

Figure 1A. The graph shows the relationship between AVM volume in the ordinate and rCBF in the abscissa (expressed by mL/100 g/min). rCBF is depicted by a dot for the area adjacent to the AVM, by an x for the ipsilateral hemisphere, and by a triangle for the contralateral hemisphere in each patient. As described in the text, rCBF is generally lower than the average for normal individuals (without AVMs). However, note the trend that the younger patients have rCBF higher than the older individuals regardless of AVM sizes. Each number at the top of a group of symbols indicates the age of the patient. *Continued.*

The mean values of the normal regional gray matter blood flow (F_1) are shown in Figure 1. The regional F_1 values for each patient were calculated in percentages relative to the normal values of the same age group (Figure 1A). To determine the statistical significance of the results, the authors selected nine patients who underwent both preoperative and postoperative blood flow studies. F_1 (rCBF) versus AVM volume were plotted in the graph (Figure 1B).

For the preoperative studies, mean values were as follows:

Adjacent to the AVM site:
81.8% ± 5.7%

In the ipsilateral region:
85.6% ± 7.6%

In the contralateral region:
89.1% ± 7.1%

For the postoperative studies mean values were as follows:

Adjacent to AVM site:
87.5% ± 6.5%

In the ipsilateral region:
87.7% ± 7.6%

In the contralateral region:
94.0% ± 8.3%

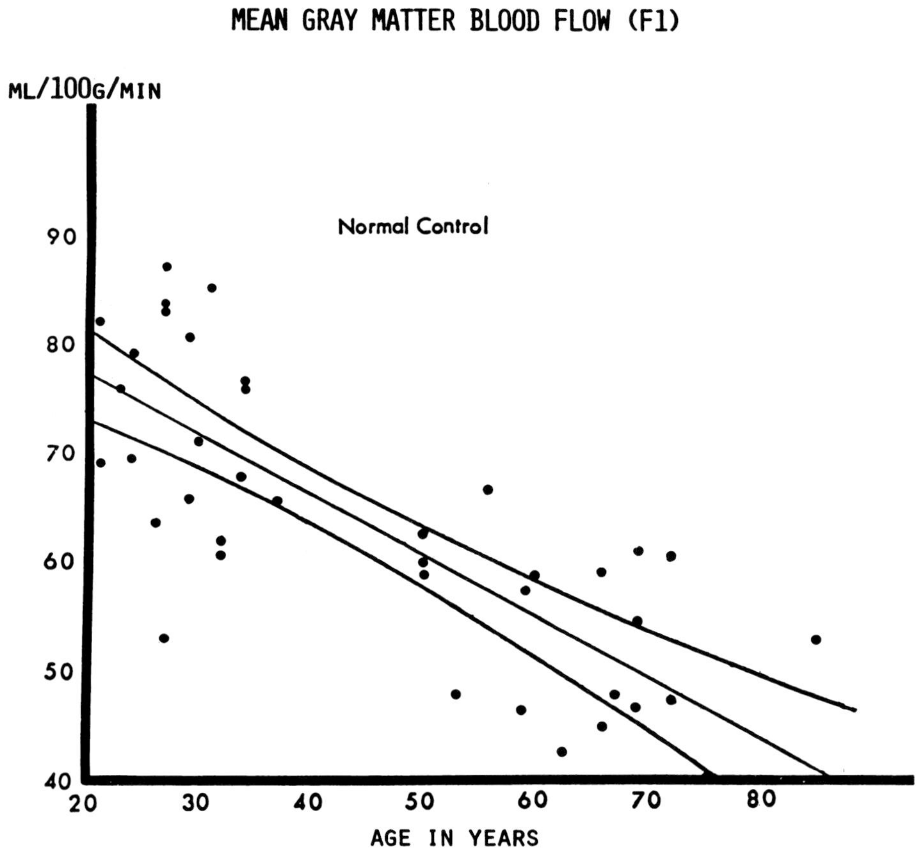

Figure 1B. Relationship between the rCBF and patient age in normal individuals.

There are some significant differences between the following groups:

1. Preoperative regional F_1 of the AVM area was less than that of the ipsilateral hemisphere (F value is 1%).
2. Preoperative mean F_1 of the ipsilateral hemisphere was less than that of the contralateral hemisphere (F value is 5%). Note that the mean F_1 value of the contralateral hemisphere was also less than normal value.
3. Postoperative regional F_1 of the AVM area was greater than that of the preoperative regional F_1 of the same area (F value is 1%).
4. Postoperative regional F_1 of the AVM area was still less than the postoperative F_1 of the contralateral hemisphere (F value is 1%).

Discussion

Preoperative regional F_1 was lower in patients with AVMs than in normal individuals. The decrease in the flow in the ipsilateral and contralateral hemispheres can be explained by arterial blood steal, as inferred from the blood flow through the AVM. The presence of preoperative hemorrhages, verified at operation, may support the concept that preoperative blood flow in the area adjacent to the AVM was markedly decreased, in comparison to the other areas, due to vasospasms secondary to hemorrhage.

These data also demonstrated that following removal of the AVM, there was an increase in F_1 toward normal levels. In addition, all 16 patients showed clinical improvement in their neurological function postoperatively.

In conclusion, several possibilities exist as the cause of neurological dysfunction: (1) low blood flow due to blood diversion into the AVM from the surrounding cerebral vessels; (2) compressive effects of the pulsatile AVM core against the surrounding brain; (3) hemorrhage around the AVM as a cause of brain compression; (4) vasospasms associated with hemorrhage; (5) cerebral edema with resultant compression and ischemia; and (6) cerebral venous thrombosis associated with that of AVM venous loops, which often follows AVM rupture; (7) increased intravenous pressure surrounding the AVM, secondary to blood flow from the AVM core to the surrounding cerebral veins through communicating venules.

From our rCBF studies, the brain receives adequate blood flow to maintain oxidative metabolism. An rCBF of 81%–89% of normal rarely reaches the penumbral level. Meyer et al.[10] studied blood flow around AVMs and reached a similar conclusion.

Section 2

Total Blood Flow to Arteriovenous Malformations

Shokei Yamada, MD, PhD, Brian Yamada, BA, and Lloyd Dayes, MD, PhD

Transcranial Doppler sonography, which is capable of measuring flow velocity, and the recent development of a computer model to measure middle cerebral artery blood flow,[1] enabled the authors to calculate the blood flow through each feeding artery and the total blood flow to the AVM. This section is a summary of a previously published article.[22]

Materials and Methods

Details of blood flow calculations have been previously published. Briefly, the equation, blood flow (mL/min) = A × FV × 60, was used to calculate flow velocity (cm/sec) on transcranial Doppler sonography ($A = \pi r^2$, where A is the area of the blood flow column and r is the internal radius of the artery). The radius of each artery was measured as previously mentioned.

Nine of the 10 patients (7 women and 3 men ranging in age from 20 to 47 years) in the study presented with focal, sensorimotor, or visual seizures characteristic of the lesions. The exception was one patient with an occipital AVM who had a history of subarachnoid and intracerebral hemorrhage, loss of consciousness, and partial visual field defect.

The three major (anterior, middle, and posterior) cerebral arteries were divided into three categories: (1) dominant feeding artery; (2) supportive feeding artery; and (3) nonfeeding artery. Any of these three major cerebral arteries may have branches that provide blood supply to the AVM. These major arteries were conventionally termed feeding arteries, although in a strict sense, their branches should be termed the feeding arteries.

The dominant feeding artery was determined by two factors: (1) angiographic demonstration of the fastest blood flow to the AVM, and (2) the greatest blood flow among these three arteries. The dominant feeding artery of a sensorimotor area AVM was always the middle cerebral artery, and the dominant feeding artery of a visual area AVM was either the posterior cerebral or the middle cerebral artery.

The supportive feeding arteries were also determined by angiography, which showed evidence of fast shunting to the AVM and a much greater blood flow than the normal blood flow (but slower than that in the dominant feeding artery). The supportive feeding arteries of a sensorimotor area AVM were the anterior cerebral arteries on the ipsilateral and contralateral sides, or the anterior cerebral arteries and the posterior cerebral artery on the ipsilateral side. Supportive feeders of a visual area AVM were either the posterior, middle, or anterior cerebral artery, or two or three of them. Nonfeeding arteries were those

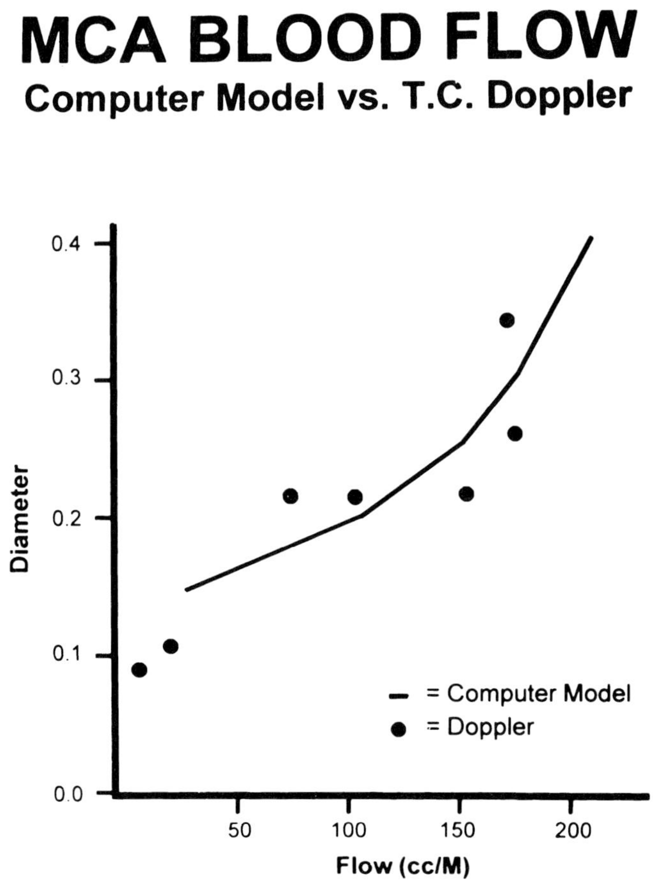

Figure 2A. Middle cerebral artery blood flow was plotted in relation to the diameter of each cerebral artery in normal individuals (shown with dots). The blood flow is represented in the ordinate and diameter in the abscissa. The curve represents the computer model blood flow of the middle cerebral arteries modified by Austin and Gaskell. *Continued.*

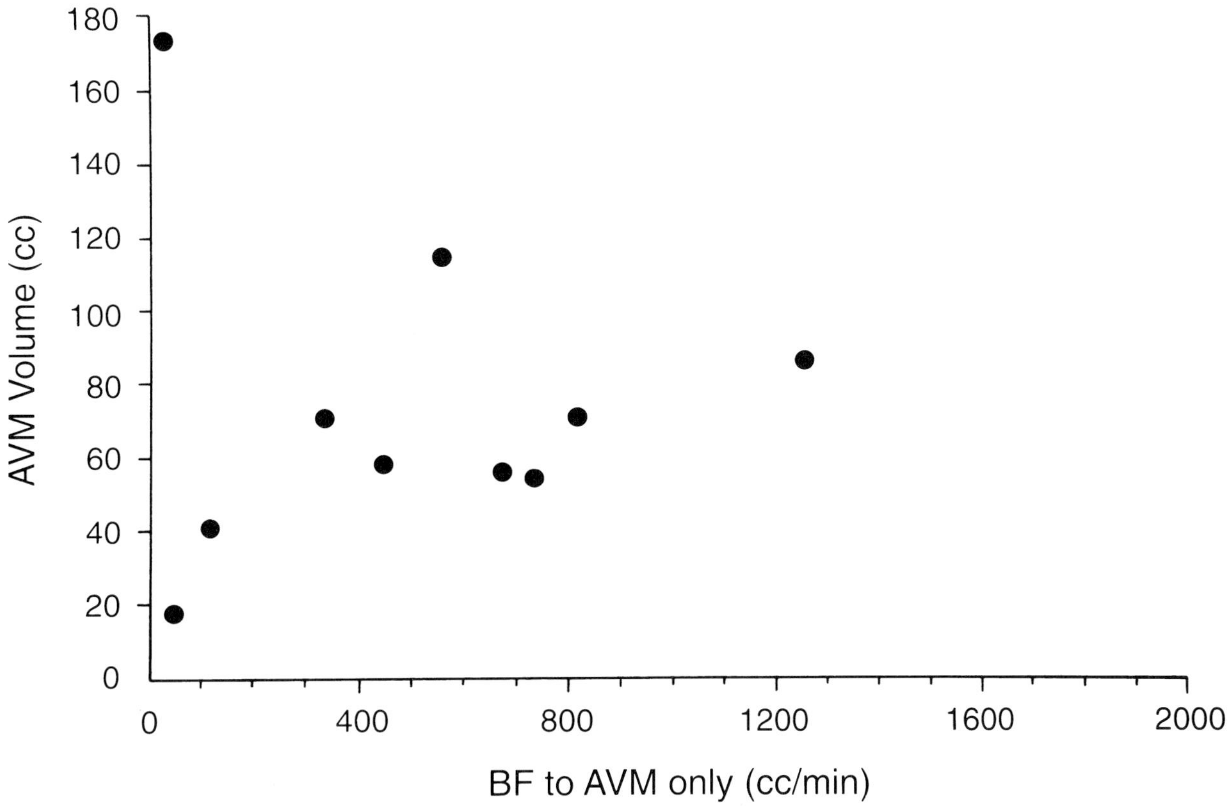

Figure 2B. The total blood flow through the AVMs in functional areas was plotted in the graph in relation to the AVM volume. The greater the AVM volume, the greater the AVM blood flow except in one case.

that failed to feed the AVM angiographically and whose blood flow was approximately at the level of normal blood flow.

Controls were obtained from patients who had an incidental aneurysm or small brain tumor that did not influence any angiographic blood flow pattern. Data obtained from these patients were comparable to the data calculated in the computer model of the middle cerebral artery by Austin and Gaskell.[1]

The blood flow from each of the feeding arteries to the AVM was calculated using the following equation: $BF_{AVM} = BF_{artery} - BF_{computer}$; where BF_{AVM} is the blood flow to each feeding artery in the AVM patient, BF_{artery} signifies blood flow through each feeding artery, and $BF_{computer}$ indicates the blood flow value of the computer model artery with the same diameter by interpolation in the blood flow curve shown in Figure 2A. The sum of the calculated blood flow of the feeding arteries was considered to be the total blood flow to the AVM.

Results

Based on the AVM location, the patients were divided into two groups: (1) a sensorimotor group – 6 cases, and (2) an occipital group – 4 cases. One of the six sensorimotor area AVM patients had bilateral AVMs (the left lesion being larger than the right) and was listed separately from the other five. The mean values of blood flow through the three types of arteries in the five patients with a sensorimotor area AVM are shown in Table 1.

The blood flow through the dominant feeding artery was three times that of the control group, and flow through the supportive feeding arteries was two times as much as the control flow. Blood flow

Table 1
Patients with AVMs in Sensorimotor Area (n = 6)
Blood Flow of Cerebral Arteries

	Dominant Feeding Arteries	*Supportive Feeding Arteries*	*Nonfeeding Arteries*
AVM	625 ± 282	347 ± 103	127 ± 86
Control	208 ± 20	160 ± 32	136 ± 46

AVM = arteriovenous malformation.

Table 2
Patients with AVMs in Occipital Area (n = 4)
Blood Flow of Cerebral Arteries

	Dominant Feeding Arteries	Supportive Feeding Arteries	Nonfeeding Arteries
AVM	338 ± 106	237 ± 74	116 ± 58
Control	176 ± 31	144 ± 45	128 ± 37

through nonfeeding arteries was lower than the control flow.

In four patients with a visual area AVM, the mean values of blood flow through the three types of arteries are shown in Table 2.

The blood flow through the dominant feeding arteries was two times that of the control group, and flow through the supportive feeding arteries was 1.6 times as much as the control flow. Blood flow through nonfeeding arteries was slightly lower than the control flow.

The total blood flow to the AVM was calculated as follows:

Four of these 6 patients with a sensorimotor area AVM had a mean total AVM blood flow of 831 ± 285 mL/min. Four patients with a visual area AVM had a total blood flow of 373 ± 122 mL/min. Total blood flow into the AVMs versus AVM volume was plotted in the graph (Figure 2B).

Discussion

Regulation of blood flow into AVMs and the surrounding cerebrovascular bed is controlled by complex mechanisms. In the normal circulatory system, blood pressure within normal arterioles falls from 65 to 40 mm Hg, and within capillaries from 40 to 20 mm Hg.[4,21] It is anticipated that the blood pressure of arterioles is exerted into the AVM venous loops, where blood pressure falls further toward the normal venous pressure (<5 mm Hg).[4,21]

The larger the total area of the shunting arterioles (commensurate with the size of the AVM), the faster the blood flow into the AVM core. In this study, blood flow into large AVMs (>5 cm in diameter) was occasionally in excess of 800 mL/min.[9,22] In normal adults, total blood flow into the brain can be approximated by the following equation: total blood flow = (carotid flow × 2) + (vertebral flow × 2), where the blood flow through one internal carotid artery is 280 mL/min and the blood flow through one vertebral artery is approximately 98 mL/min. Therefore, average total blood flow of the entire brain is 756 mL/min (G. Austin, personal communication). A person with a 1200-g brain will therefore have a perfusion flow of 64 mL/100 g/min. Thus, large AVMs in the sensorimotor area take up to 800 mL/min of arterial blood from the intracranial circulation, which is equivalent to the total blood flow of the entire brain. Although slightly less than normal, these data clearly indicate that blood flow through nutrient (cerebral) arteries is adequate to maintain metabolic function of the brain.

How then does the cerebrovascular tree adjust in order to obtain a compensatory blood flow for the brain? The cerebrovascular tree probably dilates at the arteriolar level, competing with shunting arterioles to gain preference for normal blood supply. Increased cardiac flow in giant AVMs may be a compensatory mechanism (S. Yamada, unpublished data, 1998). Collateral circulation through arteriolar or capillary connections from remote cerebral artery branches, including perforating arteries such as the lenticulostriate, anterior choroidal, and posterior choroidal arteries, into the area adjacent to the AVM may also play a role in compensatory blood flow.

Changes in the AVM core size and its pulsation were observed with controlled hypotension during surgery.[18] Angiographically, Pertuiset[13] observed a marked decrease in blood flow into the AVM during controlled hypotension, while the cerebral blood flow was maintained. This observation can be explained from the following data. Under normotension, the pressure gradient between the shunting arterioles (40–60 mm Hg systolic pressure) and capillaries (20–40 mm Hg)[4,18] is smaller than the gradient between the shunting arterioles and draining veins (<10 mm Hg).[11,12,15,18] This allows preferential blood flow to the AVM over the cerebrovascular tree. Under controlled hypotension (50 mm Hg mean systemic arterial pressure, i.e., two-thirds of normal), those pressure gradients become almost equal. This reduces preferential flow to the AVM.

Another factor that may contribute to reduced flow to the AVM is that the shunting arterioles have a muscular layer, which, although attenuated, may be more capable of contracting against hypotensive arterial pressure than against the full pressure exerted under normotension.[17,21]

Redox (reduction/oxidation ratio) studies by noninvasive in vivo reflectance spectrophotometry during controlled hypotension have shown small transitions to increased reduction in cytochrome a, a_3, without compromising adenosine 5'-diphosphate (ADP) phosphorylation and energy preservation.[19,20] This finding was supported by stable somatosensory evoked potentials during hypotension with mean systemic blood pressure lowered to 40 mm Hg.[20] These observations suggest that the brain surrounding the AVM can still receive adequate blood flow to maintain brain function in patients who show a normal life pattern except for having seizures. After removal of an AVM, however, redistribution of blood flow to the cerebrovascular bed becomes necessary.

Normal perfusion pressure breakthrough[3,15,16] has been reported after AVM resection. A pressure increase in the arteries supplying the previously ischemic area was considered to be the underlying mechanism of cerebral edema and hemorrhage as a complication of surgical obliteration of feeding vessels to the AVM. The authors have not encountered this so-called breakthrough phenomenon in their series.[17,18] The uniqueness of the authors' AVM resection technique includes interruption of only shunting arterioles and communicating venules (50–200 μm) directly connected to the venous loops of the AVM core. This permits appropriate circulatory redistribution of the cerebrovascular tree and prevents transient or permanent ischemia, which may be induced by clipping the feeding arteries demonstrated on angiography. Multistaged embolization or resection of large AVMs also allows stepwise adjustment of the cerebrovascular bed circulation.[7,13–15,17,18] Manchola's[9] data on the total blood flow into the AVM concur with the authors' previously published findings.

Section 3

Blood Flow to Feeding Arteries

Shokei Yamada, MD, PhD, and Shwan Kim, MD

In the previous section, total blood flow to AVMs 4–5 cm in diameter was calculated to be 800 mL/min. This flow equals the blood flow into the entire brain of normal individuals. In this section, the blood flow to the AVM feeding arteries was calculated preoperatively and compared with the blood flow through the same arteries after total resection of the AVM. Comparison of these flow values may elucidate some mechanisms of the redistribution of blood flow to the cerebrovascular bed, particularly those related to normal perfusion pressure breakthrough.

Materials and Methods

As described in the previous section, 10 patients (7 males and 3 females) with AVMs of different sizes (18–173 cm^3) were included in this study. The age of the patients ranged from 20 to 47 years. Locations of the AVMs were the sensorimotor area in 7 patients and the visual occipital area in 3 patients. The blood flow to each feeding artery was calculated as described in Section 2.

Results

Total blood flow through all of the feeding arteries was calculated in the manner described above. AVMs of >4 cm in diameter usually have more than three feeding arteries. The flow values and the AVM size are listed in Table 1, and blood flow into the feeding arteries versus AVM volume was plotted in graphs (Figures 3 and 4). A marked decrease in blood flow through a group of dominant and supportive feeding arteries in each patient was noted (each dot was shifted to the left as seen when Figure 3 and Figure 4 are compared).

AVMs of $\geq$40 cm^3 had extremely high blood flow, except in 1 case; there were 9 cases with large AVMs (>65 cm^3) and 1 case of a medium-sized AVM (>40 cm^3), and another case with a medium AVM (<40 cm^3). The flow volume seemed to correlate with the rapidity of angiographic demonstration of the AVM core and draining veins. In one case of a large AVM (172 cm^3), only a mild increase in blood flow was demonstrated (correlated with angiographic slow flow from the AVM core into the draining veins). In one case of a small AVM surrounded by a hematoma, the blood flow through the feeding arteries was slightly increased after AVM resection. A decrease in blood flow through the preoperatively feeding arteries after AVM resection indicates appropriate blood redistribution to the cerebrovascular bed.

Discussion

Large or giant AVMs have the increased risk of severe postoperative edema and bleeding; however, none of the authors' 10 cases had this type of complication. High volume blood flow through the AVM's feeding arteries corresponded angiographically with rapid flow into the AVM core (nidus) and draining veins. For this reason, early obliteration of draining veins in a large AVM could easily result in cerebral edema, partly due to congestion of the cerebral venous system that was connected to the major draining veins and partly to inadequate decreases in feeding artery blood flow after resection of the AVM. To minimize the postoperative cerebral normal perfusion pressure breakthrough, the blood flow to the feeding arteries to the ischemic brain surrounding large AVMs must be adjusted appropriately. To prevent normal perfusion pressure breakthrough, it is important to minimize overflow to the brain surrounding an AVM by: (1) interrupting shunting arterioles and communicating venules (50–200 μm); and (2) staged resection or staged embolization and resection to avoid congestion of the venous system around the AVM. The autoregulation in the cerebral arteries of the patients with cerebral AVMs, as mentioned in an earlier section, is maintained quite adequately. Appropriate redistribution of blood flow in the arterial branches to the brain after AVM resection can establish autoregulation with the cerebral metabolism greater than in the preoperative stage.

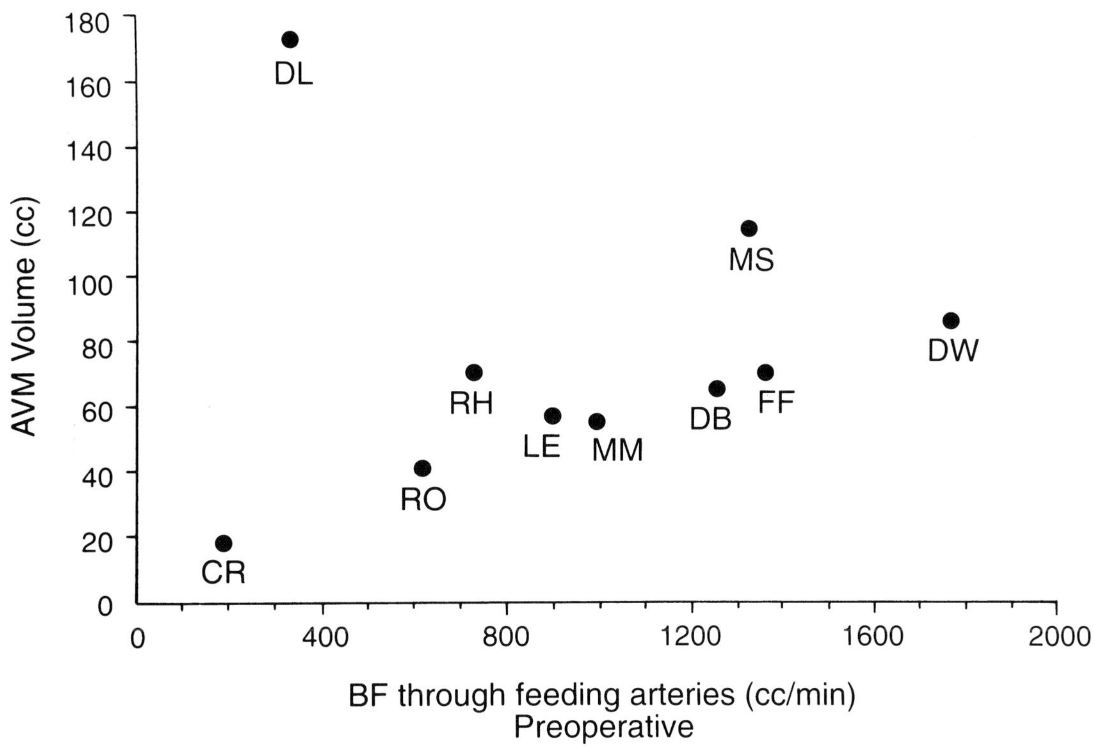

Figure 3. Preoperative blood flow through feeding arteries was plotted in relation to the AVM volume. The greater the AVM volume, the greater the feeding artery blood flow.

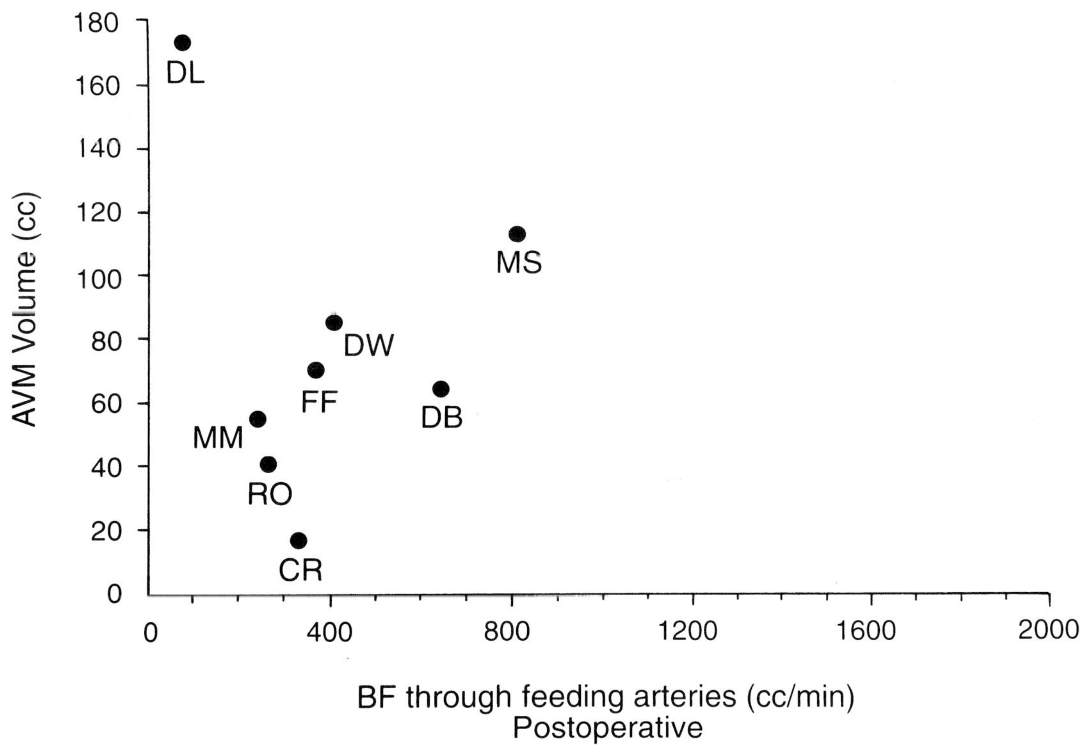

Figure 4. Blood flow through the preoperative feeding arteries after total AVM resection was plotted in relation to the AVM volume. A marked postoperative shift of the blood flow to the left was noted.

Section 4

Arteriovenous Malformation Blood Flow Correlated with Cerebral Perfusion of HM-PAO by SPECT

Shokei Yamada, MD, PhD, James B. Slater, PhD, and Jerry D. Slater, MD

Severe cerebral edema and hemorrhage after resection or embolization of larger AVMs has been explained by normal perfusion pressure breakthrough. Because normal perfusion pressure breakthrough was hypothesized to result from impairment of the blood-brain barrier (BBB) and additional increase in blood pressure and blood flow, the authors studied the uptake hexamethylpropyleneamine oxime (HM-PAO) using single photon emission computed tomography (SPECT) to evaluate blood flow and the BBB before AVM surgery. Large (>5 cm) and medium-sized (3–5 cm) AVMs were surrounded by a defect in HM-PAO uptake, indicating BBB impairment.

SPECT using HM-PAO (Ceretec) is useful for

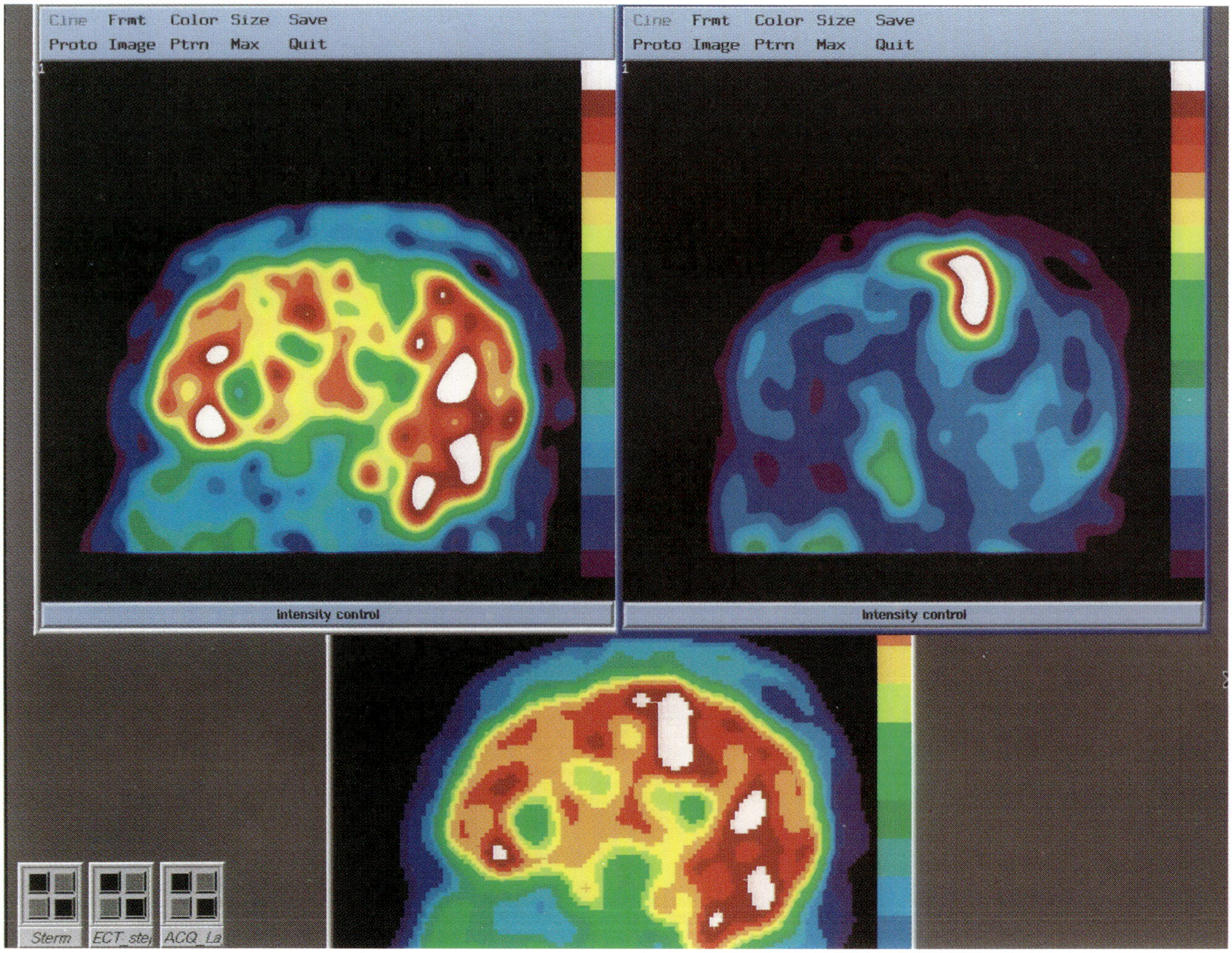

Figure 5A. *Upper right:* High Tc 99m RBC flow into the large AVM (78 mL) is indicated by the white area. *Upper left:* Marked decrease in Ceretec uptake is demonstrated in the AVM area and surrounding brain. Note that the Ceretec defect surrounds the AVM (outlined by the dotted lines), indicating BBB impairment in this area. *Bottom:* Tc 99m RBC flow and Ceretec are superimposed by computer imaging. *Continued.*

evaluating the BBB. This substance has unique features: (1) it is attracted to brain tissue because of its lipophilic nature; and (2) it is captured in the brain because of its rapid change to lipophilic chemicals outside the BBB.

The clearance rate of Ceretec from the blood compartment to the tissue signals rCBF under the assumption that Ceretec freely passes the BBB in any brain location.[1,3,6,7,9,10] This study tested the hypothesis that Ceretec passage through the BBB was impaired in the cerebral areas around an AVM.[2,4,6,8,9] Blood flow in the same areas was evaluated by measuring technetium(ta)-tagged red blood cells (RBCs)[11] simultaneously with the Ceretec uptake.[12]

Materials and Methods

Seventeen patients (3 males and 14 females) with AVMs received two injections: (1) Tc 99m-labeled Ceretec was injected prior to a SPECT scan; and (2) after the SPECT scan, Tc 99m RBCs were administered without moving the patient. A SPECT scan was taken and Ceretec-uptake defects were compared with RBC-uptake.

Results

Eight of 17 patients had large AVMs (>5 cm), 5 had medium-sized AVMs (3–5 cm), and 3 had small AVMs (<3 cm). Perfusion defects surrounded the entire circumference of the large AVMs (Figure 5A). Defects were also located posterosuperior to the medium AVMs, i.e., only on the peripheral side of the feeding arteries (Figure 5B). No defects were found around the small AVMs.

Discussion

Previous studies of rCBF or local CBF have shown the following: (1) rCBF in the brain adjacent

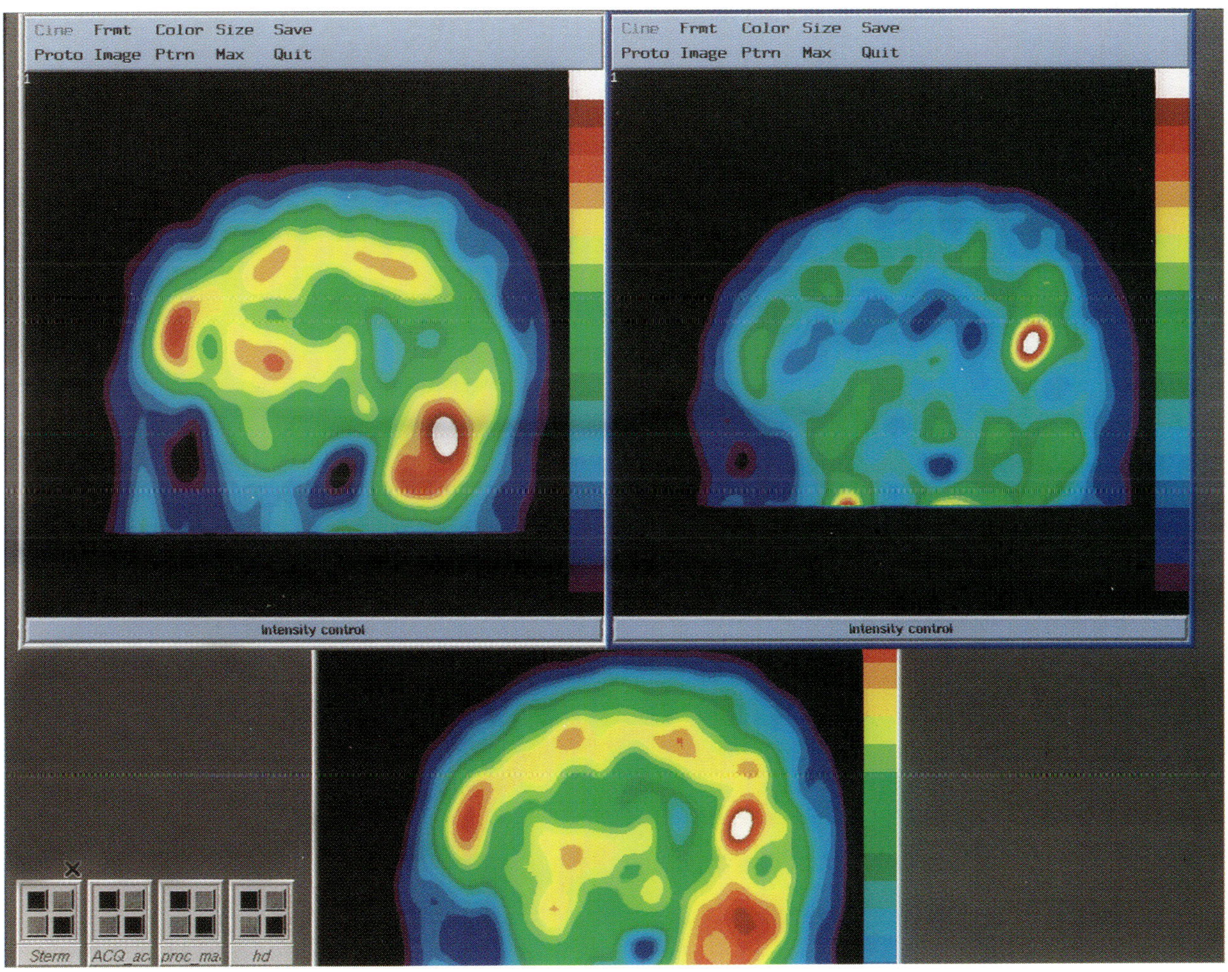

Figure 5B. RBC flow is shown in the upper right and Ceretec uptake on the upper left. Decreased Ceretec uptake is only located posterosuperior to the high RBC flow.

to the AVMs was 81.8% of normal; (2) rCBF in the ipsilateral hemisphere was 85.6% normal; and (3) rCBF in the contralateral hemisphere was 89.1% of normal.

The total blood flow to AVMs (>4 cm in diameter) was 800 mL/min,[13] which is equal to the blood flow to the entire brain in normal individuals. Our presentation of blood flow demonstrated by the SPECT studies with Tc 99m RBCs corresponded to the above-mentioned data. Despite such a large amount of steal in AVMs, cerebrovascular circulation is regulated to a reasonable degree to maintain adequate brain function in the majority of cases.

In the SPECT study, the authors conclude that there is significant BBB impairment in large AVMs, which is a potential source of postoperative normal perfusion pressure breakthrough. The perfusion defects may be attributed to low rCBF and the compressive effects of pulsatile AVM venous loops against the surrounding brain tissue. Kato et al.[5] also showed a defect in Ceretec uptake after AVM resection, and their results support our findings from the HM-PAO SPECT study. Since resection or embolization of AVMs further impairs the BBB, every effort must be taken to induce redistribution of the cerebral circulation and limit BBB impairment.

Section 5

Scanning Electron Microscopy of Arteriovenous Malformations

Shokei Yamada, MD, PhD, and Boleslaw Liwinicz, MD, PhD

AVMs are known to have direct communication between arteries and veins forming a cluster of anomalous vessels without intervening capillaries. However, schematic drawings failed to show the junctions of these arteries and veins clearly in the AVMs.[8] It was believed that an equal number of anomalous arteries and veins were entangled in the AVM. Hamby[1] was the first to schematically depict the transition between the arteries and veins, and to include spiral vessels in the AVM. Using microsurgery techniques, Yamada[5] described the exact points of junctions between the arterial and venous systems, and showed that the main portion of the cluster of anomalous vessels (the core) consists of venous loops (some of them having an arterialized wall).[3,6] Arterial blood is supplied through shunting arterioles (50–250 μm) or type 2 final feeding arteries (250–300 μm), and occasionally type 1 final feeding arteries, which are angiographically demonstrable in size. Another new finding was that communicating venules of 20–200 μm connect the AVM core and the surrounding cerebral veins.[2,6,7] The new observations are confirmed by SEM of AVM specimens that were preserved, including shunting arterioles and communicating venules in their natural configuration as they connect to the AVM loops.

Materials and Methods

During surgical dissection of the AVM, shunting arterioles and communicating venules were identified, cauterized, and sectioned using the surgical microscope. Endoscopy-assisted microsurgery was performed to confirm the identification of the shunting arterioles and communicating venules.

Six AVM specimens were examined by both light and scanning microscopy. A portion of the resected specimens was removed and fixed in formalin and studied with light microscopy to identify the presence of arterial and venous components. Another part of each specimen was cut into smaller pieces (5 mm in diameter) to undergo SEM.[4] Each piece was mounted on a polished aluminum peg with adhesive liquid (silver paint, silver paste, conductive epoxide, or saturated porlodion in amyl acetate). The surface of the specimen was cleansed by rinsing with an enzymatic solution. Shunting arterioles and communicating venules preserved during AVM dissection were identified using SEM and photographs were taken.

Results

Shunting arterioles (diameter 200 to 250 μm) were identified directly connected to the AVM core venous loops (Figure 6). The walls of these shunting arterioles were found to be 10% as thick as the diameter of the arterioles. Shunting arterioles of 50 to 100 μm were difficult to preserve at their junctions to the venous loops due to their small size and effects of shrinking by fixation. Shrinking of communicating venules that occurred during cauterization made it difficult to demonstrate the lumen of their sectioned ends at their connection to the venous loops of the AVM core. Additionally, many tributaries of these venules formed a venous plexus around the AVM loops.

Discussion

The complexity of AVMs was due partly to the lack of understanding as to where the junctions of arterial phase (efferent) and venous phase were. Yamada and associates have found that shunting arterioles are connected directly to the venous loops of the AVM core as the source of arterial blood, and that communicating venules connect the core loops and the surrounding cerebral veins.[5–7] They also noted that interruption of all shunting arterioles markedly reduced the AVM pulsation and changed the color of the draining veins from red to bluish red or blue. Although these small vessels were clearly identified with surgical microscopy and endoscopic-assisted microsurgery, histological demonstration was considered to be necessary to prove these surgical observations. The current SEM study has verified the connections of these arterioles and venules to the core vessels, and enhanced the understanding of the hemodynamic anatomy of the AVM.

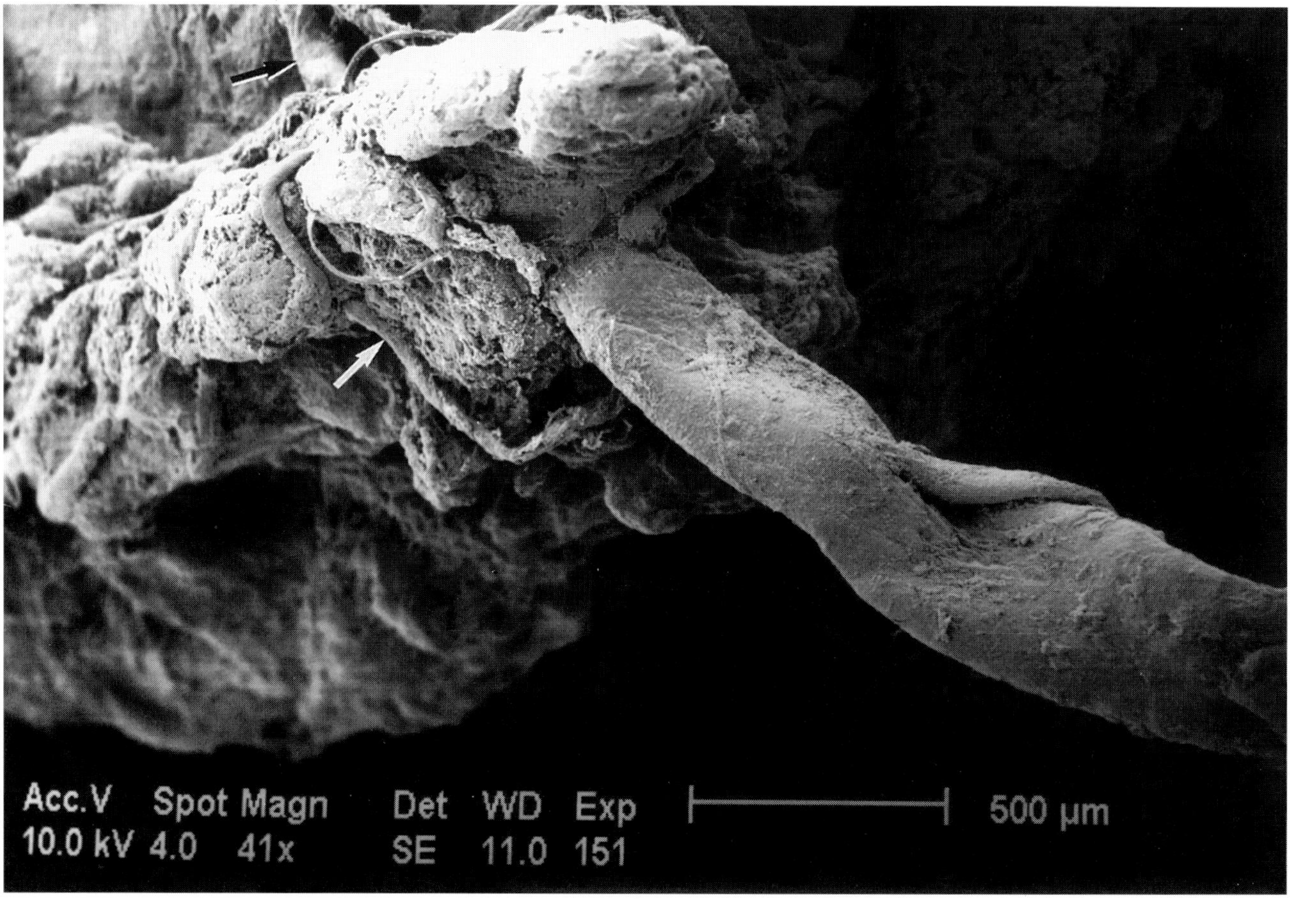

Figure 6. SEM of an AVM selectively demonstrates a shunting arteriole with 250 μm outer diameters and venules 20 μm (white arrow) and 50 μm (black arrow). The inner diameter of the arteriole was 225 μm.

References

Introduction and Sections 1, 2, 3: Blood Flow References

1. Austin GM, Gaskell R. Quantitative middle cerebral artery flow in normal and vasospastic artery. Neurol Res Suppl 14:192–196, 1992.
2. Austin GM, Hayward W, Laffin D. Modification of cerebral ischemia by microsurgical intracranial anastomosis. In Austin GM (ed): Microneurosurgical Anastomosis for Cerebral Ischemia. Springfield, IL: Charles C. Thomas, 1976, pp 327–338.
3. Awad IA, LeBlanc R, Little JR. Blood flow measurements in intracranial arteriovenous malformations. In Barrow DL (ed): Intracranial Vascular Malformations. Park Ridge, IL: American Association of Neurological Surgeons, 1990, pp 91–97.
4. Barron DH. The pressure gradient and pulse in the vascular system. In Ruch TC, Fulton JF (eds): Medical Physiology and Biophysics. Philadelphia: W.B.Saunders, 1980, pp 667–690.
5. Bederson JB. Pathophysiology and animal models of dural arteriovenous malformations. In Awad IA, Barrow DL: Dural Arteriovenous Malformations. Park Ridge, IL: American Association of Neurological Surgeons, 1993, pp 23–33.
6. Feindel W, Yamamoto L, Hodge C. Reversal of cerebral steal during surgery of arteriovenous malformations; evidence from fluorescein angiography and focal cortical blood flow measurement. Presented at annual meeting of American Association of Neurological Surgeons, paper #12, Toronto, Canada, 1977.
7. Hassler W, Steinmetz H, Gawlowski J. Cerebral hemodynamics in angioma patients: an intraoperative study. J Neurosurg 67:822–831, 1987.
8. Malis L. Arteriovenous malformations. In Youmans JR: Neurological Surgery, edition 2. Philadelphia: W.B. Saunders, 1982, pp 1786–1806.
9. Manchola IF, De Salles AAF, Foo TK, et al. Arteriovenous malformation hemodynamics: a transcranial Doppler study. Neurosurgery 33:556–562, 1993.
10. Meyer B, Schaller C, Fenkel, et al. Physiological steal around AVMs of the brain is not equivalent to cortical ischemia. Neurol Res 20:S13–S17, 1998.
11. Nornes H. Quantitation of altered hemodynamics. In Wilson CB, Stein BM: Intracranial Arteriovenous Malformations. Baltimore: Williams and Wilkins, 1984, pp 32–43.
12. Nornes H, Lundar T, Wikeby P. Cerebral arteriovenous malformations; results of microsurgical management. Acta Neurochir 50:243–257, 1978.
13. Pertuiset B. Ancri D, Sichez JP, et al. Radical surgery in cerebral AVM-Tactical procedures based upon hemodynamic factors. In Krayenbuhl H (ed): Advances and Technical Standards in Neurosurgery. Wien: Springer, 1983, Vol 10, pp 81–143.
14. Spetzler RF, Martin NA. A proposed grading system for arteriovenous malformations. J Neurosurg 65:476–483, 1986.
15. Spetzler RF, Martin NA, Carter LP, et al. Surgical management of large AVMs by staged embolization and operative excision. J Neurosurg 67:17–28, 1987.
16. Spetzler RF, Wilson CB, Weinstein P, et al. Normal perfusion pressure breakthrough theory. Clin Neurosurg 25:651–672, 1978.
17. Yamada S. Arteriovenous malformations in the functional area: Surgical treatment and regional cerebral blood flow. Neurol Res 4:283–322, 1982.
18. Yamada S, Brauer FS, Knierim DS. Direct intervention of arteriovenous malformations in functional areas of a cerebral hemisphere. J Neurosurg 72:418–425, 1990.
19. Yamada S, Brauer F, Knierim D, et al. Can somatosensory evoked potential monitoring predict energy dynamics during controlled hypotension. Neurol Res 14: 325–329, 1992.
20. Yamada S, Brauer F, Knierim D, et al. Safety limits of controlled hypotension in humans. Acta Neurochir Suppl 42:14–17, 1988.
21. Yamada S. Cojocaru T. Arteriovenous malformations. In Wood J (ed): Cerebral Blood Flow. New York: McGraw-Hill, 1987, pp 580–590.
22. Yamada S, Thio S, Iacono RP, et al. Total blood flow to arteriovenous malformation. Neurol Res 15:376–383, 1993.

Section 4: SPECT References

1. Anderson AR, Friberg HH, Schmidt, et al. Quantitative measurements of cerebral blood flow using SPECT and (99mTc)-d, I-HM-PAO compared to xenon-133. J Cereb Blood Flow Metab 8:569–581, 1988.
2. Devous MD Sr. Instrumentation , radiopharmaceuticals, and technical factors. In Ven Heertum RL, Tikofsky RS (eds): Cerebral SPECT Imaging. New York: Raven, 1989, pp 3–20.
3. Fujita H, Higano S. Linearization correction of 99mTc-labeled hexamethyl-propylene amine oxime (HM-PAO) image in terms of regional CBF distribution: Comparison to C15 O_2 inhalation steady-state method measured by positron emission tomography. J Cereb Blood Flow Metab 8:552–560, 1988.
4. Hayashida K, Nishimura T, Imakita S, et al. Filling out phenomenon with technetium 99m HM-PAO brain SPECT at the site of mild cerebral ischemia. J Nuclear Med 30:591–598, 1989.
5. Kato Y, Sano H, Nomomura K, et al. Normal perfusion pressure breakthrough syndrome in giant arteriovenous malformations. Neurol Res 19:117–123, 1997.
6. Lassen NA, Anderson AR, Frieberg L, et al. The retention of (99mTc)-d, 1 HM-PAO in the human brain after intracarotid bolus injection: A kinetic analysis. J Cereb Blood Flow Metab 8:513–522, 1988.
7. Lassen NA, Astrup J. Ischemic penumbra. In Wood JH (ed): Cerebral Blood Flow. New York: McGraw-Hill, 1987, pp 458–466.
8. Lassen NA, Blasberg RG. Technetium 99m-d, I-HM-PAO, the development of a new class of 99mTc-labeled tracer: an overview. J Cereb Blood Flow Metab 8:51–53, 1988.
9. Lear JL. Initial cerebral HM-PAO distribution compared to lCBF: Use of a model which considers cerebral HM-PAO trapping kinetics. J Cereb Blood Flow Metab 8:531–537, 1988.

10. Matsuda H, Oba H, Seki H, et al. Determination of flow and rate constants in a kinetic model of (99mTc) hexamethyl-propylene amine oxime in the human brain. J Cereb Blood Flow Metab 8:561–568, 1988.
11. Neirinckx RD, Burke JF, Harrison RC, et al. The retention mechanism of technetium 99M-Hm-PAO: intracellular reaction with glutathione. J Cereb Blood Flow Metab 8 Suppl 1:S4–S12,1988.
12. Yamada S, Slater JB, Iacono RP, et al. AVM blood flow correlated with cerebral perfusion of HM-PAO (Ceretec). Presented at annual meeting of the American Association of Neurological Surgeons, Orlando, April 22–27, 1995, pp 42–43, poster 1063.
13. Yamada S, Thio S, Iacono RP, et al. Total blood flow to arteriovenous malformations. Neurol Res 15:376–383, 1993.

Section 5: Scanning Electron Microscopy References

1. Hamby WB. The pathology of supratentorial angiomas. J Neurosurg 15:65–75, 1958.
2. Lonser R, Yamada S, Liwnicz B, et al. Scanning EM demonstration of shunting arterioles in arteriovenous malformations (AVMs). Presented at annual meeting of the Congress of Neurological Surgeons. poster #66. September 22–October 2, 1997, pp 282–283.
3. McCormick WF. Pathology of vascular malformations of the brain. In Wilson CB, Stein BM (eds): Intracranial arteriovenous malformations. Baltimore: Williams & Wilkins, 1984, pp 44–63.
4. Motta PM, Murakama T, Fujita H (eds). Scanning electron microscopy of vascular casts: methods and applications. Boston: Kluwer Academic Publishers, 1992.
5. Yamada S. Arteriovenous malformations in the functional area: surgical treatment and regional cerebral blood flow. Neurol Res 4:282–322, 1982.
6. Yamada S, Brauer FS, Knierim DS. Direct approach to arteriovenous malformations in functional areas of the cerebral hemisphere. J Neurosurg 72: 418–425, 1990.
7. Yamada S, Brauer F, Iacono RP. Surgical importance of venous channels in arteriovenous malformations. In Hakuba A (ed): Surgery of the Intracranial Venous Syatem. Yokya: Springer, 1996, pp 499–505.
8. Yasargil MG. Microneurosurgery, Vol IIIA. AVM of the Brain, History, Embryology, Pathological Considerations, Hemodynamics, Diagnostic Studies, Microsurgical Anatomy. New York: Thieme, 1993, pp 376–383.

Chapter 4

Anesthesia Requirements for Arteriovenous Malformations in Functional Areas of the Brain

Floyd S. Brauer, MD

Introduction

Surgery for arteriovenous malformations (AVMs) located in functional areas of the brain has recently become practical with the advent of careful microscopic approaches that interrupt only communicating venules and shunting arterioles of less than 200 μm in diameter. This technique for resection of large AVMs usually requires staged surgical approaches with deliberate hypotension, but has almost eliminated the problem of normal perfusion pressure breakthrough and permanent neurological deficit.

The anatomy and physiology of functional AVMs (discussed elsewhere in this book) dictate an anesthetic approach that will allow the surgeon to approach the AVM microscopically with vision unobstructed by bleeding and with subdued pulsatile movement in the vessels of the AVM itself. Thus, the basic requirements are:

1. A perfectly still patient.
2. The avoidance of hypertensive spikes.
3. Deliberate hypotension as required by the surgeon.
4. Careful positioning and padding in view of prolonged procedures.
5. Careful monitoring.
6. The ability either to awaken the patient smoothly and rapidly for immediate neurological monitoring, or provision for prolonged postoperative anesthesia with blood pressure control and artificial ventilation.

The majority of patients presenting for AVM surgery have had minimal initial hemorrhage and thus present at surgery without the usual intracranial mass problems seen with cerebral tumors and massive intracranial hemorrhage. Intracranial pressure is not usually elevated, nor are there major neurological deficits. The patients are essentially neurologically intact. The primary anesthesia objective is providing the surgeon with optimal operating conditions. This usually translates into control of even minor amounts of bleeding, which obliterate exposure in a microscopic field. Measures to control intracranial pressure are usually not needed.

Premedication

The primary goal of premedication is relief of anxiety. These patients have more than average presurgical anxiety. They have been seen and referred by several doctors, including the neurosurgeon. They have had various radiological studies including CT scan and/or magnetic resonance imaging. They have had extended discussions of the risks and benefits of the surgery versus no surgery. Therefore, they come to the operating room very apprehensive and often hypertensive. Oral midazolam (0.5 mg/kg) in syrup or coke is very helpful in children. In adults, intramuscular midazolam is given on the ward. The calming effect that midazolam produces is appreciated by patient, family, neurosurgeon, and anesthesiologist, and it affords a smoother induction. However, in

From Yamada S (ed): *Arteriovenous Malformations in Functional Areas of the Brain.* © Futura Publishing Co, Inc, Armonk, NY, 1999.

some adults, if very good rapport has been established, and the patient objects to premedication, all premedicants may be titrated intravenously as soon as the patient arrives in the operating theater. While not usually given on the ward, analgesia is provided by titrated small boluses of fentanyl intravenously after the patient arrives in the operating theater. Analgesics titrated to a slowed respiratory rate of 10–12/min prior to insertion of the arterial line are prophylactic against hypertensive spikes. An arterial catheter is routinely placed prior to induction of anesthesia and endotracheal intubation. Inasmuch as these patients usually do not have increased intracranial pressure, very adequate premedication is safe.

Induction Agents

Thiopental

Thiopental has for many years been the standard agent used to induce neuroanesthesia. The barbiturates afford a pleasant induction for the patient. They also lower $CMR0_2$ and CBF in a dose-dependent manner that is especially helpful if an increase in intracranial pressure does exist. Thiopental is usually given slowly in increased amounts above average doses of 4–6 mg/kg to doses of 6–8 mg/kg of body weight.

Propofol

Propofol produces effects on $CMR0_2$ and CBF that are very similar to those of thiopental. The reduction in mean arterial pressure (MAP) may even be greater than with thiopental, which is beneficial in selected cases. Care must be taken to obtund the irritation effect in small veins that produces pain. Intravenous alfentanil or lidocaine immediately prior to the propofol is usually efficacious.

Etomidate

Etomidate has been popular in cardiac surgery and has been recommended as an induction agent for neurosurgery in patients having significant cardiac disease. It often produces movement, however, and we have found it is rarely indicated.

Any one of the induction agents described above (thiopental, propofol, etomidate) is suitable for induction of anesthesia for an AVM, but we favor thiopental. With titration of IV fentanyl prior to induction of anesthesia, placement of an intra-arterial catheter can be accomplished in an awake patient without undue anxiety or pressor response if local anesthesia around the vessel is accomplished. The use of a somewhat larger than average dose of induction agents results in good control of the hypertensive response often seen with endotracheal intubation. Intubation should not be rushed. The goal is to prevent any hypertensive spikes in MAP. A period of 5–7 minutes prior to intubation with administration of additional fentanyl and/or volatile anesthetic agent (isoflurane) will almost always accomplish this. In a patient particularly at risk for aspiration, continuous cricoid pressure by an assistant during this time should be applied at a level of 40 newtons.[1–3]

Anesthetic Management

Monitoring

All patients have the following monitors: urinary output, peak airway pressure, ECG with a modified VS technique, intra-arterial blood pressure with arterial blood gases as indicated, central venous pressure, pulse oximeter, capnograph, and esophageal temperature. We use somatosensory evoked potentials to monitor the cerebral effects of hypotension or brain retraction.

In selected cases we add a pulmonary artery catheter, oxidative metabolic studies, and cerebral flow probes. Following induction and intubation, one must be alert to sympathetic stimulating procedures such as positioning head pin placement, skin incision, and use of electrosurgery in scalp muscle. Often additional increments of fentanyl are administered just prior to these events.

Positioning

All of our surgeries have been performed in the recumbent position using the supine, prone, or lateral positions, depending on the location of the AVM. We have found that these positions offer adequate exposure and have not noticed increased bleeding due to positioning. The sitting position in neurosurgery is controversial. Its touted benefits are primarily for the surgeon (less bleeding and a more relaxed brain). These side benefits do not appear to be significant in AVM surgery with the possible exception of a patient who has had a rather massive bleed preoperatively. The chief disadvantage of the sitting position is that of air embolism, which at times can be very significant. Reports from the Mayo Clinic and others have shown that with adequate monitoring, the sitting position does seem to be safe if venous air embolism can be detected early and a means is in place to remove air.[4,5] However, from our experience, we, like some others, strongly encourage the use of the recumbent position.[6]

Anesthesia Maintenance

Several techniques of maintenance are acceptable. We have found that isoflurane and oxygen with moderate hyperventilation produce good operating conditions. With the administration of midazolam and fentanyl for insertion of the arterial line, then additional fentanyl to a total of 6–8 μg/k prior to intubation, and an additional 100–200 μg just prior to insertion of head pins or scalp electrocautery, protection from hypertensive episodes in the early part of the surgery is assured. Additional fentanyl is usually not administered for maintenance, as stimulation once the brain is exposed is minimal. Isoflurane in air-O_2 provides good maintenance conditions. Prevention of movement during the microscopic parts of the procedure is achieved with cisatracurium 0.15 mg/kg for intubation followed by an infusion of 1–2 mcg/kg/min throughout the procedure. A low-dose cisatracurium infusion usually preserves four twitches with a twitch monitor after the intubating dose has dissipated. Isoflurane at 1.5% with hyperventilation and this low-dose atracurium infusion has prevented coughing or bucking during maintenance despite four twitches. In a minority of AVM patients, the procedure can be accomplished in one stage. In this situation, the AVM, even though in the functional area, is small and there has been little bleeding during the procedure. In these cases, the surgeon will want the patient to awaken smoothly and fairly quickly without bucking or coughing, because an awake patient is the best neurological monitor. This smooth awakening can be accomplished by stopping the atracurium infusion and tapering off the isoflurane, allowing the patient to resume spontaneous respiration. The fentanyl will still have some desired analgesic effect but no reversal of the opioid or the muscle relaxant is needed. Usually, however, the complete extirpation of a large AVM in the functional area requires several stages of surgery separated by 2–3 months intervals. In these patients, we reload the patient with fentanyl and a long-acting muscle relaxant and they are sent to a neurosurgical critical care unit on the ventilator with continuous monitoring of blood pressure.

Other factors of importance during the maintenance period are fluid administration, hypothermia, and controlled hypotension.

Fluid Administration

Only full-strength polyionic salt solutions are administered during AVM surgery, as is customary for all intracranial procedures. The primary difference in fluid administration is quantity. During AVM surgery, normally calculated fluid administration tends to cause hemodilution, which decreases the ability of platelets and RBCs to aggregate and close off small punctures, thereby creating increased blood loss. This blood loss, albeit small, interferes with microscopic exposure. Therefore, fluid administration is restricted to approximately 100–125 mL/hr. If major blood loss is incurred, we have found it helpful in obtaining hemostasis to not administer fluids or blood during the acute period of loss. Rapid administration of blood or fluids enlarge the vessels in the AVM, causing increased pulsation with increased blood loss. When the surgeon achieves hemostasis, transfusion can begin with the blood being given slowly unless it is a dire emergency. Blood transfusion is not administered if hemoglobin remains more than 10 g/L. In acute bleeding, blood loss is often utilized as an adjunct method of obtaining hypotension.

We do not use blood expanders of any kind because they all tend to interfere with platelet function. In the vast majority of cases, blood loss is not significant from a hemodynamic standpoint, but it is troublesome from an operative point of view.

As far as urinary output is concerned, we feel that any urinary output above 20 mL/hr is adequate. With our rule of thumb, to infuse full-strength polyionic salt solutions at a rate of approximately 100 cc/hr, we have not had problems with renal insufficiency following these procedures.

Hypothermia

Mild hypothermia practically always occurs during the first 30–45 minutes of the case, with core temperature dropping from approximately 37°C to 34°–35°. This is considered beneficial as it reduces metabolic activity, thus affording additional brain protection. With draping, no further heat loss is seen. Deep hypothermia is not used for these patients.

Controlled Hypotension

Regarding the history of hypotension for neurovascular surgery, in the past it was almost universally practiced. In recent years it has fallen into more disuse in cerebral aneurysms with the development of temporary clipping of feeding vessels and with the concern regarding organ damage from hypotension. However, in AVM surgery, hypotension often means the difference between success and failure due to the fact that pulsation in the AVM itself interferes with successful AVM surgery and this pulsation can be reduced significantly through the use of hypotension.

Controlled hypotension has been the keystone adjutant to anesthesia and surgery of AVMs in the functional area. The goals of controlled hypotension are:

1. Reduction of pulsation in the vessels of the AVM.
2. Prevention from rupture of the vessels in the AVM.
3. Minimize microscopic blood loss during surgery to preserve exposure.

A MAP of approximately 60–70 mm Hg is considered ideal for most of the surgical procedure. During a certain period of time as dissection is being carried out on feeding arterioles, the MAP is reduced to approximately 50 mm Hg. Should a vessel rupture or become loose, MAP has been reduced to 40 mm Hg for short periods of time until control can be obtained. In order to assure ourselves that the lowering of MAP to these levels was safe, somatosensory evoked potentials (SSEP) along with oxidative metabolic studies were used extensively. These oxidative metabolic studies (mitochondrial oxygenation) are described elsewhere by Yamada. Findings have been that both studies show parallel degradation at certain critical MAP levels that vary slightly with each patient. Because of the agreement in these studies, oxidative metabolism studies are not now routine. Each patient serves as his own control. However, in general, no patient has shown degradation in either SSEP or oxidative metabolism in critical brain areas at a MAP in excess of 50 torr. This is true even if the patient has a history of chronic hypertension. The vast majority of patients will tolerate for short periods of time (10–15 minutes) a mean pressure of 40 torr. With major blood loss in three of our patients, blood pressures of 30 torr for a period of approximately 5–10 minutes produced no postoperative neurological deficit or perioperative myocardial infarction, in spite of the fact that there was some degradation of the oxidative metabolic studies during this period of time.

Agents used to achieve controlled hypotension during neurosurgery have ranged from arfonad to nitroglycerine to nitroprusside to beta blockers. We have not used arfonad due to its tendency to tachyphylaxis and ganglionic blockade. Nitroglycerine (tridil) has proven to be difficult to titrate to predetermined MAP levels and maintain these levels. Beta blockers have produced somewhat inconsistent results and, again, are very difficult to maintain a specific desired pressure. Sodium nitroprusside administered by infusion pump has provided the degree of accuracy and safety that is needed. With a steady state of isoflurane anesthesia, nitroprusside has routinely produced the desired levels of hypotension in levels far below that needed to produce cyanide toxicity. Levels have been low enough to avoid any significant problems with pulmonary shunting. We have been able to achieve predetermined levels of pressure (40–60 torr) by an infusion of less than 1 μg/kg/min. Even at infusions at this rate, it is best to monitor arterial pH after the first hour. The cerebral vasodilating effects of nitroprusside have not been clinically significant in our practice. We have lowered the blood pressure gradually early in the case with other agents, such as the isoflurane, fentanyl, and small doses of labetalol. Then fine-tuning is done with the sodium nitroprusside infusion. The mechanism of action for both nitroprusside and nitroglycerin is thought to be vasodilatation produced by nitric oxide, which activates the enzyme, guanylatecyclase, which in turn results in increased concentrations of cyclic GMP in the vascular smooth muscle, which causes the vasodilatation of veins and arteries.

The major breakthrough in mortality and morbidity in surgery for AVMs in the functional areas of the brain has occurred as a result of interrupting only communicating venules and shunting arterioles of less than 200 μm in diameter. This has almost completely eliminated the problem of hyperemia and edema of the brain postsurgically, which has been labeled normal perfusion pressure breakthrough. We believe that staging of the operation allows the brain to compensate for the redistribution of cerebral blood flow. Blood flow through a large AVM may approach or exceed the total normal cerebral blood flow due to the low resistance in the AVM. If this blood flow is diverted suddenly, the brain has a difficult time in adjusting to this major disruption in blood flow. Marked hyperemia and edema are the result. We have not seen this complication in over 250 cases. Should normal perfusion breakthrough occur, the treatment of choice is hypervolemia, hypertension, hemodilution (Triple H) therapy,[7,8] providing bleeding does not complicate the picture.

References

1. Vanner RG. Mechanisms of regurgitation and its prevention with cricoid pressure. Int J Obstet Anesth 2:207, 1993.
2. Vanner RG, O'Dwyer JP, Pryle BJ, et al. Upper esophageal sphincter pressure and the effect of cricoid pressure. Anaesthesia 47:95, 1992.
3. Vanner RG, et al. Upper aesophageal sphincter pressure and the intravenous induction of anaesthesia. Anaesthesia 47:371, 1992.
4. Matjasko MJ, et al. Anesthesia and surgery in the seated position: Analysis of 554 cases. Neurosurgery 17:695, 1985.
5. Black S. et al. Outcome following posterior fossa craniectomy in patients in the sitting or horizontal position. Anesthesiology 69:48, 1988.
6. Standefer M, et al. The sitting position in neurosurgery: A retrospective analysis of 488 cases. Neurosurgery 14: 649, 1984.
7. Awad IA, Carter LP, Spetzeler RF, et al. Clinical vasospasm after subarachnoid hemorrhage: Response to hypervolemic hemodilution and arterial hypertension. Stroke 18:365–372, 1987.
8. Solomon RA, Fink ME, Lennihan L. Early aneurysm surgery and prophylactic hypervolemic hypertensive therapy for the treatment of aneurysmal subarachnoid hemorrhage. Neurosurgery 23:699–704, 1988.

Chapter 5

Arteriovenous Malformations in Functional Areas

John P. Girvin, MD, PhD

History

The initiation of neurosurgical attempts to treat arteriovenous malformations (AVMs) of the brain began in the middle of the 20th century. In the light of present-day knowledge, these attempts were inadequate. At this time AVMs were considered by many to be solid tumors that were simply vascular in nature. Some of the initial surgery was aimed at occluding the major feeding arteries to these "vascular tumors." These surgical approaches were bold and commendable when first conceived and of cours their failure to provide any reasonable treatment is now well recognized. There has been an evolution since that time in the treatment of AVMs, primarily because of the marked improvement in angiography, the understanding of their pathophysiology, and the response, or lack of response, to various types of treatment. Up until the 1970s, most medium or large AVMs, i.e., those greater than 3 or 4 cm in size, were considered to be inoperable if they were located in eloquent functional cortical areas such as the speech area or the central sensorimotor area. Hereafter, such AVMs will be referred to as "eloquent AVMs" or AVMs in "eloquent cortex."

Most of the early reports in the literature on cerebral AVMs were either anecdotal in nature or they consisted of highly selected groups of cases. Many contained no reference to eloquent area AVMs. Frequently this was because such AVMs were not considered operable. Thus, the literature has not provided much direction for the contemporary surgeon in management schemes of such AVMs.

The discipline of interventional neuroradiology arose out of attempts, often by surgeons, of embolizing AVMs. Many of these were rather ingenious innovations at the time, although at the present time, they pale by comparison to the tremendously sophisticated endovascular technology that has developed subsequently. In London, Ontario, we had the advantage of the expertise of Dr. Gerard Debrun. He brought to London the cutting edge of the expertise of balloon embolization—the basis upon which the present discipline of interventional neuroradiology, or endovascular therapy, was founded. He left London but not without leaving a legacy of a strong interventional group whose publications and reports speak for themselves.

In the early and middle 1970s, Drs. Fox and Vinuela were attempting to occlude AVMs with the advancing technology of the time. This was carried out by catheters through the transfemoral route. Two patients in a large series had near complete embolizations of their AVMs and when repeat angiography was carried out some months later, it had been found that the remaining AVM had spontaneously thrombosed over that period of time. Figure 1A is a preoperative angiogram of one of the patients. Figure 1B discloses the remaining AVM 1 week following intraoperative embolization. Figure 1C is the angiogram 6 months later, demonstrating spontaneous disappearance of the remaining AVM during the intervening 6 months. This was interpreted as resulting from spontaneous thrombosis caused by a "reaction" to the embolizing glue, isobutyl cyanoacrylate (IBCA).

Based on the enthusiasm generated by the foregoing two cases along with the very prevalent practice in London of operating upon patients under local anesthesia, a group of the so-called large central "in-

From Yamada S (ed): *Arteriovenous Malformations in Functional Areas of the Brain.* © Futura Publishing Co, Inc, Armonk, NY, 1999.

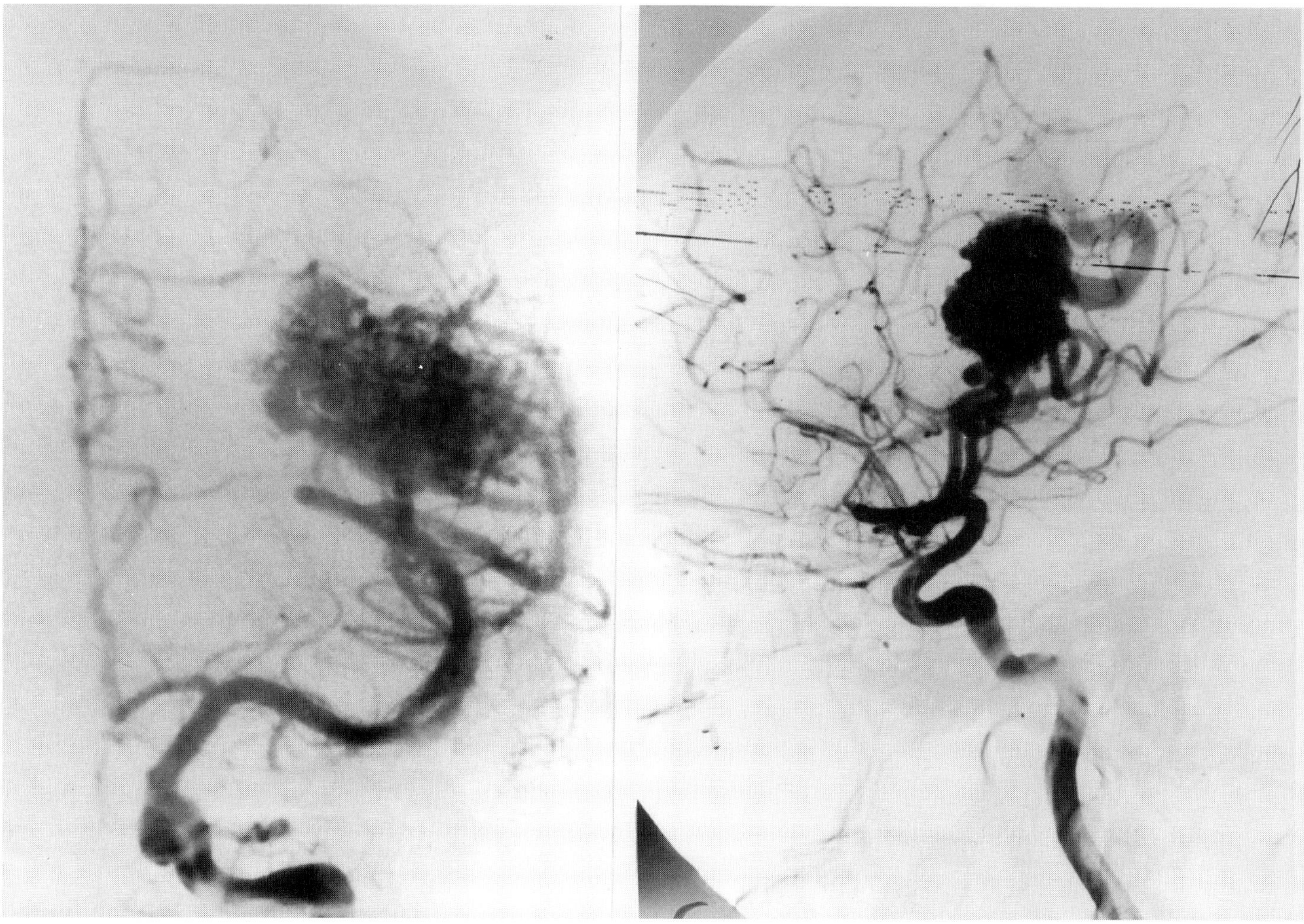

Figure 1. Angiograms of a 37-year-old housewife who presented with simple partial motor seizures, affecting her lower right face, and dysphasia, later going on to secondary generalization. **A.** Pre-embolization angiograms disclosing an AVM in the left central, suprasylvian region. *Continued*

operable" AVMs were treated by multivessel occlusion intraoperatively. Over the ensuing 2 or 3 years, 14 or 15 patients were operated on, with their feeding vessels identified, cannulated, and then using the best superselective angiography of the day, embolized with IBCA.[7] In this group of patients, the best estimates were that somewhere between 75% and 95% of the nidus of AVM had been obliterated in each. It was hoped at this time that two objectives might be realized. First, as already noted, it was eagerly anticipated that some of these patients would go on to disclose completion of the obliteration of the AVM by spontaneous thrombosis. Second, it was hoped that the obliteration of the majority of the AVM would lead to some protection from recurrent hemorrhage, although certainly we were very guarded in our thoughts in this regard.

Some very difficult lessons were learned from this initial series of patients. By the end of 2 or 3 years, this whole group had postoperative angiography. In not one patient was there any clear-cut evidence of obliteration of the AVM with the passage of time. In some cases there appeared to be some further reduction of the nidus; in others there was an increase. The same was true for flow through the AVMs. Thus, it became obvious that our initial enthusiasm and optimism regarding the spontaneous obliteration of the remaining AVM in such patients was unjustified. Perhaps more predictable, but every bit as lamentable, was the fact that these individuals also appear to have gained nothing from the point of view of protection against recurrent bleeding. At least three of the patients have re-bled and one has died in the intervening 8 years. Thus, as with incomplete surgical obliteration,[1] similarly there would appear to be no protection with incomplete endovascular oc-

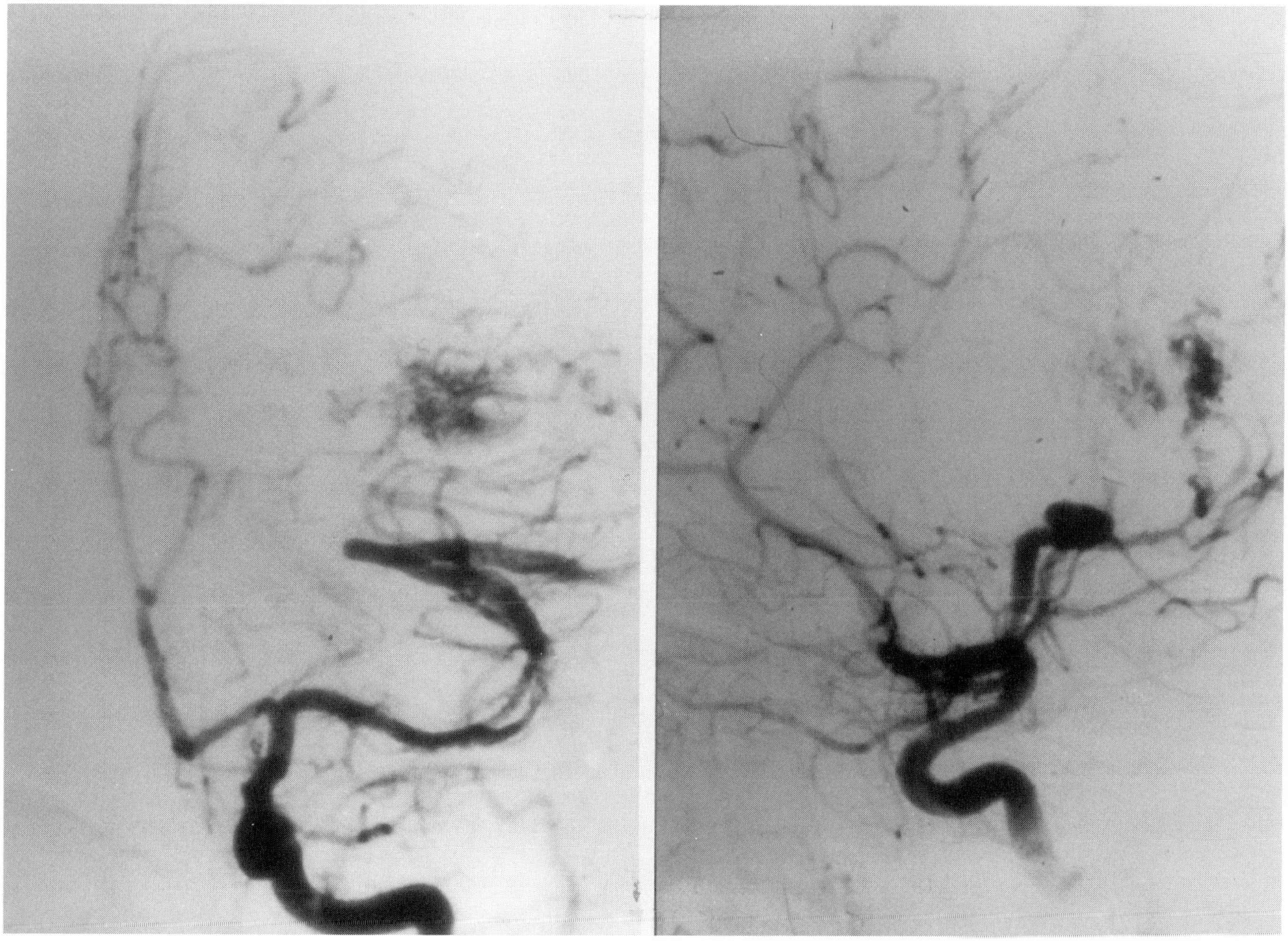

Figure 1B. Angiograms 24 hours after intraoperative embolization of the two major MCA arterial feeders. *Continued*

clusion, even though a very significant portion of the nidus had seemingly been obliterated. This simply stood as a further reinforcement of the fact that the *only* treatment for an AVM is complete obliteration or, better, its complete removal.

Over the past decade Spetzler and his colleagues have embarked upon the staging of removals of large eloquent AVMs. This ambitious undertaking consists of more than one operation, days to weeks or even months apart, during which meticulous microsurgical technique is utilized to gradually remove the AVM. Although the results have not been uniformly successful, nevertheless they provide a basis for some optimism in this group of very difficult cases.[9]

Theoretical and Practical Considerations

Time of Development of AVM

AVMs are congenital, originating sometime during fetal life. It is the notion of this author that these probably occur during the period of organogenesis somewhere around 4–6 weeks of fetal age. Thus, intuitively one might expect that if these were small and they shunted little blood, they would have little effect on the surrounding cortex with respect to its function. On the other hand, based on the same intuition, it would be predicted that if they were large they might well be associated with an alteration in the function of the surrounding cortex. Thus, it has become well recognized that large AVMs may occur in some central areas where they almost certainly occupy a part of the cortex that would normally be expected to be involved with some type of eloquent function and yet that function is remote from where it would have been anticipated to have been found.

Frequently in such cases the phenomenon has been explained by the "displacement" of the functional cortex. As already stated, my own view is that this is not so much a matter of "displacement" as it is of "development" in another location (this may be purely semantic). It is well known that over the latter

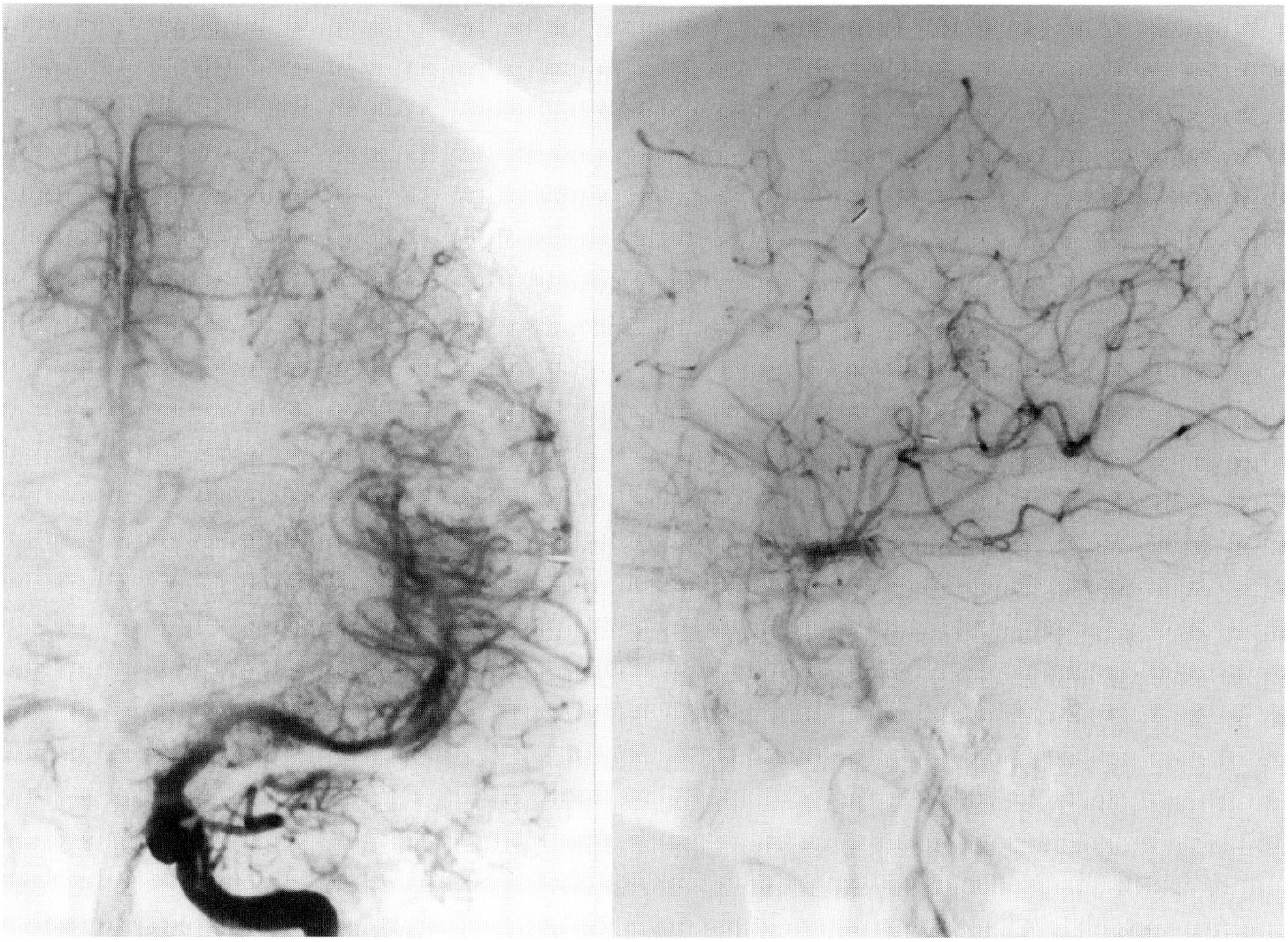

Figure 1C. Angiogram 6 months following the embolization. Postoperatively she had a hemiparesis and expressive dysphasia and then a massive swelling of the hemisphere with alteration in consciousness 2 weeks later with subsequent complete recovery except for her continuing seizures.

part of gestation and the initial few years of life there can be a transfer of speech from one hemisphere to another. Thus, there is no doubt that the possibility of "displacement" exists pathophysiologically. Quite irrespective of whether this is displacement or simply development remote from a usual location, the fact is that eloquent areas of cortical function may be found outside of the topographical reasonable limits of normal in some cases where the areas are occupied by medium or large AVMs.

Location/Angiographic Appearance of AVMs

AVMs in and around the central area may frequently be seen within the rolandic, or central, fissure. This fissure normally does not run in a coronal plane, but rather obliquely to it. Thus, AVMs can be found *within* the fissure, per se, and yet on the typical anterior-posterior (AP) and lateral angiograms, it may look spherical or elliptical in shape. The interpretation, therefore, is that the AVM is in fact a sphere and of necessity, involves not only the subarachnoid space and/or the cortex but the underlying white matter in the area as well. Stereoscopic or oblique x-rays will help sort this out, if it is suspected. This is more common in the case of medium-sized AVMs where it may become an important issue with respect to operability. Thus, an AVM within the rolandic fissure, which occupies only the fissure and hence is extracortical, can be removed, and yet this may not be appreciated on routine AP and lateral angiograms.

Investigation of Language

If an AVM occurs in an area where speech might normally be found, then it might be deemed inoperable. On the other hand it clearly might be operable if it was known that the speech center had transferred to the other side. Can such a transfer be confirmed? The traditional intracarotid amytal test for speech[11,12] has been the traditional preoperative method for localizing speech. However, its use is extremely difficult in the presence of AVMs with significant flows. AVMs that are large enough to beg the question of whether there has been transfer of speech will be large enough to shunt amytal through them without any significant narcotization of the surrounding area. Having experienced the disappointment of this on so many occasions 25 years ago, I am convinced that the best information can be gained not by performing the amytal test on the side of the lesion but on the opposite, or contralateral, side!

If the contralateral intracarotid injection of amytal leads to the typical transient paralysis and hemianopia without any evidence of alteration in language, then speech has not been transferred. In this case the clear negative response is informative and definitive. However, if in fact there is some speech alteration then there will be very definitely some niggling concern about whether all speech or only part of speech (i.e., one area only) has been transferred. Experienced neuropsychologists may aid greatly in this determination. In these cases, an ipsilateral carotid amytal test might possibly add some information with respect to specific items, but the likelihood is it will be of no further benefit. In these cases, therefore, the presence or absence of speech in association with the AVM may be able to be appreciated only with operation under local anesthesia.

Normal Perfusion Pressure Breakthrough Bleeding

Spetzler and colleagues described so-called "normal perfusion pressure breakthrough" bleeding (NPPB), which occurred after the resection of some AVMs.[10] The theory is that NPPB is associated with the abrupt occlusion of flow through an AVM and the subsequent readjustment of the normal surrounding microvasculature and brain to that occlusion. It is theorized that the perfusion of the latter has been deficient for some period of time, in association with a diversion of blood through the adjacent AVM, and that when the perfusion is returned to normal, this may exceed the ability of the adjacent cerebral microvasculature to compensate for the increase with normal autoregulation. Thus, while the cerebral perfusion may be equal to that of the normal brain, this normality represents a marked increase over what was present prior to the excision of the AVM. This normal perfusion amounts to a transient pathological perfusion pressure which, in the absence of normal autoregulation, results in hemorrhage.

Spetzler and colleagues outlined the positive correlative (risk) factors for NPPB as being: (1) size; (2) high flow; (3) paucity of filling of the surrounding "normal" cerebral vasculature; (4) vascular "steal" from the vertebrobasilar or contralateral carotid circulation; (5) extensive contribution from the external carotid artery; and (6) clinical findings of a progressive or fluctuating neurological deficit.[9]

Anesthesia and Cortical Functional Mapping

Choice of Anesthesia

There is controversy regarding the use of local anesthesia in many neurosurgical operations. This author advocates its use for many reasons, quite apart from surgical operations for epilepsy. The comfort of the surgical team (surgeon, anesthetist, operating room staff, etc.) will in large part determine the frequency with which it is used and the ease of its use. In centers where its use is prevalent, it represents nearly a "routine" when utilized in the case of a patient harboring an AVM. If its use is only very infrequent, then perhaps it is unwise to use it in the case of a patient with an AVM. As outlined previously,[7] the appearance of vomiting, rupture of the malformation, lack of cooperation of an apprehensive patient, or a generalized seizure can be a major, and even at times catastrophic, event to the team that is unfamiliar with dealing with patients under local anesthesia. The importance of an experienced anesthetist who is capable of early recognition for, and the use of, readily available syringes of sodium pentothal, dimenhydrinate, and diazepam cannot be overestimated. In spite of the foregoing, this author considers that the safety of the procedure to the patient is sufficiently enhanced that its use is indispensable in many cases of AVMs in eloquent areas.

The use of bupivacaine hydrochloride with 1: 200,000 epinephrine as a local anesthetic has revolutionized procedures carried out under local anesthesia. The duration of this local anesthetic in the concentration of 0.5% with added epinephrine allows anesthetic blockade for as long as 8–12 hours following injection. The initial concern about the use of epinephrine in patients with AVMs has faded with the passage of time. One milliliter of typical injectable bicarbonate solution added to the 20 mL vial greatly decreases the discomfort of the injections.

The supraorbital, zygomatico-temporal, auriculo-temporal, lesser occipital, and greater occipital nerves can be blocked in various combinations in order to provide the appropriate anesthesia of the scalp. These injections are usually made 1–2 hours prior to the patient going to the operating room. This allows good stable diffusion of the anesthetic to occur, the patient to have behind him/her the injections that may be associated with discomfort, and reduction of the likelihood of toxicity from the further local anesthesia that will be used in the scalp flap later in the operating room.

After the patient is taken to the operating room, he/she is placed in the lateral position on a double sponge mattress with pillows between the legs and behind the back for support. The head is placed as comfortably as possible on a padded headrest. The scalp, which has usually already been clipped of hair, is prepared aseptically and then usually 50–60 mL of 0.33% bupivacaine with 1:200,000 (or 1:300,000) epinephrine are used to infiltrate subcutaneously the proposed scalp incision. The drapes are then sewn in place around the wound over some type of a plastic adhesive drape in order to decrease the likelihood of irrigation fluid escaping beneath the drapes into the ear or onto the face of the patient.

The scalp incision is made and if the injection of local anesthetic was appropriate, then hemostasis is easily achieved with only bipolar coagulation of the galeal vessels and packing of the contiguous portions of the flap and scalp with peroxide gauze for a few minutes. The insentient bone can be drilled and sawed without incident, but the underlying dura mater with its nerves following the course of the middle meningeal artery must be narcotized with local anesthetic during the procedure of its separation from the overlying bone. The choice of this anesthetic is arbitrary. The author has used a mixture of equal parts of 1% lidocaine and 0.25% bupivacaine without epinephrine. Good anesthesia of the dura can be obtained by injecting small amounts of this between the leaflets in the dura (the adequacy of such an injection can be judged by the appearance of a pale bleb over the dural surface). Once the bone is removed, the dura is once again injected with the mixture which will last as long as 2–5 hours. With the exception of operations at the base of the middle fossa or at the midline (superior sagittal sinus and falx) no further anesthesia would ordinarily be required during a craniotomy. If a temporal lobectomy forms a part of the operative procedure, then injections into the free edge of the tent, just behind the petrous bone, may be necessary.[4] Operations that involve the midline may well require injections of the superior sagittal sinus and the falx. Familiarity with the innervation of the dura, sagittal sinus, and falx facilitates the placement of these injections.[3,4,8]

Functional Cortical Mapping

Functional mapping of the cortex is routinely carried out with electrical stimulation. The parameters of stimulation may include frequencies in the range of 25–50 hertz, pulse durations in the range of 200–500 microseconds, and train durations of 2–3 seconds. The usual waveforms now are rectangular and in this acute stimulation, it is inconsequential whether they are biphasic or monophasic. Most stimulation now is isolated capacitatively or optically. Although the balanced biphasic stimulating pulse is the ideal noninjurious waveform for use in chronic stimulation, it is not necessary in the case of acute stimulation. In a likewise fashion although constant current is the ideal output for biological stimulation, on the other hand, if the electrode impedance is relatively constant, which is certainly the case with the larger electrodes used for cortical stimulation, then constant voltage is equally efficacious. Finally, unifocal or bifocal stimulation may be used. The author prefers the former. Using the stimulus parameters noted above, responses from stimulation in the lower threshold areas (precentral gyrus, postcentral gyrus, Broca's area) can be obtained with 1–2 ma current (5–10 volts with electrode impedances of 2–5 kilohms).

The likelihood of producing focal motor seizures from AVMs in the rolandic region is greater than in any other type of cortical pathology. This in and of itself is of no consequence. However, it very definitely is consequential should the focal seizure go on to secondary generalization. There are a number of measures that can be taken that will decrease the likelihood of this possibility. First, the alert anesthetist will have immediately at hand a syringe of pentothal (or propofol). If secondary generalization appears to be imminent, then 50–100 mg of pentothal will nearly always abort the secondary generalization and leave a patient who will be awake again within a matter of a few minutes. Second, the exploratory stimulation should not be done in sequential topographical order. Rather it should be somewhat random around the area that is being explored by the stimulation i.e., stimulation should not be carried out continually in a line over a single gyrus. If after discharge (AD) occurs and one is not recording from the stimulated point at the time, then the surgeon will be unaware of such discharge. With stimulation of immediately adjacent points there is an increased probability that ADs will summate and give rise to a seizure that would not otherwise have been produced had the AD disappeared in the immediately adjacent point prior to stimulation. Thus, stimulation should be carried out by "jumping around" the area in order to avoid this complication. Third, once the lower threshold areas have been stimulated and mapped, one should not return to these areas with any further stimulation that might therefore be very much suprathreshold.

Following these guidelines, the area in question can usually be mapped with relative safety. As has been pointed out previously, the threshold for identification of the temporoparietal (Wernicke) speech area may be very much higher than that of the lower rolandic region.[4]

Resection Guidelines

A full discussion of the guidelines regarding resection in functional areas is beyond the scope of this article. It has been discussed recently.[6] In brief, resection around the eloquent areas of language or sensory motor function should be carried out with monitoring of that neurological function by an experienced individual in the operating room. Such an individual (e.g., anesthetist) becomes very adept at describing motor movements, inquiring from the patients as to sensory experiences, and picking up subtle abnormalities in speech. This of course is the raison d'etre of operations under local anesthesia. Whereas such operations are very easily controlled in the case of the surgery for epilepsy or tumors, this cannot be applied necessarily to cases of AVMs where occasionally resection may be more determined by intraoperative hemorrhage than by the neurological monitoring of function. Therein, of course, lies the decision to resect, or not to resect!

In general, the closer the resection is carried to the functional area, the greater and more prolonged will be the transient interference with that particular function postoperatively. The leeway in the rolandic area is much greater frontally in the precentral sulcus than posteriorly in the post-central sulcus.[6]

Management

Overview

Although the evolution of the management of AVMs is dynamic, given the ongoing improvements and increasing sophistication in the technologies of both surgery and endovascular therapy, in London, Ontario, there is a reasonable, albeit not necessarily always unanimous, consensus with respect to treatment of most AVMs. Thus, what may be reasonable and accepted today might well take second place tomorrow. A proposed scheme of management is outlined below. The factor of age is not considered for each category in a specific way.

Considering what is known about the natural history of AVMs and the mortality and morbidity from surgery in the hands of the surgeon, there is some age beyond which the potential risks of operative intervention outweigh the natural historical risks of the lesion. Chovanes and colleagues have depicted this mathematically.[2] This must be factored into any decision concerning potential surgery of AVMs and a certain amount of individualization must occur in the decision making in the case of a given patient.

The second variable that is not considered specifically within the management scheme of each AVM outlined below is the question of the flow through the AVM. High-flow AVMs are obviously more dangerous from both the points of view of natural history as well as surgically. The quantification of flow through an AVM probably cannot be determined with certainty at the present time. However, the qualitative judgments of high and low flow within the AVM is valid and again must be factored into the formula for decision making with respect to potential surgical intervention. (It is the high-flow AVMs where a sudden obliteration may result in NPPB bleeding.)

Small AVMs (<2–3 cm)

Small AVMs can usually be removed surgically with very little mortality or morbidity. Our own preference is to remove these under local anesthesia but certainly the majority of them can be carefully removed under general anesthesia. Figure 2 is the angiogram of a 12-year-old boy who had a single focal cerebral seizure with secondary generalization, whose investigation disclosed the presence of a dominant rolandic AVM. As would have been predicted, this was an easily removed surface AVM which in fact lay over his motor hand area.

Less predictable is the AVM shown in Figure 3. This AVM was in a 28-year-old woman who had had focal cerebral motor seizures involving her face just before menstruating for 12 straight months. Her AVM was located entirely within the rolandic fissure. It was extracortical, even though this would not have been appreciated when looking at the straight AP and lateral views. It was removed under local anesthesia

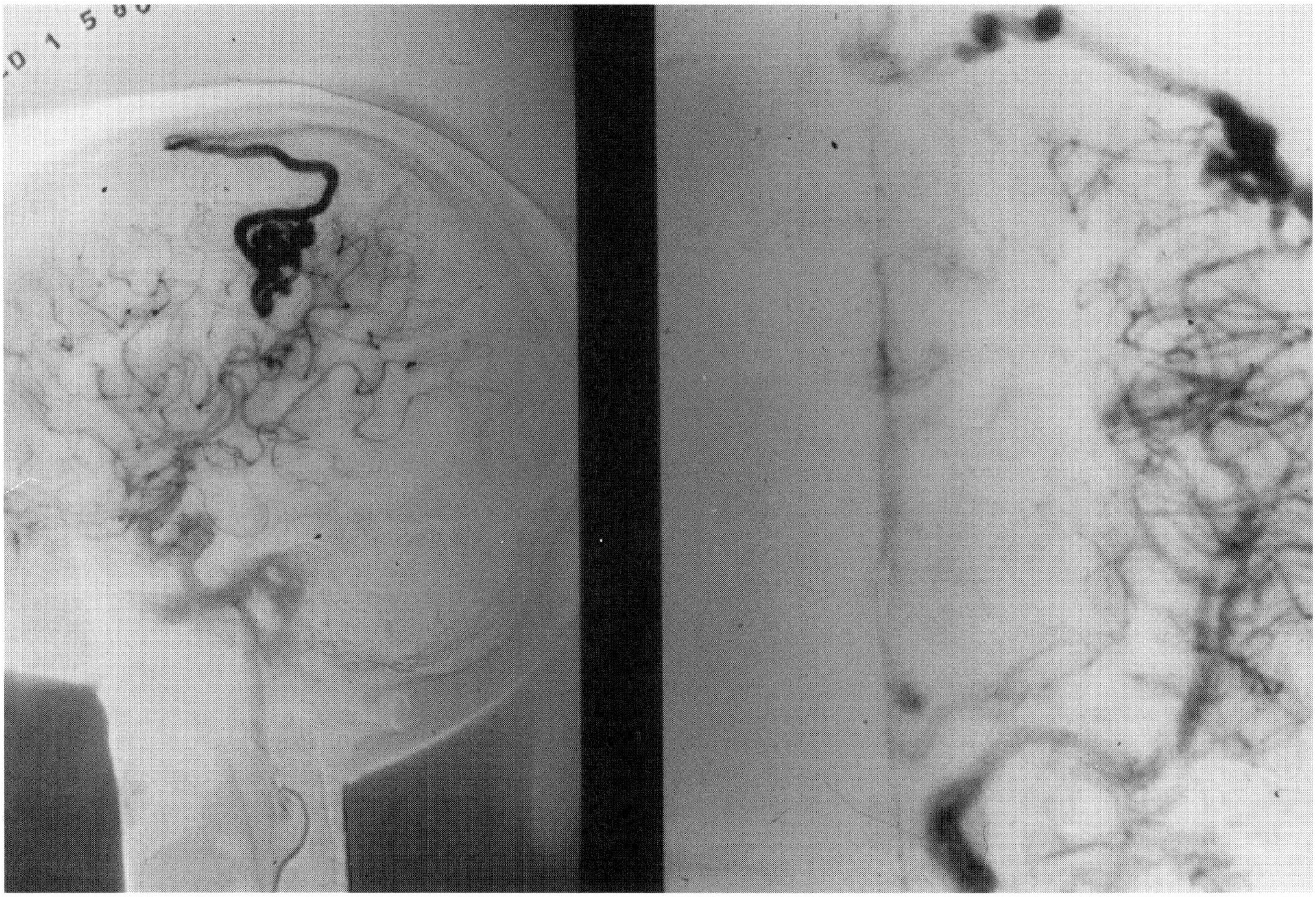

Figure 2. Angiogram of a 12-year-old boy who had a single simple partial motor seizure of the right hand with secondary generalization.

after opening up the rolandic fissure. Neither of these two patients had any postoperative deficit. It was experience with cases such as these that has taught us that such cases could have been operated on under general anesthesia with similar results.

Medium-Sized AVMS (2.5–5 cm)

In these AVMs, as in the rolandic AVM shown in Figure 3, stereoscopic angiography may help to sort out whether or not the malformation is planar. Thus, even preoperatively, if such is the case, then there is reasonable predictability that it is operable. This is very important information preoperatively. Preoperative information about language through the use of the intracarotid amytal test, as noted earlier, may also aid in planning the operation. The operation is then preferably carried out under local anesthesia, particularly when there is a reasonable possibility or likelihood that there has been an alteration in the expected location of eloquent cortical function. If the AVM is extracortical or if the area of cortex involved in the eloquent function is separated from the area of cortex contained in the AVM, then the removal is quite straightforward. If the AVM is intimately involved with the eloquent function, involving a number of so-called "en passage" vessels that cannot be stripped of feeders to the AVM, then removal may not be possible.

Small and medium-sized AVMs in the dominant posterior perisylvian region have frequently been found to reside entirely within the posterior and medial aspects of the sylvian fissure and have been just as easily resectable as the AVM of the rolandic region noted in Figure 3. Figure 4 depicts an AVM in a 65-year-old woman who presented with simple and complex partial seizures. Her AVM was located in the most posteromedial aspect of the dominant sylvian fissure. A number of AVMs have been removed from this area and the interesting aspect to these has been

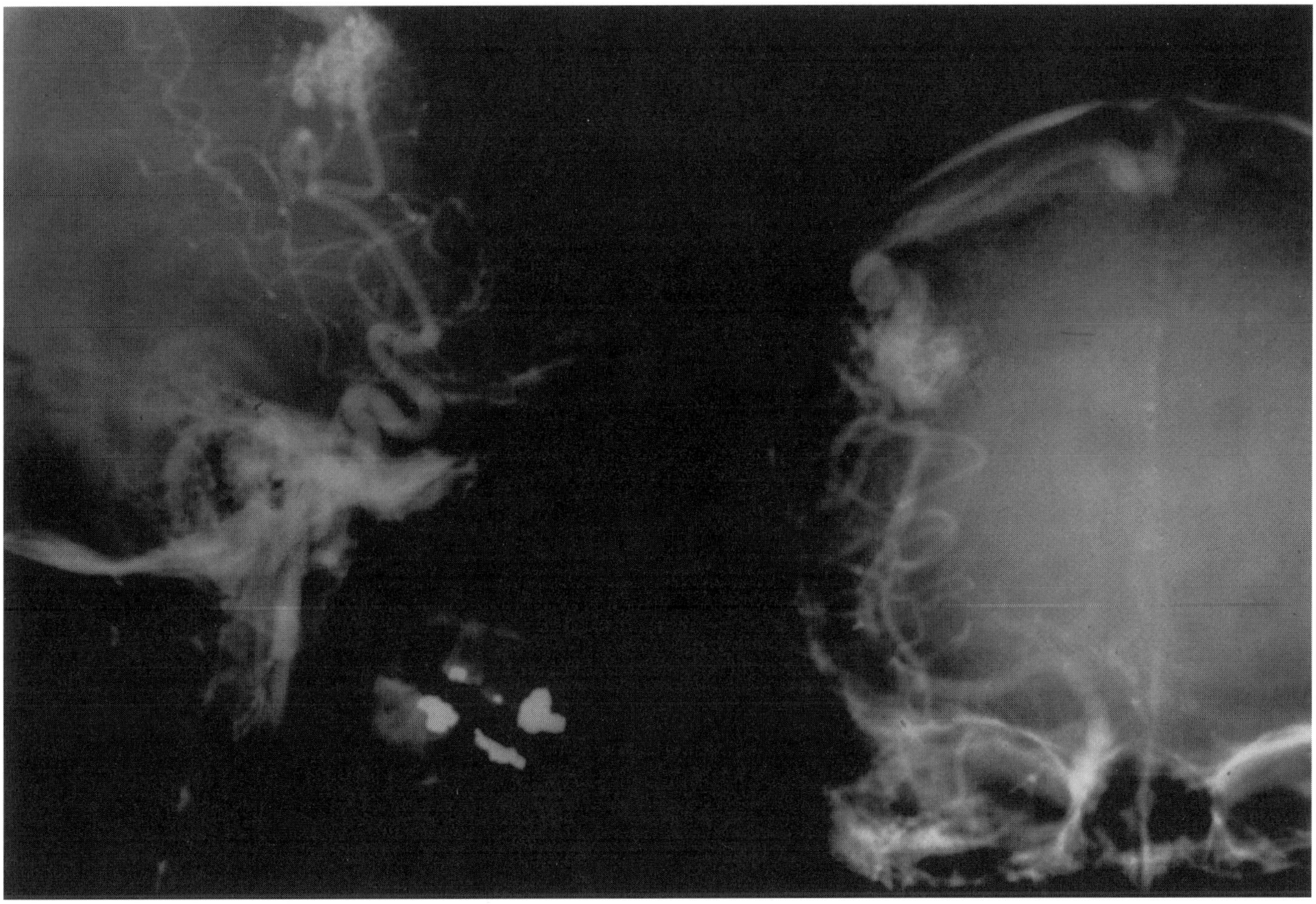

Figure 3. The angiogram of a 28-year-old woman who presented with simple partial motor seizures of her left face in association with menstrual periods over the course of a year. Postoperatively she had a transient mild left hemiparesis that cleared within 10 days. Her seizures ceased.

their primary extracortical location, and also that at the depth of the posterior fissure there is frequently no more than 2 or 3 mm of cerebral mantle between the base of the fissure and the ventricle. The latter has often been opened in those cases in which the vessels seem to involve the parenchyma. In these cases the parenchymal involvement has always been deep in the fissure and the surgery has resulted in no deficit. These cases were initially done under local anesthesia but as with the small AVMs, the majority of them could probably be removed quite safely under general anesthesia.

Large AVMs (>5 cm)

Very large AVMs may be inoperable; they may be treated by staged removals or may be operated on with preceding endovascular therapy, or may be treated by endovascular therapy alone.

Many of the very large AVMs involving eloquent cortex and more particularly in the dominant hemisphere are clearly inoperable. In our own experience the natural history of such AVMs is more characterized by a dynamically accelerated neurological deficit and increasingly intractable seizures than rebleeding. This increasing deficit, either from presumed ischemic changes in the associated functionally important cortex or from repeated hemorrhages may change the criteria for operation with the passage of time. Thus, the individual who has become hemiplegic no longer faces the risk of this deficit from surgery. Again, individualization of therapy must occur in such cases. When operation is undertaken, this may be done in stages, as noted earlier, or may involve some type of endovascular therapy preoperatively or intraoperatively.

Based on our experience over the last 15 years, endovascular therapy (embolization) is now used

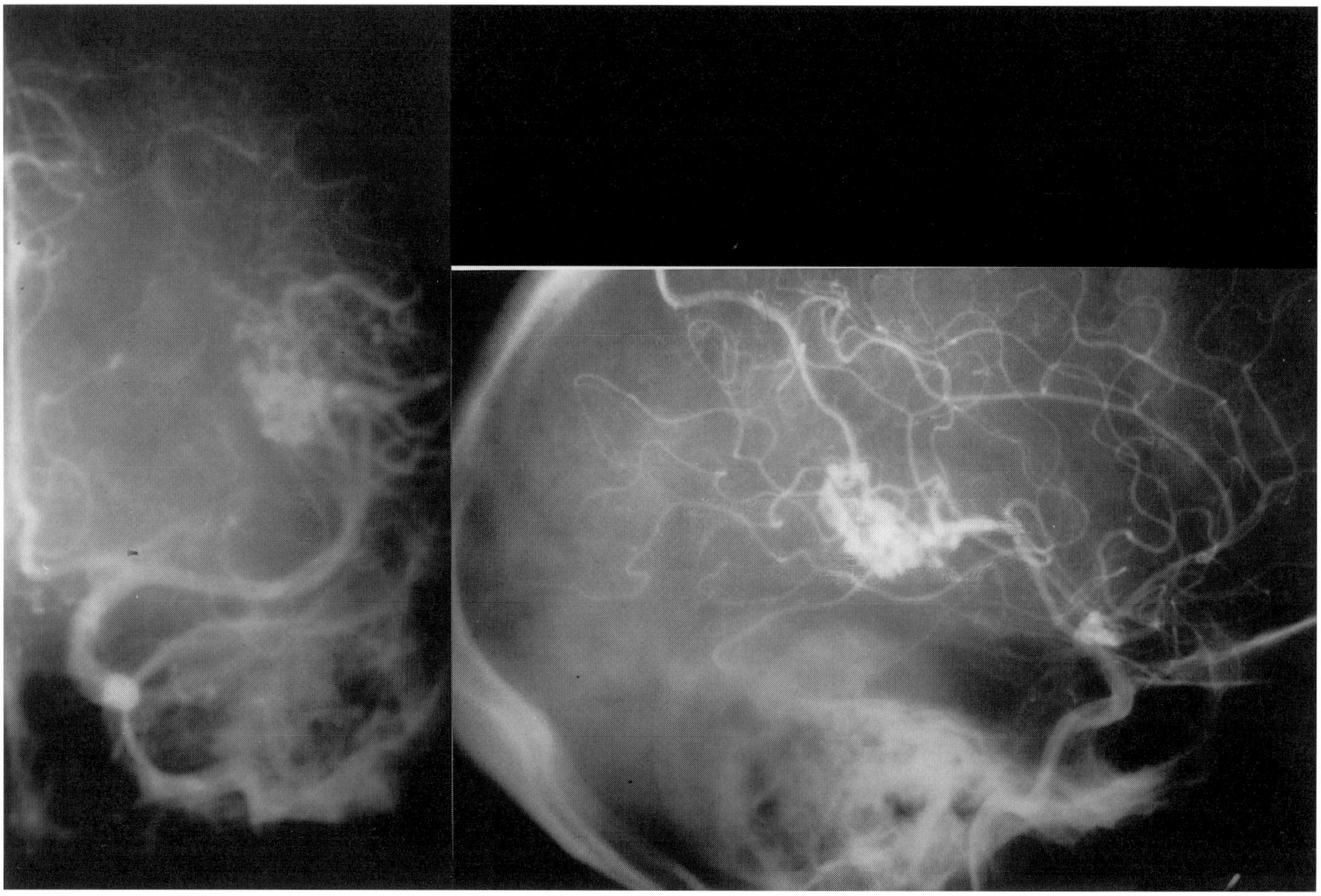

Figure 4. Angiograms of a 65-year-old woman who was admitted with a 40-year history of pounding left parietal headaches lasting usually for several minutes and associated with visual and auditory hallucinations and occasional nausea and vomiting. These seizures had considerably worsened over the previous 3 years and were accompanied by dizziness, disorientation, inappropriate behavior, and memory impairment. At operation, there was a clearly evident fistulous nidus that contained two or three middle cerebral incoming arterial feeders and the outgoing large draining superior anastomotic vein. In this regard, therefore, it was not unlike a vein of Galen aneurysm.

only in specific instances. First, it may be used in the case of high-flow AVMs where the "steal" phenomenon is implicated in the production of the neurological symptomatology. In such circumstances it may be used alone simply in order to reduce the steal or it may be used as an adjunct to surgery. The primary aim of its use is to reduce flow as much as possible in order to decrease the likelihood of breakthrough bleeding at the time of definitive resection. Second, it may be used simply as an adjunct to surgery alone in which case it may be used preoperatively or incorporated into the operation per se. Although within our group of neurosurgeons there has been some controversy as to its value, nevertheless I have found it to be a highly valuable adjunct to surgery. The avascularity of the operative procedure has often made me question whether there has not been complete thrombosis of the AVM between the time of embolization and angiography and the time of operation.

Conclusion

Small AVMs should be able to be removed safely from eloquent areas. A number of medium-sized AVMs justify preoperative attempts at determining operability (specialized angiography or intracarotid amytal testing) and usually justify operative exposure under local anesthesia to determine the relationship of the AVM to associated eloquent cortex. Large AVMs are less likely to be effectively treated surgically. In some instances, absolutely nothing can be done that would be justified at the outset. However, combinations of endovascular therapy and surgery are being increasingly utilized and their indications will increase as the severity of frequent rebleeding, intractable seizures, and/or increasing neurological deficit occur.

In all of these cases, this author considers that local anesthesia is a benefit, either being able to be used for the whole of the operation or the initial part of the operation during which mapping of functional cortex may be undertaken. It is precisely the use of local anesthesia that has taught us that it is not necessary in all cases.

Finally, in the treatment of AVMs, there are many confounding variables, the two most important perhaps being age and the flow of blood through the AVM which necessitate the individual tailoring of management in any given case. However, added to this list must be the experience of the operating team, the backup in the associated neurological disciplines, and the expertise of the surgeon's neuroradiological interventional colleagues.

Acknowledgments: The author thanks Mrs. Willa Harding for her capable typing of this manuscript.

References

1. Amacher AL, Allcock JM, Drake CG. Cerebral angiomas: The sequelae of surgical treatment. J Neurosurg 37:571–575, 1972.
2. Chovanes GI, Buchheit WA, Kenning JA. Medical vs.surgical treatment of unruptured arteriovenous malformations using life expectancy as a basis for comparison. 1987 (personal communication).
3. Feindel W, Penfield W, McNaughton F. The tentorial nerves and localization of intracranial pain in man. Neurology 10:555–563, 1960.
4. Girvin JP. Neurosurgical considerations and general methods for craniotomy under local anesthesia. Int Anesthesiol Clin 24:89–114, 1986a.
5. Girvin JP. Resection of intracranial lesions under local anesthesia. Int Anesthesiol Clin 24:133–155, 1986b.
6. Girvin JP. Complications of epilepsy surgery. In Luders H (ed): Epilepsy Surgery. New York: Raven Press, 1991, pp 653–660.
7. Girvin JP, Fox AJ, Vinuela F, et al. Intraoperative embolization of cerebral arteriovenous malformations in the awake patient. Clin Neurosurg 31:188–247, 1984.
8. Penfield W, McNaughton F. Dural headache and innervation of the dura matter. Arch Neurol Psychiatr 44: 43–75, 1940.
9. Spetzler RF, Martin NA, Carter LP, et al. Surgical management of large AVMs by staged embolization and operative excision. J Neurosurg 67:17–28, 1987.
10. Spetzler RF, Wilson CB, Weinstein P, et al. Normal perfusion pressure breakthrough theory. Clin Neurosurg 25:651–672, 1978.
11. Wada J. A new method for the determination of the side of cerebral speech dominance: A preliminary report on the intracarotid injection of sodium amytal in man. Igaku to Seidutsugaki. Medicine and Biology 14: 221–222, 1949 (In Japanese).
12. Wada J, Rasmussen T. Intracarotid injection of sodium amytal for the lateralization of cerebral speech dominance: Experimental and clinical observations. J Neurosurg 17:266–282, 1960.

Chapter 6

Cavernous Malformations of the Brain Stem

Thomas M. Wascher, MD, and Robert F. Spetzler, MD

Introduction

Cavernous malformations represent 8% to 15% of all intracranial vascular malformations and are reported to occur in 0.1% to 0.5% of the general population.[14,18,45,46,61,63] Previously published series indicate that 10% to 30% of all intracranial cavernous malformations are located within the brain stem and cerebellum and are more frequently symptomatic than their supratentorial counterparts.[43] Clinically, cavernous malformations are thought to compose a significant percentage of "angiographic occult cerebral vascular malformations."[7,10–12,17,18,26,38,48,49,66,70,78]

Thought to be congenital, two forms of cavernous malformations are recognized: familial and sporadic. Recent studies indicate that up to 50% of patients show a strong family history consistent with an autosomal dominant inheritance pattern, particularly in families of Hispanic descent.[5,6,8,18,28,35,42,50,58,64] Many of the familial patients are affected by multiple lesions (up to 90%), compared to the 10% to 16% incidence of multiplicity observed in sporadic cases.[14,60,61,63,84] Symptomatic lesions have been described in all age groups, with an onset of symptoms between the third and fifth decades without a sex predominance.[41,43,56,77] The mean age of presentation (approximately 25 years) seen with familial cases is 10 to 12 years younger than that observed with sporadic cases.[14,61,84]

Cavernous malformations of the brain stem have a distinctive clinical presentation and characteristic course once they become symptomatic, often resulting in severe neurological impairment when left untreated. This chapter discusses the pathology, clinical course, diagnosis, surgical indications, and the appropriate surgical management of cavernous malformations involving the brain stem.

Pathology

On gross inspection, a cavernous malformation appears as a lobulated, well-circumscribed, mulberry-like lesion that varies from several millimeters to several centimeters (Figure 1).[47,63] The characteristic microscopic appearance is that of abnormally dilated, sinusoidal vascular channels without intervening brain parenchyma (Figure 2).[47,63] The walls of the sinusoidal spaces are composed of a single layer of flattened endothelial cells, without smooth muscle, and are separated from each other by collagenous hyalinized or fibrous tissue (Figure 3). Elastic fibers in the walls of the vascular spaces are characteristically absent.[44,63,67] Evidence of prior hemorrhage is a frequent finding, while thrombosis, organization, inflammatory changes, and calcification may be seen centrally in larger lesions.[6,44,62,63] The lesion may be surrounded by a variable degree of gliosis that may also extend from the periphery toward its center. The surrounding vasculature is typically normal, and an arterial supply is rarely visualized; however, dilated capillaries are often found in the adjacent brain. Recent literature supports an association of proximity between cavernous and venous malformations, a relationship that has primary surgical significance (discussed below).[59,86]

Clinical Presentations and Natural History

Cavernous malformations of the brain stem present with progressive neurological deficits secondary

From Yamada S (ed): *Arteriovenous Malformations in Functional Areas of the Brain.*

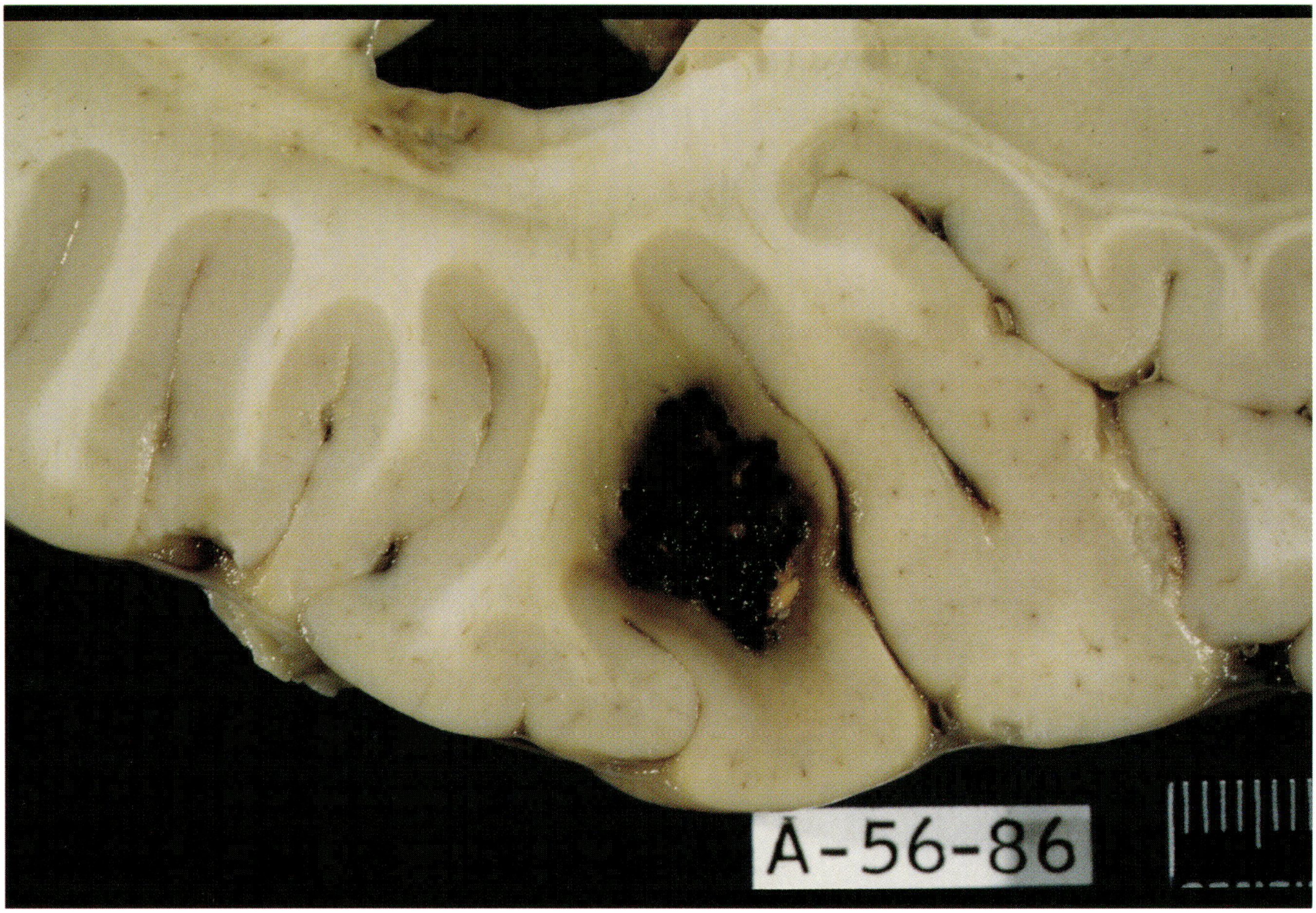

Figure 1. Autopsy specimen demonstrating the typical appearance of a cavernous malformation. The lesion is lobulated and sharply demarcated from the surrounding brain. Note the appearance of blood breakdown products both within and immediately surrounding the lesion.

to mass effect on adjacent brain stem tracts and/or nuclei or with the sequelae of hemorrhage. Because of their location within an exquisitely eloquent region, even small brain stem cavernous malformations are likely to be associated with neurological deficits. As with other lesions in this region, neurological signs and symptoms can be predicted based on clinico-anatomic correlations, depending on the neural pathways affected. The most common signs and symptoms associated with brain stem cavernous malformations are facial pain or hypesthesia, hemiparesis and spasticity, hemisensory deficits and dysesthesias, disorders of ocular motility (especially dysconjugate gaze and nystagmus), and severe headaches. Other findings include VII-VIII cranial nerve neuropathies, neuropathies of the IX-X-XI cranial nerve complex, dysarthria and tongue weakness secondary to XII cranial nerve neuropathy, involvement of cerebellar tracts including ataxia and dysmetria, signs and symptoms of hydrocephalus, and Parinaud's syndrome (Table 1).

Hemorrhage into a cavernous malformation is marked by acute onset of headache, vertigo, nausea, vomiting, and the new onset or exacerbation of existing neurological deficit(s). In contrast to arteriovenous malformations, cavernous malformations of the brain stem rarely bleed into the subarachnoid space or into the ventricular system; we have found this to be a useful differentiating feature preoperatively.[86] More commonly, these lesions bleed into the sinusoidal space of the malformation itself, resulting in acute enlargement and neurological signs and symptoms due to acute mass effect.

The natural history of cavernous malformations is only now being elucidated with the widespread use of magnetic resonance (MR) imaging. Preliminary reports indicate that supratentorial nonfamilial cavernous malformations hemorrhage at an annualized

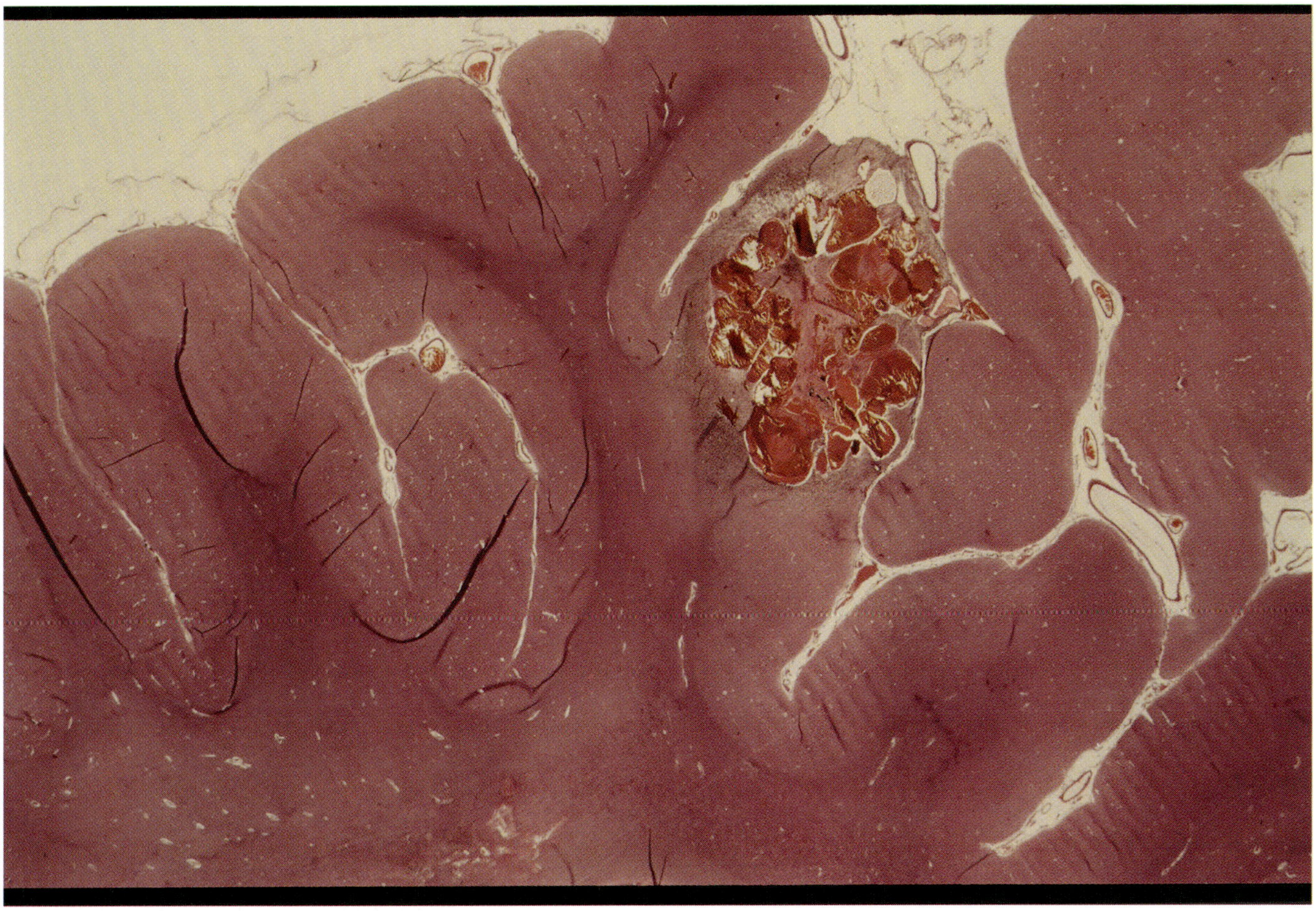

Figure 2. Photomicrograph of a cavernous malformation, demonstrating the abnormally dilated, sinusoidal channels without intervening brain parenchyma.

rate of 0.25% to 0.7%.[14,85] This figure appears to be significantly higher (6.5% per patient per year) in patients with the familial form of the disease.[84] Likewise, worsening of neurological signs and symptoms is also more frequent in the familial group, occurring in more than 15% per year.[84]

In addition, evidence indicates that these lesions are dynamic, with changes in number, size, and MR imaging signal characteristics. The appearance of new lesions may represent the growth of very small lesions without symptomatic hemorrhage. Mechanisms purported to cause growth and MR imaging signal changes include the following: (1) progressive ectasia of vascular channels and budding of capillaries from cavernous spaces resulting in growth of the vascular nidus; (2) recurrent "external" microhemorrhages or red blood cell diapedesis with thrombosis, followed by organization, fibrosis, and calcification; (3) acute gross hemorrhage resulting in acute size increase; and (4) cyst formation from "internal" hemorrhage that ruptures septae between adjacent sinusoids.[54,86] Further growth and perifocal edema may be related to secondary microhemorrhages and fluid exudation from the neocapillary membrane in the cyst capsule.[54]

Cavernous malformations of the brain stem, once symptomatic, appear to pursue an aggressive clinical course marked by progressive neurological deterioration, often with interspersed episodes of acute exacerbation.[19,60,83,86] Although hemorrhage into a cavernous malformation is rarely massive, the sequelae of any brain stem bleeding, however slight, can be disastrous. However, if the limited tolerance of the brain stem to accommodate an acute expansion of an intrinsic mass lesion is not exceeded, hematoma resorption may result in gradual neurological improvement with substantial recovery.

Diagnostic Studies

The angiographic findings of a cavernous malformation include the presence of an avascular region

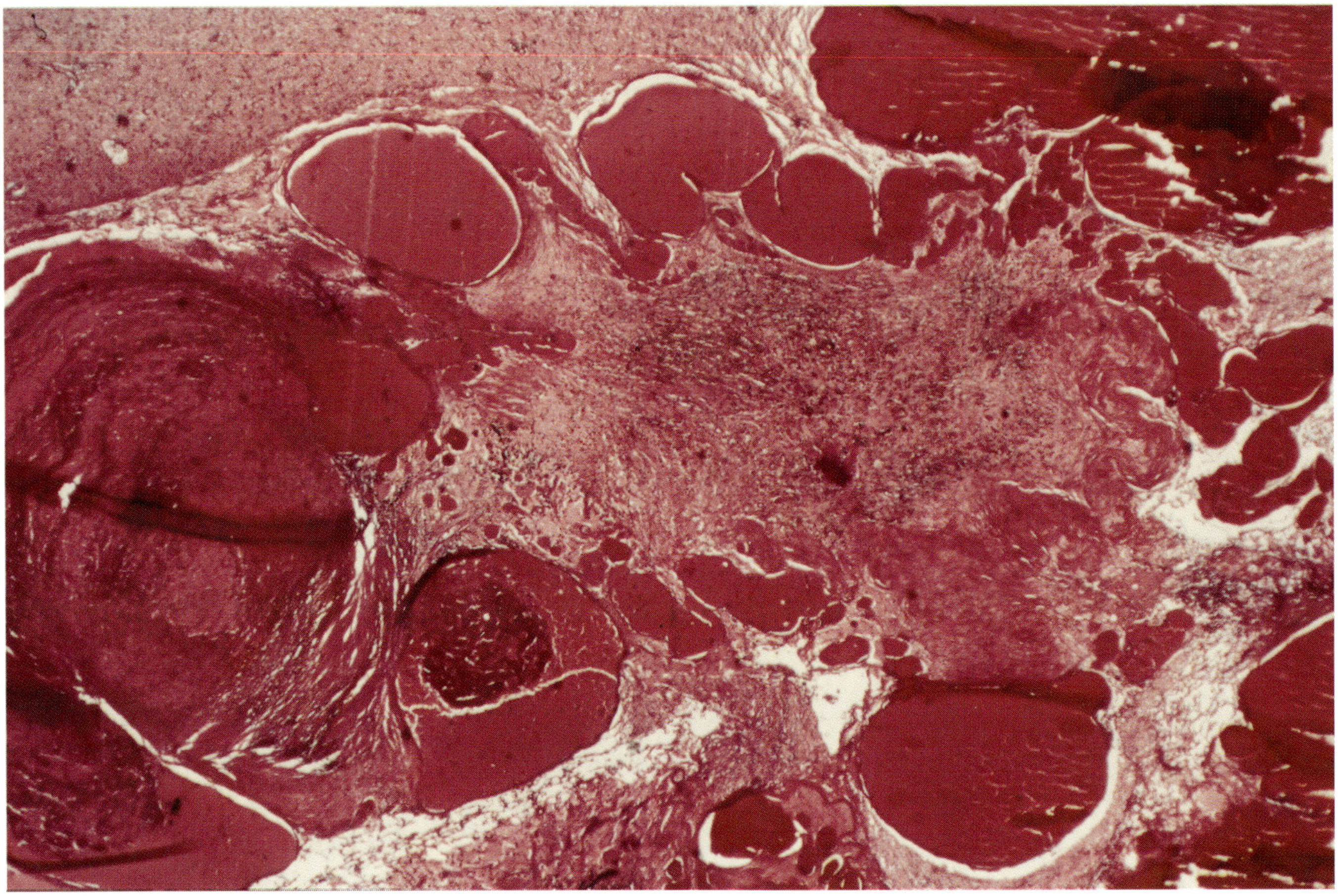

Figure 3. Photomicrograph of the same lesion as in Figure 2 but at high power (hematoxylin and eosin stain). The walls of the dilated vascular channels are characteristically thin-walled without smooth muscle or elastic fibers. Gliotic and fibrotic tissues are present in the center of the lesion along with deposits of hemosiderin. Normal brain tissue intervenes between these channels at the periphery.

Table 1

Preoperative Neurological Signs and Symptoms in 21 Patients with Brain Stem Cavernous Malformations

*Signs and Symptoms**	*Number of Patients*
Facial pain/hypesthesia	12 (57%)
Hemiparesis	10 (48%)
Disorder of ocular motility	10 (48%)
Severe headaches	10 (48%)
Hemisensory deficit/dysesthesias	8 (38%)
VII, VIII cranial nerve neuropathy	6 (29%)
IX, X, XI, XII cranial nerve neuropathy	6 (29%)
Ataxia, dysmetria	3 (14%)
Parinaud's syndrome	2 (10%)

* A patient may display more than one sign and/or symptom.

in the capillary phase, at times with mass effect, exhibiting a dense venous pooling pattern.[57,75,77] These findings are too nonspecific and infrequent to be of use in specific diagnosis. In comparison, although enhanced computed tomography (CT) appears to be more sensitive in the detection of cavernous malformations, the findings are insufficiently specific to allow a presumptive preoperative diagnosis in more than half of the cases.[57,74,76]

Before the advent of MR imaging, the diagnosis of cavernous malformation required surgical confirmation. However, the MR imaging appearance has proven to be highly characteristic, allowing an accurate diagnosis without invasive testing or the risks of surgical extirpation.[57] This characteristic appearance is due to magnetic susceptibility effects related to field heterogenicity that is more conspicuous on high-field imaging, related to the presence of hemosiderin and methemoglobin deposits.[57]

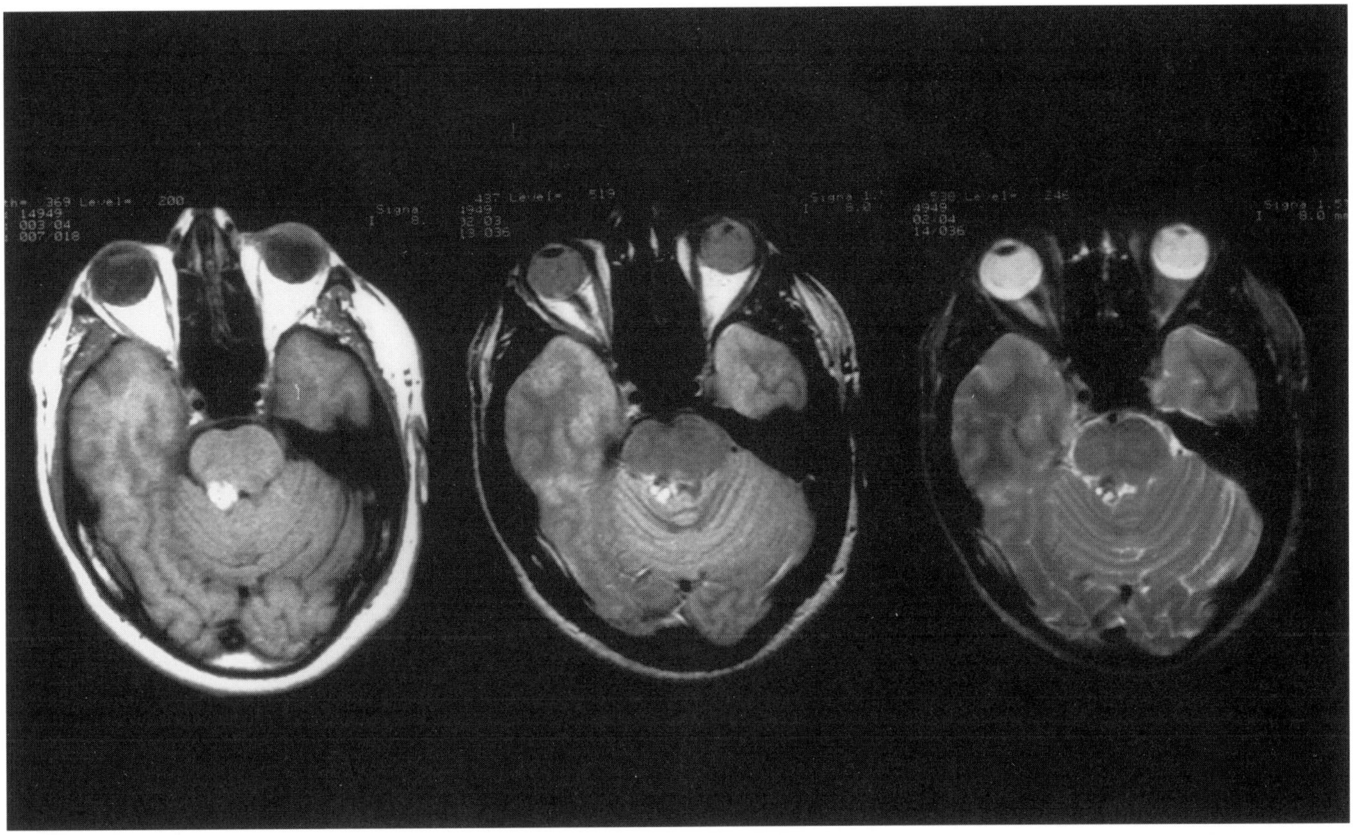

Figure 4. Magnetic resonance imaging appearance of brain stem cavernous malformation. **A.** From left to right: axial T1-weighted TR (repetition time) 450 ms; TE (echo time) 16 ms; intermediate-weighted (TR, 2500 ms; TE, 30 ms); and T2-weighted (TR, 2500 ms; TE, 90 ms) images of a small cavernous malformation involving the right pontine tegmentum. Note the increasingly apparent hypointense rim from hemosiderin deposition in and around the lesion with T2-weighting. *Continued*

On T2-weighted MR imaging, the appearance of a reticulated core of mixed signal intensity with a surrounding rim of decreased signal intensity is classic for diagnosis of a cavernous malformation (Figures 4A and B).[57] Smaller lesions exhibit focal areas of decreased signal intensity without a core of different signal (Figure 5). MR imaging, especially with the gradient-refocused echo technique, has proven to be both sensitive and specific for the detection of cavernous malformations and appears to be the imaging modality of choice for identification, diagnosis, and follow-up.[20,57,58,61]

Surgical Indications

Several reports indicate poor results (due primarily to rehemorrhage and brain stem compression) when accessible brain stem cavernous malformations are not treated aggressively.[67,86] Therefore, appropriate management of symptomatic brain stem lesions is safe excision whenever possible. Important factors to consider in surgical intervention include the following: (1) the neurological condition of the patient; (2) the past behavior of that particular offending lesion (single versus multiple hemorrhages, extent of symptomatology); (3) proximity to the brain stem surface; and (4) the presence of a surgical avenue for resection that spares eloquent brain tissue.

Specific recommendations regarding the appropriate time to wait after an ictus before intervening surgically are best individualized. Most patients with an apoplectic event due to a brain stem cavernous malformation will show remarkable recovery as the hematoma resorbs. It appears appropriate to follow such patients until their condition improves sufficiently to permit safe excision.

Evidence now suggests that the subset of cavernous malformations (symptomatic or asymptomatic) entirely surrounded by functional eloquent brain stem parenchyma is best treated by close observation. However, surgical excision should be offered to patients with symptomatic brain stem lesions that are

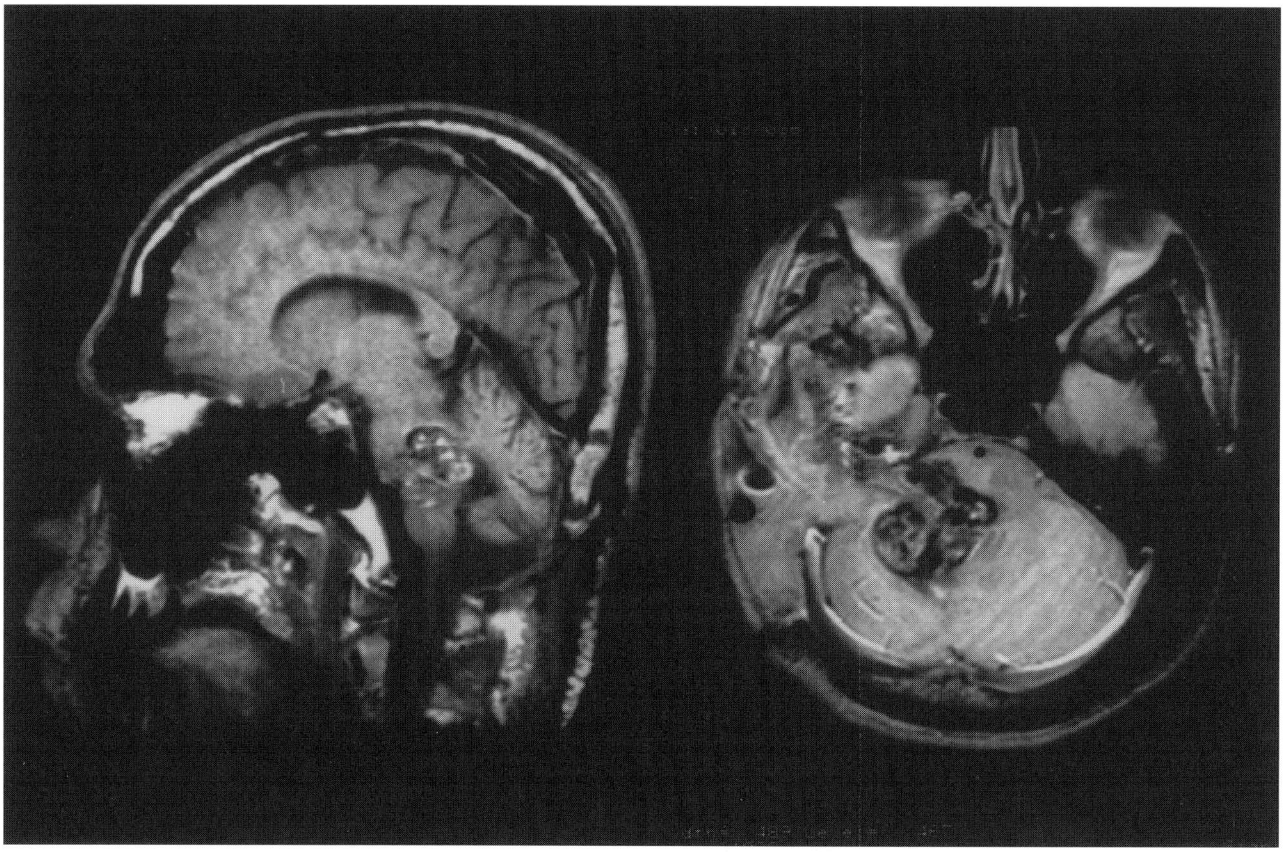

Figure 4B. Sagittal T1-weighted (TR, 700 ms; TE, 17 ms) and axial intermediate-weighted (TR, 2500 ms; TE, 30 ms) images of an extensive cavernous malformation involving the right cerebellum, middle cerebellar peduncle, and pons. The lesion exhibits the classic reticulated core of mixed signal density, which is surrounded by a rim of decreased signal intensity.

(1) superficial in location and (2) that can be exposed through an operative approach that spares eloquent brain stem neural pathways. Individual evaluation must be used to determine if the deficits resulting from surgery outweigh the risks of expectant management.

General Principles of Preoperative and Intraoperative Management

The cornerstone of successful management of brain stem cavernous malformations, as in all neurosurgical procedures, is the selection of an appropriate approach that optimizes exposure of the offending lesion with an absolute minimum of distortion of normal neurovascular relationships. A detailed and thorough knowledge of the normal neurovascular anatomy of the posterior fossa, tentorial incisura, foramen magnum region, temporal bone, and the cerebellum–brain stem is a prerequisite to suitable preoperative planning and appropriate intraoperative decision making. A complete understanding of the relationships of the neurovascular structures as well as readily identifiable reference points in the surgical field (e.g., major arterial branches, cranial nerve entry root zones, mass effect from an underlying cavernous malformation, residua from previous hemorrhage) provides confidence in relating anatomic and pathological structures and in formulating a surgical plan after exact intraoperative localization of the lesion. Stereotactically guided craniotomy, although useful for supratentorial lesions, is not as reliable for infratentorial surgery due to the required extra-axial dissection, cerebrospinal fluid (CSF) drainage required for brain relaxation, and the resulting alterations in spatial relationships between brain and skull.

After localizing the lesion, the surgeon usually encounters a cavity containing vascular spaces of the cavernous malformation and degradation products of prior hemorrhage. Unlike supratentorial malformations, lesions located within the brain stem can be extremely adherent to surrounding normal parenchyma.[86] Initial dissection should concentrate on circumferential separation of the malformation from surrounding gliosis prior to internal decompression

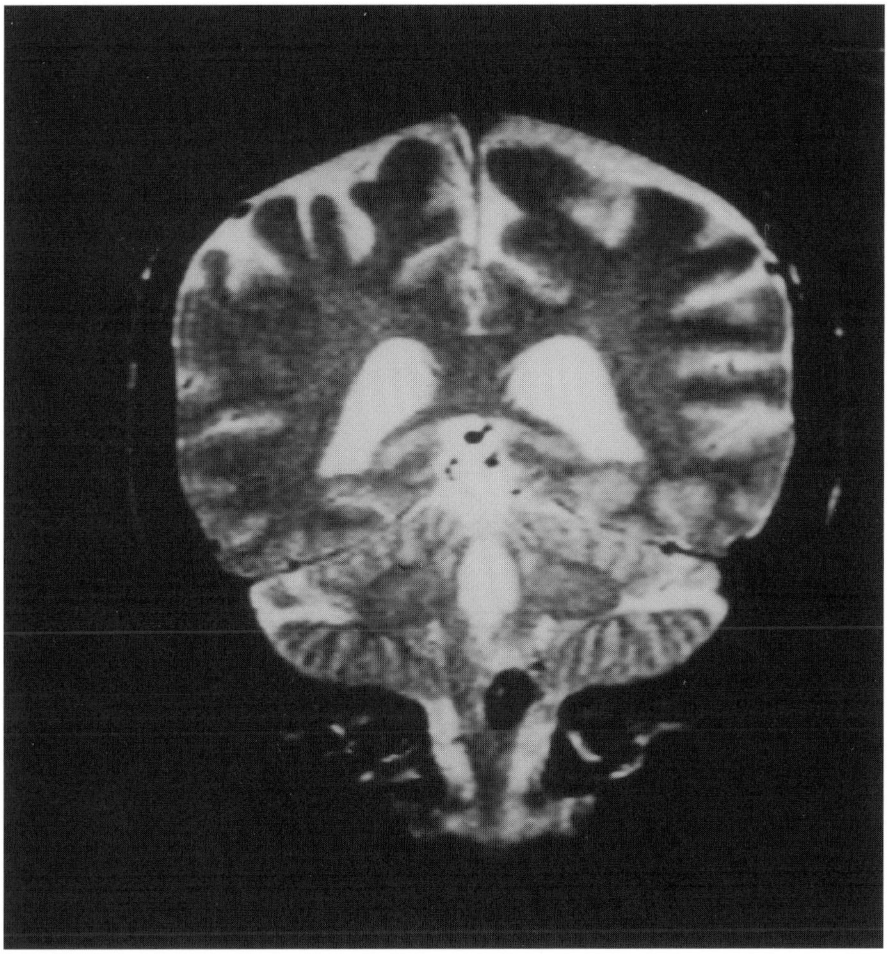

Figure 5. Magnetic resonance imaging appearance of a small cavernous malformation involving the left cervicomedullary junction. In this case, the T2-weighted image appears as a focal area of decreased signal intensity due to magnetic susceptibility effects caused by the presence of hemosiderin and methemoglobin deposits.

of the lesion, if possible. Despite the lack of apparent feeding vessels, bleeding can occasionally be brisk if the center of the malformation is entered before circumferential dissection.[81] Once devascularized, the intracapsular contents of the malformation are removed in a piecemeal fashion. The remaining portions of the lesion are then dissected from the surface of the brain stem and nerves, rather than attempting to deliver the intact malformation through a small opening. All perforating arterial vessels must be dissected meticulously and preserved.

The goal of surgery must be complete extirpation of the lesion (with reasonable attention to minimize injury to normal brain); several authors have reported symptomatic recurrences and hemorrhages after partial or seemingly complete removal.[4,86] When the cavernous malformation can be excised completely, the risk of further neurological deterioration due to further growth and hemorrhage is eliminated and a cure appears to be permanent.

Finally, the association between cavernous malformations and venous malformations, which may be as high as 16%,[4,59,86] must be remembered. Although the surgical management of cavernous malformations requires that the entire raspberry-like lesion should be removed, interruption of a venous malformation can threaten drainage from normal parenchyma and result in venous infarction.[4] Therefore, when a large venous malformation is encountered in the proximity of a symptomatic cavernous malformation, the surgical approach must be tailored to permit resection of the cavernous malformation while maintaining drainage from the venous malformation.

Surgical Approaches to Brain Stem Cavernous Malformations

The surgical approaches listed below are those that we have found useful for the surgical management of cavernous malformations involving the brain

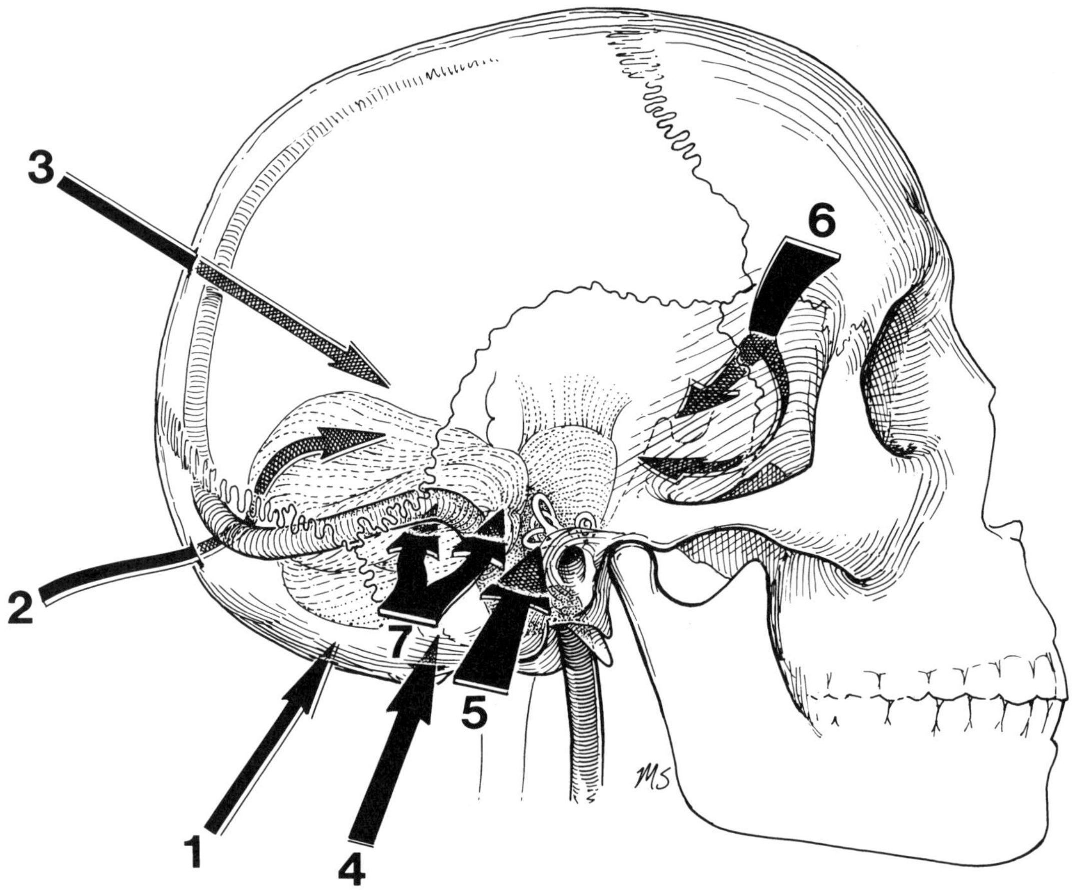

Figure 6. Summary of surgical approaches to cavernous malformations involving the brain stem. These include the (1) suboccipital approach; (2) infratentorial supracerebellar approach; (3) occipital transtentorial approach; (4) far lateral approach; (5) transtemporal approaches; (6) frontotemporal/subtemporal transtentorial approach; and (7) combined petrosal approaches. Reprinted with permission from the Barrow Neurological Institute.

stem (Figure 6). The reader is referred to individual articles for detailed descriptions of the specific operative approaches.

Suboccipital Approach

Cavernous malformations involving the floor of the fourth ventricle and dorsal medulla are easily approached through a standard suboccipital craniotomy (Figures 6, 7A and B).[13,16] Intraoperative ultrasonography may be useful to guide dissection when these lesions are within the cerebellar hemisphere and extend into the brain stem. Malformations of the floor of the fourth ventricle may require separation of the cerebellar tonsils or division of the vermis. It is imperative that the floor of the fourth ventricle be identified as the major regional landmark to avoid unnecessary dissection within the brain stem itself.[16] With this approach, cavernous malformations as far rostral as the dorsal pontine tegmentum can be exposed and resected safely after division of the cerebellar vermis. Although providing excellent exposure of midline posterior lesions, the suboccipital approach provides poor access to ventrally located lesions without significant retraction.

Infratentorial Supracerebellar Approach

The infratentorial supracerebellar approach permits exposure of malformations involving the tectum and pineal region.[71–73] Care must be taken to identify and prevent injury to the vein of Galen, the internal cerebral veins, the basal veins of Rosenthal, and the midbrain branches of the posterior choroidal arteries during dissection within the quadrigeminal cistern. If necessary, further exposure may be achieved by incising the tentorium 1 cm lateral to the straight sinus. Advantages of this approach include adequate exposure of the dorsal midbrain, without violation of normal brain parenchyma as well as avoidance of the deep venous system. The approach is limited by a superolateral extension of the malformation above the tentorium that may be difficult to reach from an infratentorial exposure.

Occipital Transtentorial Approach

The occipital transtentorial approach provides exposure of the superior cerebellar peduncles and vermis, the anterior medullary velum, the posterior third ventricle, the splenium, and the quadrigeminal plate.[33,53,55] Compared to the infratentorial supracerebellar approach, this approach provides broader exposure in the region of the tentorial incisura, without sacrificing normal neurovascular structures.[55] The superior vermis may be divided to allow entry into the fourth ventricle and to expose the superior cerebellar peduncles; opening into the suprapineal recess permits exposure of the third ventricle as far forward as the foramen of Monro.[9] However, the occipital transtentorial approach may require retraction of the occipitoparietal lobe, thereby resulting in sensory or visual field deficits.[73]

Far Lateral Approach

As elaborated by Heros[30] and modified by Spetzler[69] for vertebrobasilar junction aneurysms, the far lateral suboccipital approach provides excellent exposure of the anterior and lateral medulla, cervicomedullary junction, and associated structures. Patient positioning is extremely important to maximize exposure: a modified park-bench position with the ipsilateral mastoid process as the highest point in the operative field is preferred (Figures 8 and 9).

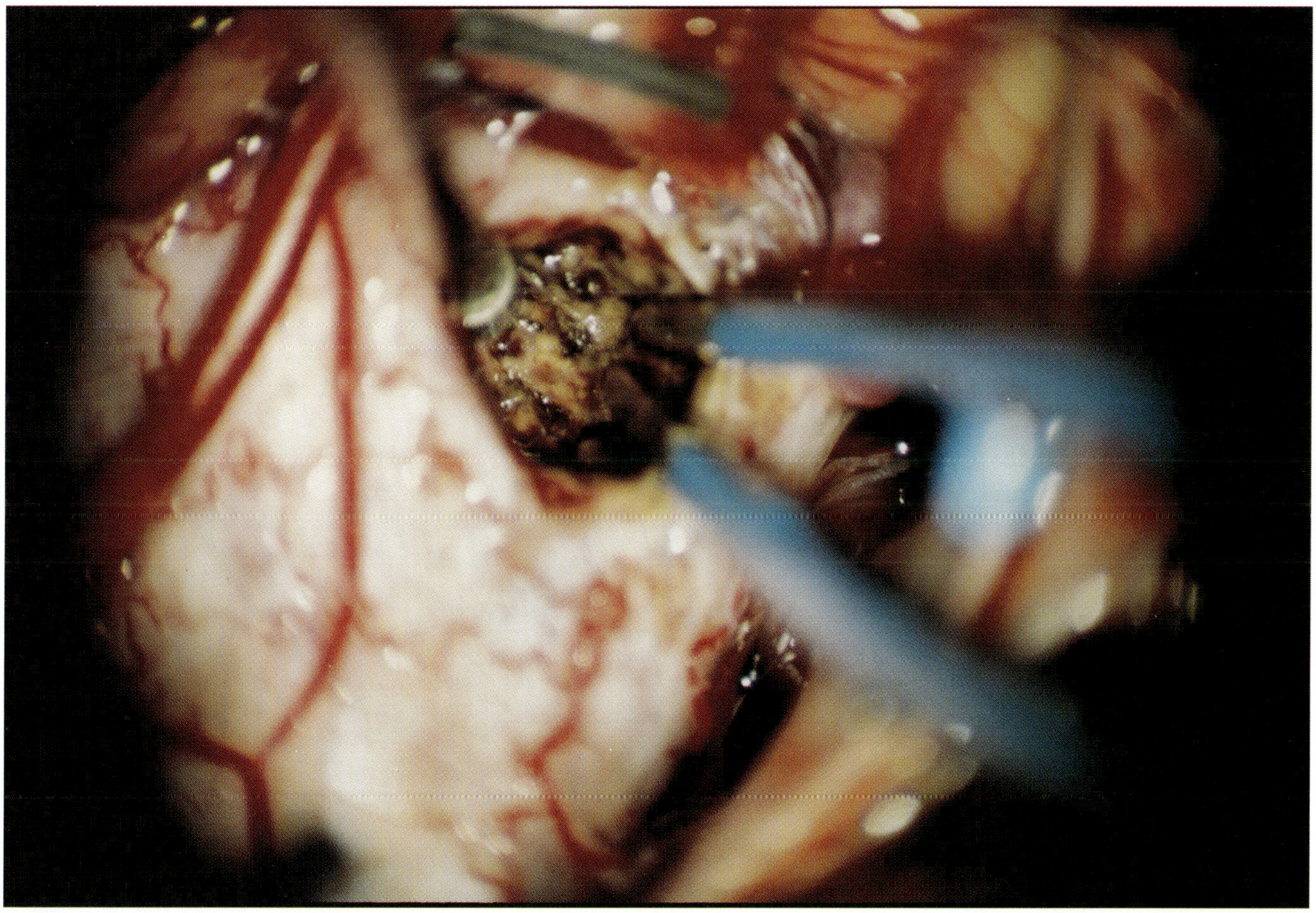

Figure 7. Intraoperative views of a cervicomedullary cavernous malformation exposed by the suboccipital approach (same patient whose magnetic resonance image study is seen in Figure 5). **A.** Initial dissection of the malformation concentrates on separation of the lesion from surrounding gliosis before internal decompression. The intracapsular contents are removed in a piecemeal fashion through as small an opening as is practical. Reprinted with permission from Thieme Medical Publishers. *Continued*

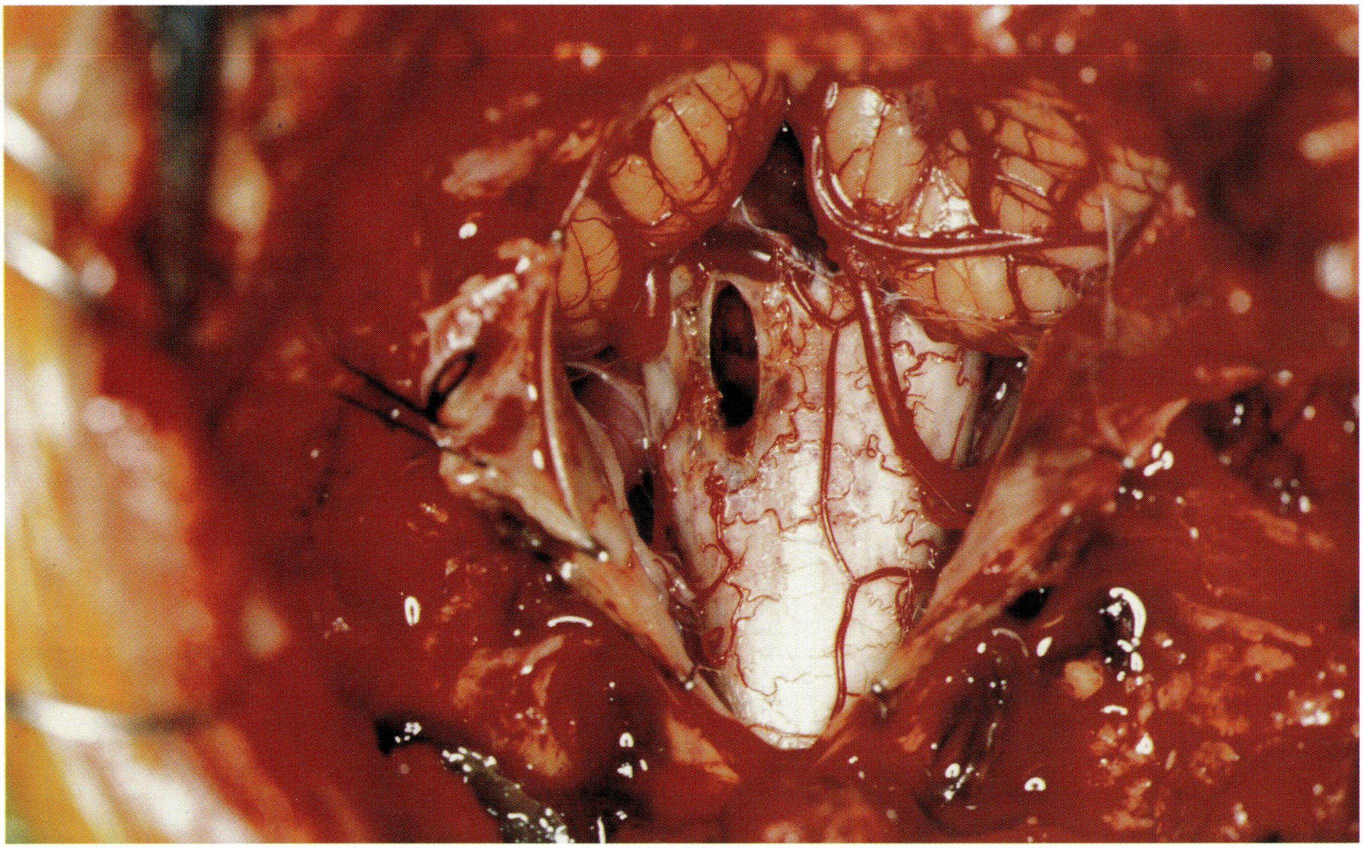

Figure 7B. Intraoperative view after completion of resection. Note the small opening into the brain stem parenchyma required for complete removal as well as the preservation of adjacent vasculature. Reprinted with permission from Thieme Medical Publishers.

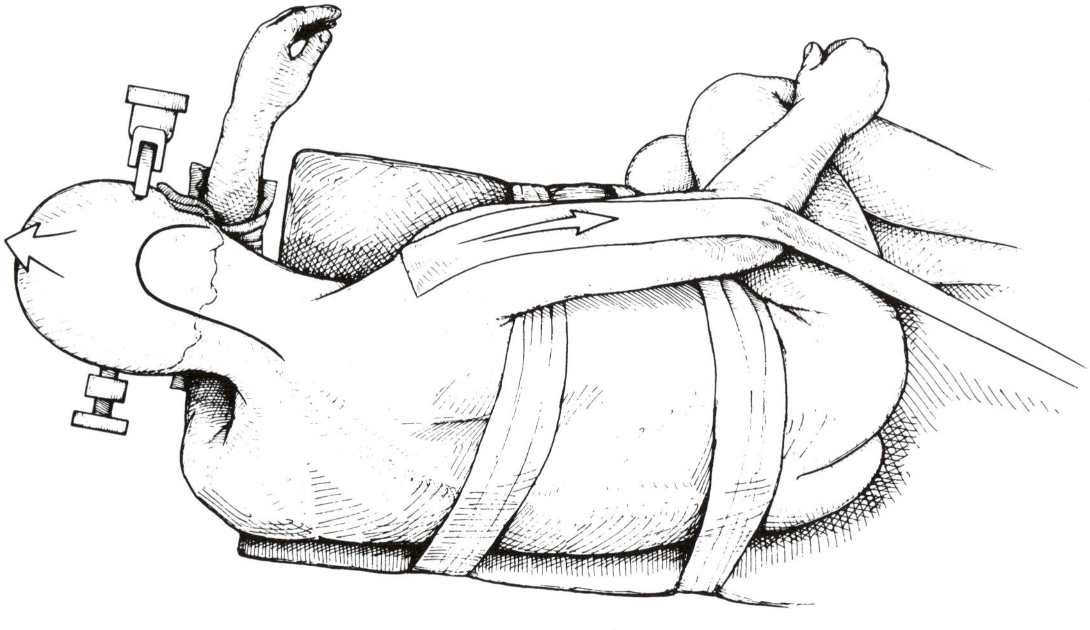

Figure 8. Positioning for the far lateral approach. View is from above (approach for a right-sided lesion). The patient is placed in a modified park-bench position with the cervical spine flexed in the anteroposterior plane, rotated 45° to the left, and flexed laterally 30° to the left. The inverted hockey-stick incision extends along the midline, following the superior nuchal line, and terminates just medial to the mastoid process. Reprinted with permission from the Barrow Neurological Institute.

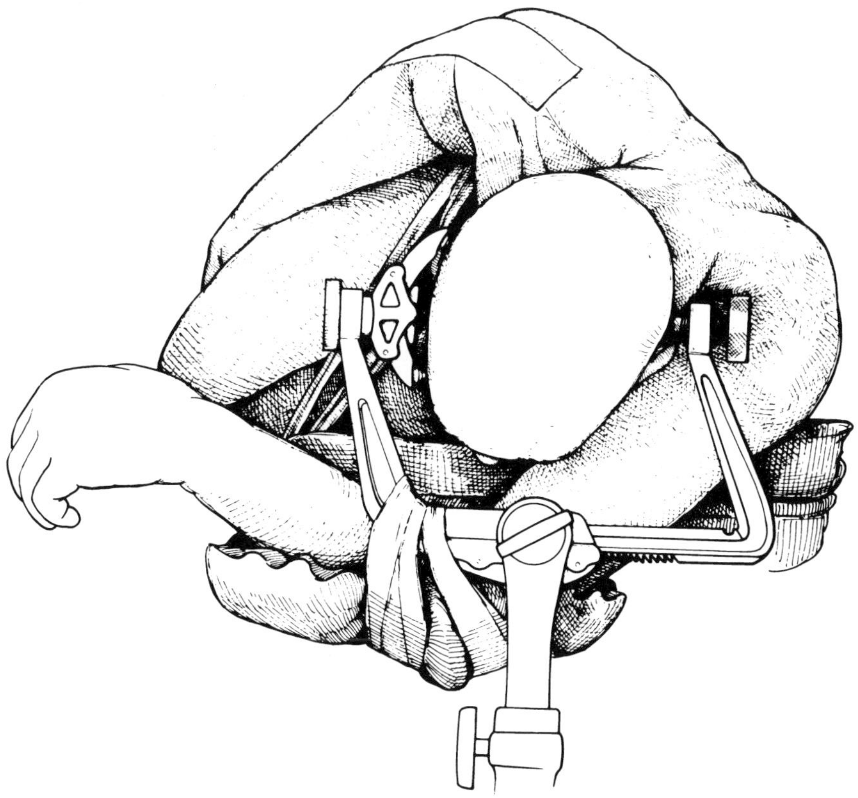

Figure 9. Positioning for the far lateral approach. View is from the cranial vertex. Note how the dependent arm has been padded and cradled beneath the Mayfield head holder. Reprinted with permission from the Barrow Neurological Institute.

In addition, the extreme lateral removal of bone from the lateral mass of C1 and the posterior third of the occipital condyle is the key to providing an unobstructed exposure of the inferior clivus, anterolateral medulla, and cervicomedullary junction without retraction (Figure 10).[30] The advantages to the far lateral approach include the following: (1) an extremely flat approach to the clivus, provided by removal of the occipital condyle, therefore allowing a wide angle of visualization along the skull base; (2) proximal and distal control of the vertebral artery and its branches; (3) excellent visualization of the inferior cranial nerves and the craniovertebral junction; and (4) no retraction of neurovascular structures. However, it is technically challenging and requires expertise with dissection around the vertebral artery.

Transtemporal (Translabyrinthine, Transcochlear, and Transotic) Approaches

The transtemporal approaches provide direct access to lesions in and around the internal auditory meatus and have been well described by Fisch,[21] King,[36] and House and Hitselberger.[32] These exposures would be ideally suited for the patient with a cavernous malformation involving the pontomedullary junction who has already lost serviceable hearing. The exposures are based on removal of bone, not cerebellar retraction, and the course of the facial nerve is identified early in the procedure to ensure its protection. These procedures can also be combined to permit access to the anterior pons or combined with a retrosigmoid approach to improve exposure of the lateral pontomedullary junction.[24] These exposures shorten the working distance to the brain stem and provide adequate exposure of the anterolateral pontomedullary junction without brain retraction or transgression of septic spaces. Disadvantages include hearing loss and temporary paralysis of the facial nerve after its transposition, as occur with the transcochlear approach.

Frontotemporal/Subtemporal Transtentorial Approach

Cavernous malformations involving the anterior midbrain–interpeduncular fossa region can be approached through a frontotemporal or a subtemporal

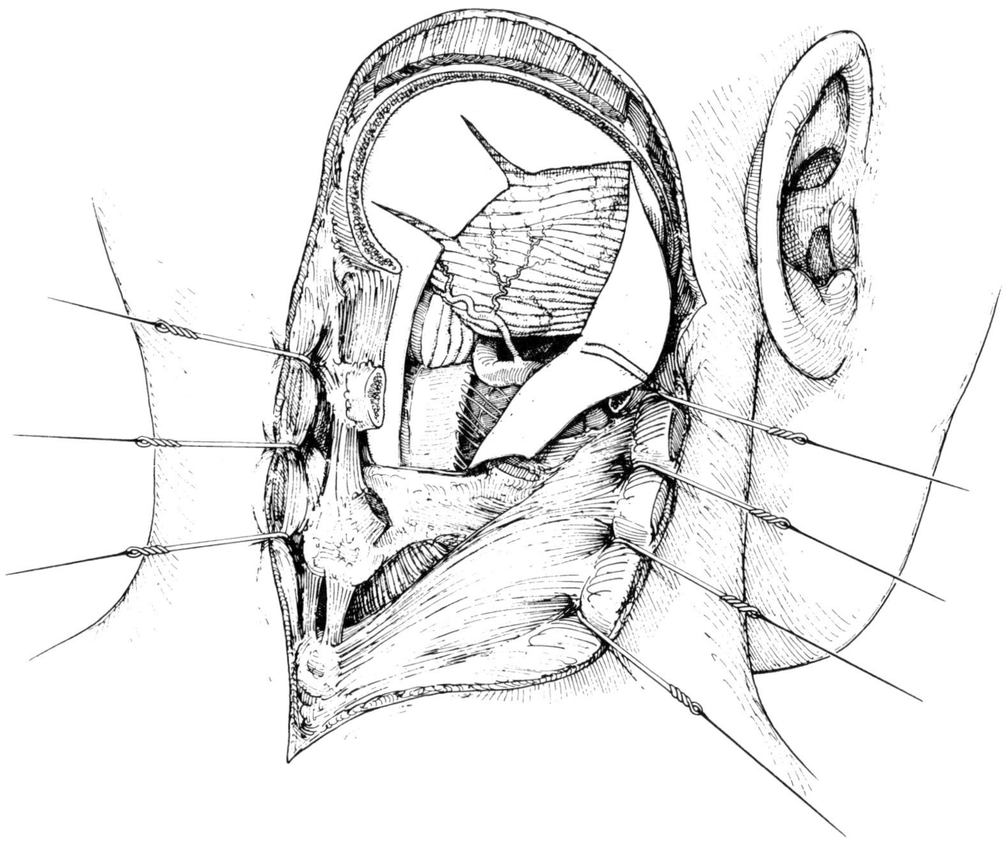

Figure 10. Intraoperative view of the far lateral approach after durotomy has been performed. Far lateral suboccipital bone removal allows for lateral retraction of the vertebral artery after the dura is tented, exposing the cerebellar hemisphere, inferior clivus, anterolateral medulla, and cervicomedullary junction with minimal retraction. Reprinted with permission from the Barrow Neurological Institute.

craniotomy, the details of which have been well described by Yasargil.[80,82] Wide splitting of the Sylvian fissure through a frontotemporal craniotomy combined with division of the medial tentorium will permit excellent exposure of the bilateral cerebral peduncles, interpeduncular cistern, posterior third ventricular floor, and associated neurovascular structures. Extended exposure of lesions located high in the interpeduncular fossa can be achieved by removal of the zygomatic arch and posterior ridge of the frontal process of the zygoma, as well as by intradural removal of the posterior clinoid process.[15,22] Although they require a certain degree of retraction, these approaches allow delineation of the cranial nerves of the anterolateral upper brain stem and associated blood supply in a direct fashion.

Combined (Petrosal) Approaches

The combined approaches include a combination of subtemporal, transtentorial, and retrosigmoid approaches that provides excellent exposure of the lateral upper two-thirds of the brain stem without retracting the brain, sacrificing hearing, or endangering the facial nerve. The approach, as originally described by Malis,[39] includes division of the sigmoid sinus distal to the vein of Labbé. As modified by Spetzler,[68] the procedure includes ligation of the superior petrosal sinus and division of the sigmoid sinus inferiorly to the sinodural angle (Figures 11–13). Therefore, to avoid venous infarction, a prerequisite to either of these maneuvers is good quality, bilateral, venous phase angiography demonstrating transverse sinuses that communicate through a widely patent torcular as well as through an intact contralateral sigmoid sinus, jugular bulb, and internal jugular vein. After the ipsilateral sigmoid sinus has been divided, the ipsilateral vein of Labbé then drains through the medial portion of the lateral sinus and across the torcular through the opposite jugular vein (Figure 11).

Mastoidectomy is initially performed followed

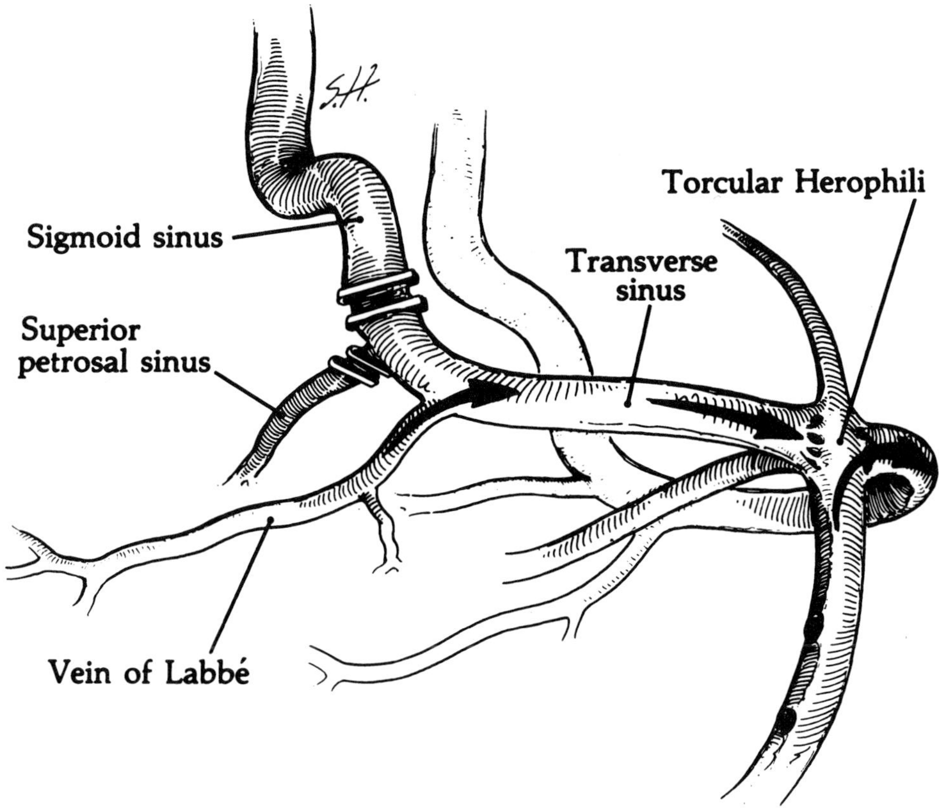

Figure 11. Schematic diagram of the major veins and dural venous sinuses to be considered in the combined (petrosal) approaches. Orientation is as seen by the surgeon; the top of the figure is inferior anatomically and the right of the figure corresponds to posterior anatomically. Before ligating the sigmoid sinus, a widely patent torcular and contralateral jugular venous system must be demonstrated angiographically. This allows the vein of Labbé to drain through the medial lateral sinus and across the torcular through the opposite jugular vein. Reprinted with permission of the Barrow Neurological Institute.

by a subtemporal–retrosigmoid craniotomy extending both above and below the tentorium. Bone is then removed over the sigmoid sinus from the sinodural angle down to the jugular bulb. After durotomy, incision of the tentorium from the superior petrosal sinus to the hiatus allows for excellent exposure of the lateral brain stem as well as of the anterior and superior surfaces of the cerebellum.

The petrosal approach, as described by Al-Mefty,[1,2] involves more extensive drilling of the temporal bone. After mastoidectomy and complete exposure of the sigmoid sinus, the superior petrosal sinus is clipped and divided. The dura is opened both posteriorly and anteriorly to the sigmoid sinus. The dural incision is then extended through the tentorium to the incisura. In this fashion, the surgeon can alter the field of view between the supra- and the infratentorial routes without transecting the sinus.

These approaches afford excellent exposure of the anterolateral brain stem down to the level of the foramen magnum (Figure 13). The advantages of these approaches, which are especially suited for large malformations involving extensive areas of the anterolateral brain stem, are as follows: (1) minimal retraction is required; (2) the operative field to the brain stem is shortened by extensive bone removal; (3) the approach permits a direct line of sight to the anterolateral brain stem; (4) the vestibular and auditory apparati are preserved; (5) the vein of Labbé is preserved; and (6) multiple angles for dissection between the cranial nerves are provided.[1]

Other Combined Approaches

Limitations of exposure associated with any one of the preceding approaches can easily be overcome by using a combination of approaches. Combined suboccipital-petrosal, retroauricular and preauricular transpetrosal-transtentorial, anterior transpetrosal-transtentorial, and suboccipital-translabyrinthine approaches, which have all been described for

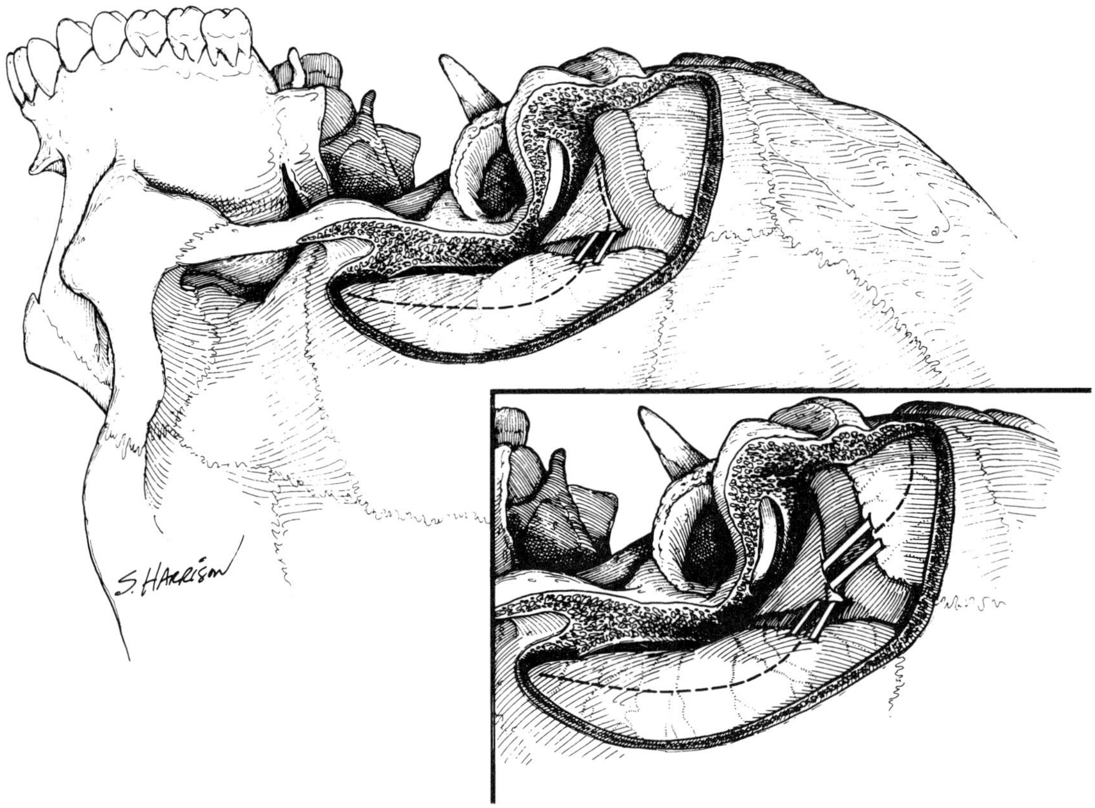

Figure 12. Right combined (petrosal) approach. After completion of craniotomy and further bone removal, a durotomy is performed along the floor of the middle cranial fossa and the superior petrosal sinus is ligated and divided. As described by Al-Mefty,[1,2] the dural opening is continued just anterior to the sigmoid sinus and the jugular bulb to the sinodural angle, preserving the sigmoid sinus. **Inset:** Alternatively, as described by Spetzler et al.,[68] if adequate collateral venous drainage can be demonstrated, the sigmoid sinus can be divided inferiorly to the sinodural angle. Reprinted with permission of the Barrow Neurological Institute.

resection of cerebellopontine angle and clival tumors to maximize exposure and to minimize brain retraction, are also applicable to cavernous malformations of the anterolateral brain.[23,25,27,31,34] With a combination of far lateral suboccipital, translabyrinthine, subtemporal, and transtentorial approaches (referred to as the *extensive combined* or the *far lateral-combined* approach), the entire anterior and lateral brain stem and craniovertebral junction with excellent exposure of the cranial nerves and associated vascular structures can be visualized (Spetzler, unpublished data).

Selection of the Appropriate Surgical Approach

Surgical management of cavernous malformations involving the deep cerebellum and brain stem remains a formidable challenge. The myriad of approaches described in the literature emphasizes that no one approach is perfect for all cases. Therefore, each approach or combination of approaches has its own advantages and disadvantages that necessitate individualization of every case.

MR imaging in the axial, coronal, and sagittal planes and (most recently) three-dimensional reconstructions utilizing computer-assisted parallel processing has proven invaluable in preoperative localization and in selection of the most advantageous surgical route. Individual evaluation must be performed to determine if a corridor to the malformation through noneloquent brain is available, if the potential resulting neurological deficits would be acceptable, and if the risks preclude operative intervention. Finally, factors such as pre-existing neurological deficits, the presence of co-existing cerebrovascular mal-

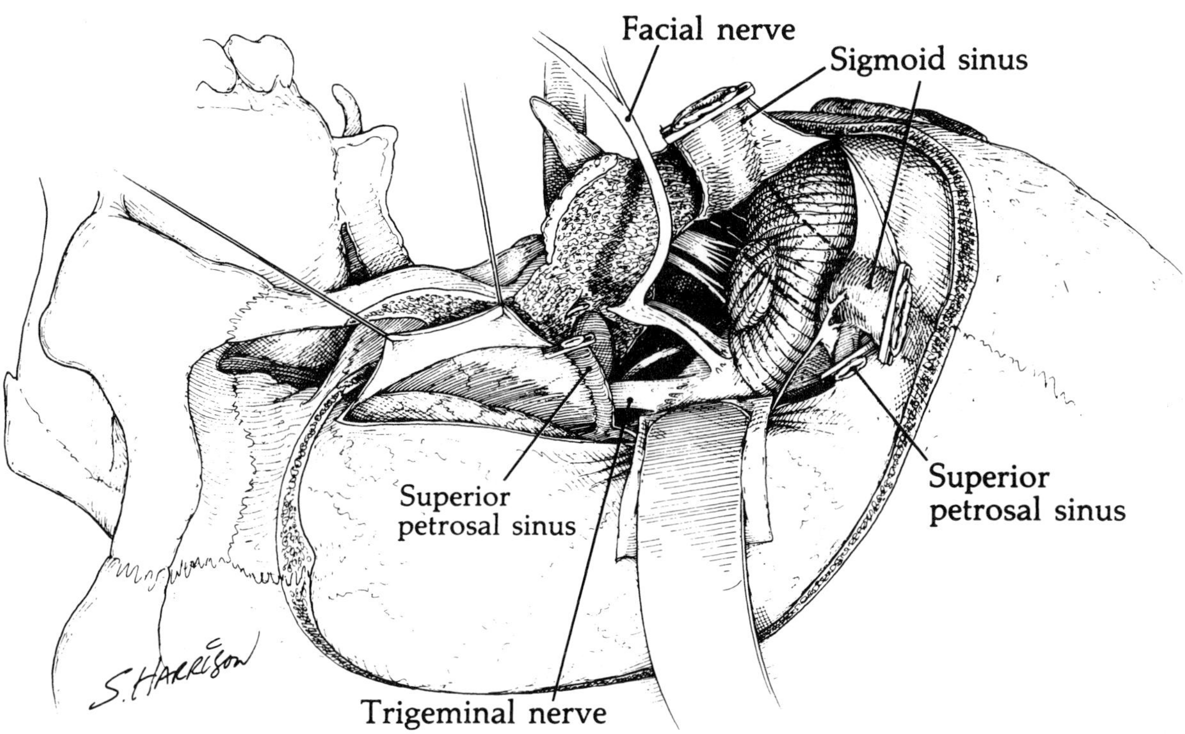

Figure 13. Right combined (petrosal) approach, after durotomy with ligation of the superior petrosal and sigmoid sinuses. Division of the tentorium allows the vein of the Labbé to be retracted superiorly with the tentorial leaflets. This affords excellent exposure of the anterolateral brain stem down to the foramen magnum with the protection of the vein of Labbé and a minimum of brain retraction. Reprinted with permission of the Barrow Neurological Institute.

formations, and the presence of existing bone defects as a result of previous procedures (as well as location, size, and relationship of the cavernous malformation to the brain stem surface) must all be considered in choosing the appropriate avenue of surgical attack.

Results of Surgical Management of Infratentorial Cavernous Malformations

Previously published reports have suggested that an aggressive surgical approach to the treatment of symptomatic cavernous malformations of the infratentorial space can provide favorable results.[3,4,19,29,37,40,48,51,52,65,75,77,79,81,83,86] Since 1985 the senior author (RFS) has operated on 64 intracranial cavernous malformations, of which 21 (31%) involved the brain stem. Operative indications for this series of patients included (1) progressive symptomatology, (2) superficial location of the malformation within the brain stem, and (3) an operative approach that could spare eloquent brain tissue.[86]

The average age of these 13 females and 8 males was 37.0 ± 13.4 years (range, 14 to 71 years). Of the 21 patients, 18 (86%) described acute onset of symptomatology suggestive of an apoplectic event. Neurological deficits at the time of operation are delineated in Table 1. Nine of these patients had at least one additional lesion scattered elsewhere throughout the neuraxis; 6 of these patients had other family members with cavernous malformations in accordance with a familial inheritance pattern.

The location of the malformations and the surgical approaches employed to effect their resection are shown in Table 2. The average size of the lesion in this series was 1.6 ± 1.1 cm (range, 0.4 to 4.0 cm). Two patients also had an associated venous angioma, which required modifying the surgical approach in one case. An arachnoid cyst and an arteriovenous malformation unrelated to the cavernous malformation were observed in one patient each. Complete resection (as judged by intraoperative findings as well as postoperative MR imaging) was possible in 18 of the 21 cases (86%). An estimated 90% to 95% resection was achieved in the remaining three cases. Histopathological examination revealed acute or subacute thrombus in 62% and hemosiderin in 90% of the sur-

Table 2
Location and Surgical Approach Used in 21 Patients with Brain Stem Cavernous Malformations

Location		*Number of Patients*
Midbrain Tectum		3 (14%)
Supracerebellar infratentorial approach	2	
Occipital transtentorial approach	1	
Midbrain Tegmentum		1 (5%)
Combined approach		
Midbrain Crura Cerebri		1 (5%)
Fronto-subtemporal transtentorial approach		
Pontomesencephalic Junction		2 (10%)
Supracerebellar infratentorial approach	1	
Fronto-subtemporal transtentorial approach	1	
Pontine Tegmentum		
A. Midline		6 (29%)
Suboccipital splitting of vermis	6	
B. Lateral		2 (10%)
Combined approach	2	
Basis Pontis		2 (10%)
Subtemporal transtentorial approach	1	
Fronto-subtemporal transtentorial approach	1	
Pontomedullary Junction		1 (5%)
Combined approach		
Medulla		1 (5%)
Far lateral approach		
Cervicomedullary Junction		2 (10%)
Suboccipital approach + C1-C2 laminectomies	2	

Table 3
Complications Related to Surgical Management of 21 Patients with Brain Stem Cavernous Malformations

Complications	*Number of Patients*
Transient	
Hemiparesis	5 (24%)
Diplopia, disorder of ocular motility	4 (19%)
VI, VII cranial nerve neuropathy	4 (19%)
Hydrocephalus, shunt failure	3 (14%)
Meningitis	2 (10%)
Lower extremity deep venous thrombosis	2 (10%)
Gait ataxia	1 (5%)
IX, X, XI, XII cranial nerve neuropathy	2 (10%)
Cerebrospinal fluid leak	1 (5%)
Permanent	
Dysmetria + internuclear ophthalmoplegia	2 (10%)
Partial III cranial nerve neuropathy	1 (5%)
Mild upper and lower extremity dysmetria	1 (5%)
Mild internuclear ophthalmoplegia	1 (5%)

gical specimens, indicating the propensity of these lesions to hemorrhage and rehemorrhage.

Median follow-up was 26 ± 22 months. Table 3 lists the neurological deficits appearing after or exacerbated by surgery. Transient complications refer to neurological deficits that resolved completely on follow-up examinations. Overall, there was no mortality, no major morbidity, and a permanent minor morbidity related to surgery of 24%. At the last follow-up, 20 of the 21 patients were significantly improved compared to their preoperative neurological status. Using appropriate individualized planning and case selection and using the surgical indications, approaches, and principles described above, symptomatic superficial cavernous malformations of the brain stem can be completely removed with minimal morbidity.

References

1. Al-Mefty O. Surgical exposure of petroclival tumors. In Wilkins RH, Rengachary SS (eds): Neurosurgery Update I. Diagnosis, Operative Technique, and Neuro-Oncology. New York: McGraw Hill, 1990, pp 409–414.
2. Al-Mefty O, Fox JL, Smith RR. Petrosal approach for petroclival meningiomas. Neurosurgery 22:510–517, 1988.
3. Bellotti C, Medina M, Oliveri G, Barrale S, et al. Cystic cavernous angiomas of the posterior fossa: Report of three cases. J Neurosurg 63:797–799, 1985.
4. Bertalanffy H, Gilsbach JM, Eggert HR, et al. Microsurgery of deep-seated cavernous angiomas: Report of 26 cases. Acta Neurochir (Wien) 108:91–99, 1991.
5. Bicknell JM. Familial cavernous angioma of the brain stem dominantly inherited in Hispanics. Neurosurgery 24:102–105, 1989.
6. Bicknell JM, Carlow TJ, Kornfeld M, et al. Familial cavernous angiomas. Arch Neurol 35:746–749, 1978.
7. Chin D, Harper C. Angiographically occult cerebral vascular malformations with abnormal computed tomography. Surg Neurol 20:138–142, 1983.
8. Clark JV. Familial occurence of cavernous angiomata of the brain. J Neurol Neurosurg Psychiatry 33:871–876, 1970.
9. Clark K. The occipital transtentorial approach to the pineal region. In Schmidek HH, Sweet WH (eds): Operative Neurosurgical Techniques. Indications, Methods,

and Results (2nd ed, vol 1), Orlando, FL: Grune & Stratton, 1988, pp 411–422.
10. Cohen HCM, Tucker WS, Humphreys RP, et al. Angiographically cryptic histologically verified cerebrovascular malformations. Neurosurgery 10:704–714, 1982.
11. Crawford JV, Russell DS. Cryptic arteriovenous and venous hamartomas of the brain. J Neurol Neurosurg Psychiatry 19:1–11, 1956.
12. Davis DH, Kelly PJ. Stereotactic resection of occult vascular malformations. J Neurosurg 72:698–702, 1990.
13. De Oliveira E, Rhoton AL Jr, Peace D. Microsurgical anatomy of the region of the foramen magnum. Surg Neurol 24:293–352, 1985.
14. Del Curling O Jr, Kelly DL Jr, Elster AD, et al. An analysis of the natural history of cavernous angiomas. J Neurosurg 75:702–708, 1991.
15. Dolenc VV, Skrap M, Sustersic J, Skrbec M, et al. A transcavernous-transsellar approach to the basilar tip aneurysms. Br J Neurosurg 1:251–259, 1987.
16. Duckworth J, Schmidek HH. Surgical management of posterior fossa tumors. In Schmidek HH, Sweet WH (eds): Operative Neurosurgical Techniques. Indications, Methods and Results (2nd ed, vol 1). Orlando, FL: Grune & Stratton, 1988, pp 653–664.
17. Ebeling JD, Tranmer BI, Davis KA, et al. Thrombosed arteriovenous malformations: A type of occult vascular malformation. Magnetic resonance imaging and histopathological correlations. Neurosurgery 23:605–610, 1988.
18. El-Gohary EM, Tomita T, Gutierrez FA, et al. Angiographically occult vascular malformations in childhood. Neurosurgery 20:759–766, 1987.
19. Fahlbusch R, Strauss C, Huk W, et al. Surgical removal of pontomesencephalic cavernous hemangiomas. Neurosurgery 26:449–457, 1990.
20. Farmer JP, Cosgrove GR, Villemure JG, et al. Intracerebral cavernous angiomas. Neurology 38:1699–1704, 1988.
21. Fisch U, Mattox D. Microsurgery of the Skull Base. New York: Thieme Medical, 1988.
22. Fujitsu K, Kuwabara T. Zygomatic approach for lesions in the interpeduncular cistern. J Neurosurg 62: 340–343, 1985.
23. Glasscock ME III, Gulya AJ, Pensak ML. Surgery of the posterior fossa. Otolaryngol Clin North Am 17(3): 483–497, 1984.
24. Glasscock ME III, Hays JW, Jackson CG, et al. A one-stage combined approach for the management of large cerebellopontine angle tumors. Laryngoscope 88: 1563–1576, 1978.
25. Glasscock ME III, Miller GW, Drake FD, et al. Surgery of the skull base. Laryngoscope 88:905–923, 1978.
26. Gomori JM, Grossman RI, Goldberg HI, et al. Occult cerebral vascular malformations: High-field MR imaging. Radiology 158:707–713, 1986.
27. Hakuba A, Nishimura S, Jang BJ. A combined retroauricular and preauricular transpetrosal-transtentorial approach to clivus meningiomas. Surg Neurol 30: 108–116, 1988.
28. Hayman LA, Evans RA, Ferrell RE, et al. Familial cavernous angiomas: Natural history and genetic study over a 5-year period. Am J Med Genet 11:147–160, 1982.
29. Heffez DS, Zinreich SJ, Long DM. Surgical resection of intrinsic brain stem lesions: An overview. Neurosurgery 27:789–798, 1990.
30. Heros RC. Lateral suboccipital approach for vertebral and vertebrobasilar artery lesions. J Neurosurg 64: 559–562, 1986.
31. Hitselberger WE, House WF. A combined approach to the cerebellopontine angle: A suboccipital petrosal approach. Arch Otolaryngol 84:267–285, 1966.
32. House WF, Hitselberger WE. The transcochlear approach to the skull base. Arch Otolaryngol 102: 334–342, 1976.
33. Jamieson KG. Excision of pineal tumors. J Neurosurg 35:550–553, 1971.
34. Kawase T, Shiobara R, Toya S. Anterior transpetrosal-transtentorial approach for sphenopetroclival meningiomas: Surgical method and results in 10 patients. Neurosurgery 28:869–876, 1991.
35. Kidd HA, Cumings JN. Cerebral angiomata in an Icelandic family. Lancet 1:747–748, 1947.
36. King TT, Morrison AW. Translabyrinthine operation for the removal of acoustic nerve tumors. In Schmidek HH, Sweet WH (eds): Operative Neurosurgical Techniques. Indications, Methods and Results (2nd ed, vol 1). Orlando, FL: Grune & Stratton, 1988, pp 685–704.
37. LeDoux MS, Aronin PA, Odrezin GT. Surgically treated cavernous angiomas of the brain stem: Report of two cases and review of the literature. Surg Neurol 35:395–399, 1991.
38. Lobato RD, Perez C, Rivas JJ, et al. Clinical, radiological, and pathological spectrum of angiographically occult intracranial vascular malformations: Analysis of 21 cases and review of the literature. J Neurosurg 68: 518–531, 1988.
39. Malis LI. Surgical resection of tumors of the skull base. In Wilkins RH, Rengachary SS (eds): Neurosurgery. New York: McGraw Hill, 1985, pp 1011–1021.
40. Mangiardi JR. The surgical management of brainstem hematomas. Perspect Neurolog Surg 2(1):33–48, 1991.
41. Martin NA, Wilson CB, Stein BM. Venous and cavernous malformations. In Wilson CB, Stein BM (eds): Intracranial Arteriovenous Malformations. Baltimore: Williams & Wilkins, 1984, pp 234–245.
42. Mason I, Aase JM, Orrison WW, et al. Familial cavernous angiomas of the brain in an Hispanic family. Neurology 38:324–326, 1988.
43. McCormick PC, Michelsen WJ. Management of intracranial cavernous and venous malformations. In Barrow DL (ed): Intracranial Vascular Malformations. Neurosurgical Topics, Park Ridge, IL: American Association of Neurological Surgeons, 1990, pp 197–217.
44. McCormick WF. The pathology of vascular ("arteriovenous") malformations. J Neurosurg 24:807–816, 1966.
45. McCormick WF. Classification, pathology, and natural history of angiomas of the central nervous system. Weekly update. Neurol Neurosurg 1(14):1–7, 1978.
46. McCormick WF. Vascular disorders of nervous tissue: Anomalies, malformations, and aneurysms. In Bourne GE (ed): Structure and Function of Nervous Tissue. Vol III, Biochemistry and Disease. New York: Academic Press, 1969, pp 537–596.
47. McCormick WF. Pathology of vascular malformations of the brain. In Wilson CB, Stein BM (eds): Intracranial Arteriovenous Malformations. Baltimore: Williams & Wilkins, 1984, pp 44–63.
48. McCormick WF, Hardman JM, Boulter TR. Vascular malformations ("angiomas") of the brain, with special reference to those occurring in the posterior fossa. J Neurosurg 28:241–251, 1968.

49. McCormick WF, Nofzinger JD. "Cryptic" vascular malformations of the central nervous system. J Neurosurg 24:865–875, 1966.
50. Mizutani T, Goldberg HI, Kerson LA, et al. Cavernous hemangioma in the diencephalon. Arch Neurol 38: 379–382, 1981.
51. Ondra SL, Doty JR, Mahla ME, et al. Surgical excision of a cavernous hemangioma of the rostral brain stem: Case report. Neurosurgery 23:490–493, 1988.
52. Pendl G, Vorkapic P, Koniyama M. Microsurgery of midbrain lesions. Neurosurgery 26:641–648, 1990.
53. Poppen JL. The right occipital approach to a pinealoma. J Neurosurg 25:706–710, 1966.
54. Pozzati E, Giuliani G, Nuzzo G, et al. The growth of cerebral cavernous angiomas. Neurosurgery 25:92–97, 1989.
55. Reid WS, Clark WK. Comparison of the infratentorial and transtentorial approaches to the pineal region. Neurosurgery 3(1):1–8, 1978.
56. Rigamonti D. Natural history of cavernous malformations, capillary malformations (telangiectases), and venous malformations. In Barrow DL (ed): Intracranial Vascular Malformations. Neurosurgical Topics, Park Ridge: IL, American Association of Neurological Surgeons, 1990, pp 45–51.
57. Rigamonti D, Drayer BP, Johnson PC, et al. The MRI appearance of cavernous malformations (angiomas). J Neurosurg 67:518–524, 1987.
58. Rigamonti D, Hadley MN, Drayer BP, et al. Cerebral cavernous malformations: Incidence and familial occurrence. N Engl J Med 319(6):343–347, 1988.
59. Rigamonti D, Spetzler RF. The association of venous and cavernous malformations: Report of four cases and discussion of the pathophysiological, diagnostic, and therapeutic implications. Acta Neurochir (Wien) 92: 100–105, 1988.
60. Robinson JR Jr, Little JR, Awad IA. The natural history of cavernous angiomas (abstract). J Neurosurg 72:333A, 1990.
61. Robinson JR, Awad IA, Little JR. Natural history of the cavernous angioma. J Neurosurg 75:709–714, 1991.
62. Runnels JB, Gifford DB, Forsberg PL, et al. Dense calcification in a large cavernous angioma: Case report. J Neurosurg 30:293–298, 1969.
63. Russell DS, Rubinstein LJ: Pathology of Tumours of the Nervous System (5th ed). Baltimore: Williams & Wilkins, 1989.
64. Rutka JT, Brant-Zawadzki M, Wilson CB, et al. Familial cavernous malformations. Diagnostic potential of magnetic resonance imaging. Surg Neurol 29:467–474, 1988.
65. Saito N, Yamakawa K, Sasaki T, et al. Intramedullary cavernous angioma with trigeminal neuralgia: A case report and review of the literature. Neurosurgery 25: 97–101, 1989.
66. Shuey HM Jr, Day AL, Quisling RG, et al. Angiographically cryptic cerebrovascular malformations. Neurosurgery 5:476–479, 1979.
67. Simard JM, Garcia-Bengochea F, Ballinger WE Jr, et al. Cavernous angioma: A review of 126 collected and 12 new clinical cases. Neurosurgery 18:162–172, 1986.
68. Spetzler RF, Daspit CP, Pappas CTE. The combined supra- and infratentorial approach for lesions of the petrous and clival regions: Experience with 46 cases. J Neurosurg 76:588–599, 1992.
69. Spetzler RF, Grahm TW. The far-lateral approach to the inferior clivus and the upper cervical region: Technical note. BNI Quarterly 6(4):35–38, 1990.
70. Steiger HJ, Tew JM Jr. Hemorrhage and epilepsy in cryptic cerebrovascular malformations. Arch Neurol 41:722–724, 1984.
71. Stein BM. The infratentorial supracerebellar approach to pineal lesions. J Neurosurg 35:197–202, 1971.
72. Stein BM. Supracerebellar approach for pineal region neoplasms. In Schmidek HH, Sweet WH (eds): Operative Neurosurgical Techniques. Indications, Methods and Results (2nd ed, vol 1). Orlando: FL, Grune & Stratton, 1988, pp 401–409.
73. Stein BM, Bruce JN, Fetell MR. Surgical approaches to pineal tumors. In Wilkins RH, Rengachary SS (eds): Neurosurgery Update I. Diagnosis, Operative Technique, and Neuro-Oncology. New York: McGraw-Hill, 1990, pp 389–398.
74. Tagle P, Huete I, Mendez J, et al. Intracranial cavernous angioma: Presentation and management. J Neurosurg 64:720–723, 1986.
75. Vaquero J, Carrillo R, Cabezudo J, et al. Cavernous angiomas of the pineal region: Report of two cases. J Neurosurg 53:833–835, 1980.
76. Vaquero J, Leunda G, Martinez R, et al. Cavernomas of the brain. Neurosurgery 12:208–210, 1983.
77. Voight K, Yasargil MG. Cerebral cavernous haemangiomas or cavernomas. Incidence, pathology, localization, diagnosis, clinical features and treatment: Review of the literature and report of an unusual case. Neurochirurgia 19:59–68, 1976.
78. Wakai S, Ueda Y, Inoh S, et al. Angiographically occult angiomas: A report of thirteen cases with analysis of the cases documented in the literature. Neurosurgery 17(4):549–556, 1985.
79. Well SM, Tew JM Jr. Surgical management of brain stem vascular malformations. Acta Neurochir (Wien) 105:14–23, 1990.
80. Yasargil MG. Microneurosurgery. I. Microsurgical Anatomy of the Basal Cisterns and Vessels of the Brain, Diagnostic Studies, General Operative Techniques and Pathological Considerations of the Intracranial Aneurysms. New York: Thieme Medical, 1984.
81. Yasargil MG. Microneurosurgery. IIIB. AVM of the Brain, Clinical Considerations, General and Special Operative Techniques, Surgical Results, Nonoperated Cases, Cavernous and Venous Angiomas, Neuroanesthesia. New York: Thieme Medical, 1988.
82. Yasargil MG, Mortara RW, Curcic M. Meningiomas of basal posterior cranial fossa. In Krayenbuhl H, Brihaye J, Loew F, et al (eds): Advances and Technical Standards in Neurosurgery (vol 7). New York: Springer-Verlag, 1980, pp 4–115.
83. Yoshimoto T, Suzuki J. Radical surgery on cavernous angioma of the brainstem. Surg Neurol 26:72–78, 1986.
84. Zabramski JM, Wascher TM, Johnson B, et al. The natural history of familial cavernous malformations: Results of an ongoing study. J Neurosurg 80:422–432, 1994.
85. Zentner J, Hassler W, Gawehn J, et al. Intramedullary cavernous angiomas. Surg Neurol 31:64–68, 1989.
86. Zimmerman RS, Spetzler RF, Lee KS, et al. Cavernous malformations of the brain stem. J Neurosurg 75:32–39, 1991.

Chapter 7

Multimodality Treatment of Vascular Malformations in Functional Brain Areas, Using Stereotactic Radiosurgery, Embolization, and Microsurgery

Gary K. Steinberg, MD, PhD, Michael P. Marks, MD, Richard P. Levy, MD, PhD, and Jacob I. Fabrikant, MD, PhD

Introduction

Arteriovenous malformations (AVMs) in noncritical cerebral locations, such as the anterior frontal lobe or anterior temporal lobe, can usually be removed using conventional microsurgical techniques with low risks and excellent outcome. However, AVMs in "eloquent" locations, including critical motor, sensory, language or visual cortical regions, brain stem, corpus callosum, thalamus, and basal ganglia, are more difficult to resect safely.[2,4,5,17–19] We have found a staged, multimodality approach using combinations of embolization, microsurgery (often with a stereotactic approach or with intraoperative cortical mapping), and focused stereotactic radiosurgery (Bragg-peak, helium ion) to be extremely useful in treating these difficult AVMs.

Angiographically occult vascular malformations (AOVMs) cause significant morbidity when located in functional brain areas.[1,12,20,22,23,27] The roles of both microsurgery and stereotactic radiosurgery for such lesions have been controversial in the past. Our previous use of both of these modalities has led us to revise our therapeutic approach to AOVMs.

Over the last 10 years, as we gained more experience using these various therapeutic techniques in different combinations, we evolved an individualized and rational approach that is now applied to each patient with an intracranial vascular malformation. We present our past experience and current methodology for treating these difficult malformations in functional brain regions.

Methods

We analyze the angiogram carefully to identify certain angiographic characteristics of AVMs that have been shown to correlate with increased risk of hemorrhage: intranidus aneurysms, central venous drainage, small size, and the absence of angiomatous change (anomalous transcortical arterial supply to the AVM).[13,14] The presence of angiomatous change is also taken into consideration for treatment modality selection, since it has a high correlation with the development of clinical "steal" neurological symptoms and signs, including progressive neurological deficit.[15] Other AVM characteristics, including size, location, and pattern of venous drainage, as well as the patient's age, presenting symptoms, neurological status, and medical condition are factored into treatment planning (since these parameters are predictors

From Yamada S (ed): *Arteriovenous Malformations in Functional Areas of the Brain.*

for risks of microsurgery or radiosurgery).[17,21,25] The patient's preference for a particular treatment modality or combination of modalities is carefully considered in selecting proper treatment.

Between 1981 and 1994 we treated over 600 intracranial vascular malformations located in functional ("eloquent") regions. Approximately 50% of the vascular malformations were located in the brain stem, corpus callosum, thalamus or basal ganglia. The remaining half of these patients had vascular malformations in critical areas of the cerebrum, including motor, sensory, language, or visual cortical areas. The AVM volumes ranged from 0.08 to 288 cm^3 (<8.4 cm diameter) with approximately one-third of the AVMs larger than 25 cm^3 (>3.7 cm diameter). The AOVMs measured between 0.1 and 18 cm^3. About half of the patients were male and half were female. Patients' ages ranged from 1 to 72 years old.

Embolization

Endovascular embolization of AVM nidus or feeding arterial pedicles was performed in approximately 150 patients, with a total of 250 separate procedures. Intraoperative embolization was used in 15 cases. Embolization materials included polyvinyl alcohol (PVA), gel foam, silk, platinum coils, and N-butyl cyanoacrylate (NBCA). Currently, we are using primarily the liquid adhesive, NBCA, for embolization.

Microsurgery

Open (nonstereotactic) microsurgery was used in about 250 cases. A stereotactic approach with the Cosman-Roberts-Wells (CRW) system was used for approximately 80 patients, when the AVM or AOVM was small or subcortical. Intraoperative cortical mapping of motor, sensory, or language areas was used for 15 AVMs, with direct cortical stimulation and EEG recording sometimes in conjunction with median nerve or posterior tibial nerve stimulation; these patients were usually anesthetized and nonparalyzed, but a few patients underwent awake intraoperative cortical mapping.

Stereotactic, Helium Ion Radiosurgery

Four hundred twenty-six patients were treated with Bragg-peak, helium ion radiosurgery (379 AVMs, 47 AOVMs), using doses of 10–45 GyE delivered to treatment volumes of 0.3–70 cm^3. Our treatment methods with the charged-particle radiosurgery method have been described previously.[6,10,11,19,20,21,24,25] Currently, we are using Bragg-peak, proton beam radiosurgery in conjunction with the Proton Facility and the Department of Radiation Medicine at Loma Linda University.

Results

Embolization Only

Eight patients with AVMs in functional areas were cured with endovascular embolization only, resulting in complete angiographic obliteration of the AVM. We have followed these patients clinically and angiographically for 1 month to 4 years after embolization. None of these patients have angiographically recanalized their AVM or suffered a hemorrhage following angiographic obliteration. Seven of these patients had improvement in their preoperative neurological symptoms and signs or remained neurologically normal following embolization; one patient suffered a new aphasia and hemiparesis, but made a good recovery over 6 months; another patient developed a quadrantanopsia following embolization that was still present at 6 months follow-up.

Microsurgery Only

Approximately 125 patients had complete resection of the AVM with microsurgery alone. These were usually small to moderate-sized AVMs (1–3 cm diameter). A stereotactic approach was used in many of these cases. Intraoperative angiography was often used to assess complete AVM resection and a postoperative angiogram, performed at 5–14 days postoperatively, confirmed complete AVM resection in all of these patients. About 85% of these patients had improvement in their preoperative symptoms/signs and remained neurologically normal or unchanged neurologically. While approximately 15% of patients were worsened neurologically by surgery, most of them made excellent recoveries over several weeks to months. No patients re-bled after complete AVM resection.

Radiosurgery Only

Approximately 300 AVM patients were treated solely with radiosurgery. Helium ion radiosurgery alone resulted in complete angiographic AVM obliteration in 80%–85% of patients followed for at least 3 years (Figure 1). Smaller AVMs (<14 cm^3) showed a 3-year complete obliteration rate of 90%–95%, while the larger AVMs (>14 cm^3) demonstrated oblitera-

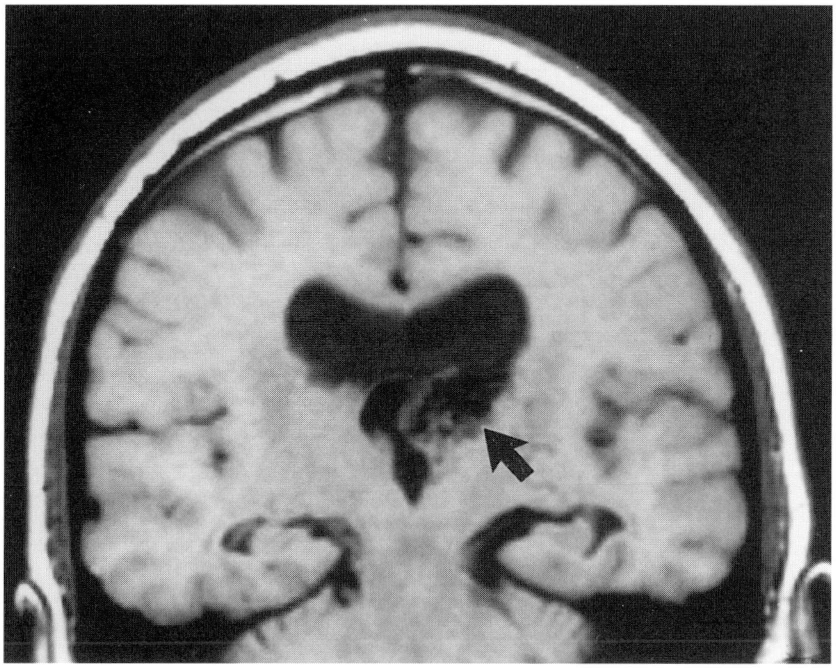

Figure 1. A 29-year-old male who suffered an intraventricular hemorrhage from a left thalamic AVM was treated with helium ion Bragg-peak radiosurgery. **A.** T1-weighted coronal image demonstrating the flow voids present in a left thalamic AVM (arrow). Mild mass effect is present with displacement of the third ventricle noted. *Continued*

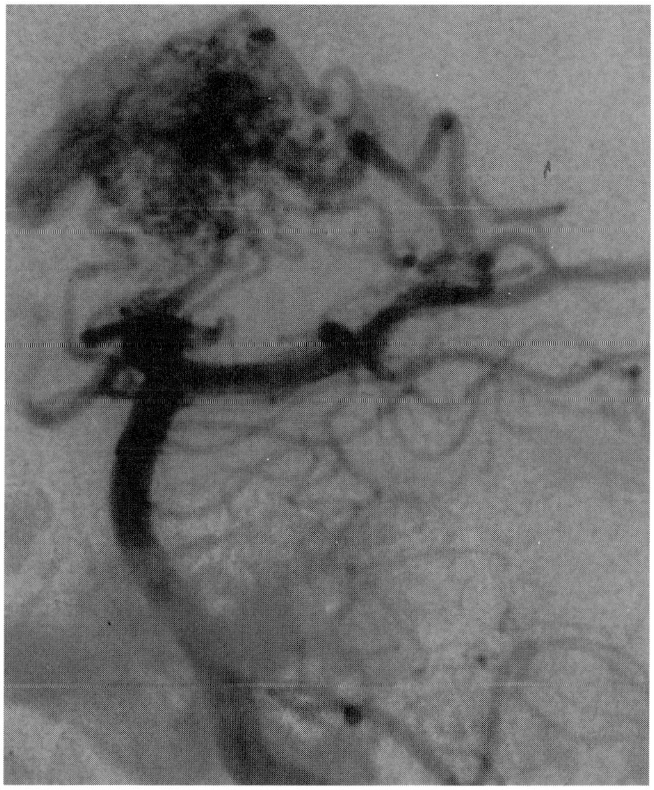

Figure 1B. Left vertebral artery angiogram lateral projection demonstrating a small high-flow AVM with early venous drainage. Multiple thalamoperforating arteries and the medial posterior choroidal artery supply the AVM. *Continued*

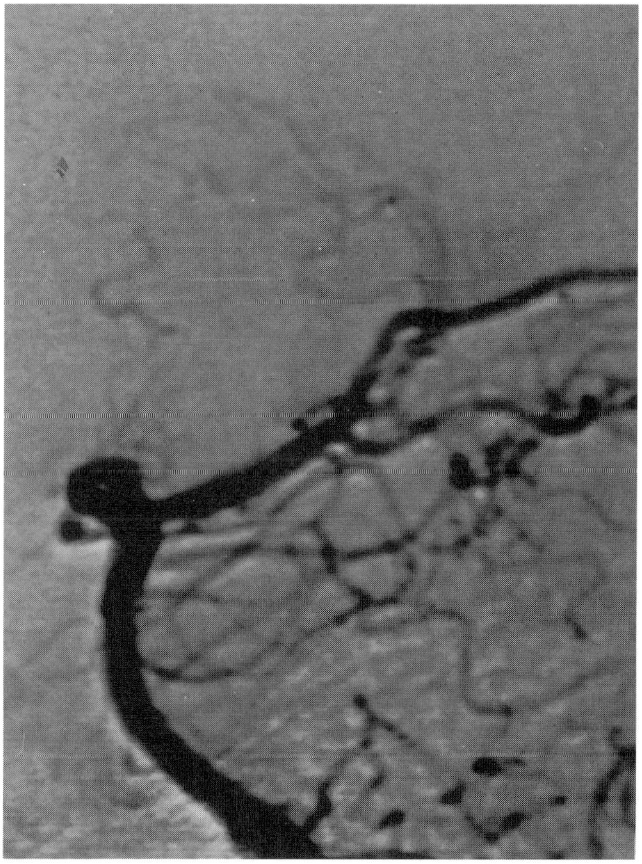

Figure 1C. Left vertebral artery angiogram lateral projection 19 months post treatment with helium ion Bragg-peak radiosurgery (20 GyE to 5100 mm^3) demonstrating complete obliteration of the AVM nidus and arteriovenous shunt. The patient remained neurologically normal.

tion rate of 60%–70% at this time point.[19,21] Obliterations occurred 11–36 months following treatment. With our current dose of 20–25 GyE, about 1%–3% of patients developed new delayed neurological deficits from radiation-induced edema or necrosis; half of these complications were transient or minor. A few patients suffered a hemorrhage from their AVMs before AVM obliteration was complete. Once complete angiographic obliteration of the AVM had been demonstrated, no patient suffered either subsequent recanalization of the AVM or subsequent hemorrhage. Our detailed results of radiosurgical treatment have been documented previously.[6,10,11,19,21]

Embolization Followed by Microsurgery

The combination of embolization followed by microsurgery resulted in complete AVM obliteration in 35 patients harboring AVMs in functional regions (Figure 2). These AVMs measured up to 6 cm diameter. In most cases, the entire AVM (embolized + nonembolized portions) was resected. However, in a few cases portions of AVM thrombosed by embolization alone were not resected. Postoperative angiography at 5–14 days following surgery confirmed complete angiographic AVM obliteration in all patients. No AVMs re-bled or showed recanalization following embolization plus microsurgical resection. Approximately 15% of patients had new neurological deficits following embolization or surgery; however, most deficits were temporary, with recovery over weeks to months.

Embolization Followed by Radiosurgery

Embolization followed by helium ion radiosurgery was used in 30 patients. Although complete long-term follow-up is not available on these patients, total angiographic obliteration was achieved in some. In all cases, only the nonembolized portion of the AVM received radiosurgery. One patient who was embolized with PVA early in our experience, recanalized a portion of the embolized but nonradiated AVM. No AVMs embolized with NBCA and subsequently radiated have recanalized in follow-up angiograms. The AVMs in the embolization/radiosurgery group measured up to 6 cm in diameter. None of the patients with complete angiographic AVM obliteration re-bled or recanalized in long-term follow-up. A few patients suffered re-bleeds after embolization and radiosurgery but before complete AVM thrombosis was achieved.

Embolization Followed by Microsurgery and Radiosurgery

Twenty-five patients underwent staged treatment using initial embolization followed by partial microsurgical resection and, finally, helium ion radiosurgery for the residual AVM. This approach was used for larger AVMs that extended to "eloquent" areas. These AVMs measured up to 7 cm in diameter. In these cases, only angiographically demonstrable residual AVM was irradiated. So far, long-term follow-up is incomplete, but some of these patients have already obliterated the residual irradiated AVM. One patient bled fatally after the combined treatment but before AVM obliteration was complete. Another patient had a minor bleed after surgery, before undergoing radiosurgery.

Microsurgery Followed by Radiosurgery

Partial microsurgical AVM resection followed by radiosurgery was used in 30 patients. The surgical procedure was performed to reduce AVM volume in noncritical areas, leaving a small to moderate-sized AVM in a functional area for treatment with radiosurgery. Some of the AVMs have been completely obliterated with this combination of modalities, but many of these patients have not yet had their 2-year follow-up angiogram.

Microsurgery Followed by Embolization and Radiosurgery

In 10 patients, after partial microsurgical resection, the residual AVM was considered too large for a good response with radiosurgery alone. These patients were treated with endovascular or intraoperative embolization prior to helium ion radiosurgery. This approach resulted in complete AVM obliteration in some patients, but most patients have not yet had their 2-year follow-up studies.

Radiosurgery Followed by Embolization

One patient with a left posterior temporal AVM and one with a thalamic AVM showed no angiographic change in the AVM 3 years after helium ion radiosurgery. Subsequent endovascular emboliza-

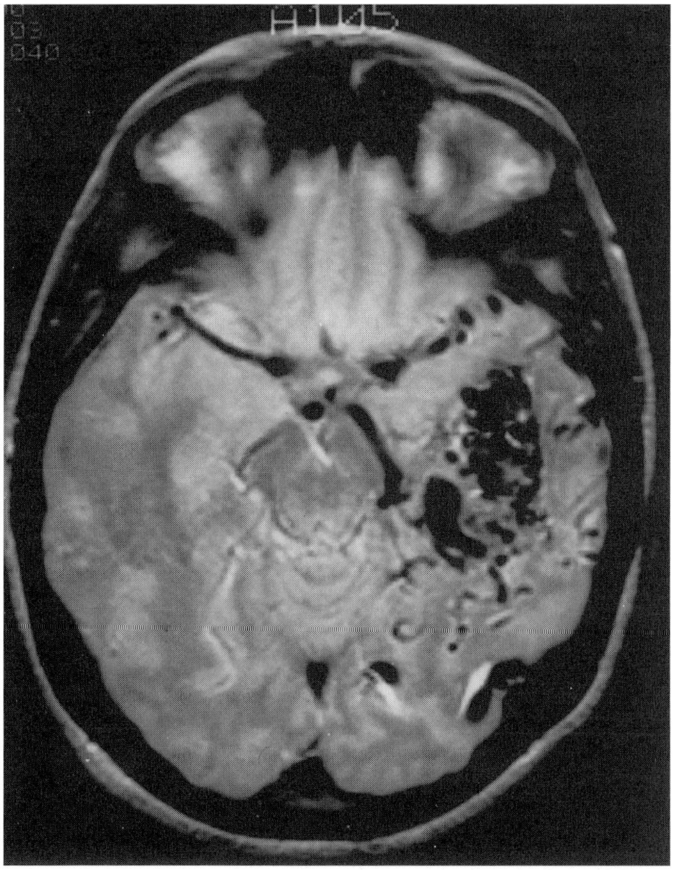

Figure 2. A 38-year-old female with medically intractable seizures and a left temporal AVM. **A.** Axial T2-weighted MRI demonstrates flow voids from the left temporal AVM nidus. The AVM was supplied predominately by the posterior cerebral artery, although the middle cerebral artery did contribute to the supply. *Continued*

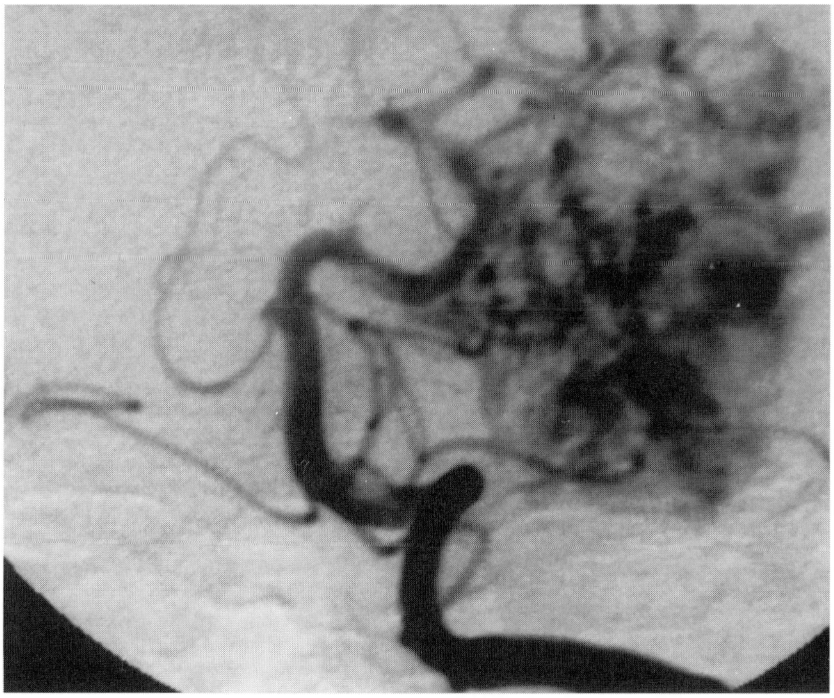

Figure 2B. AP projection from a left vertebral artery angiogram demonstrating the portion of the nidus supplied by the posterior cerebral artery. *Continued*

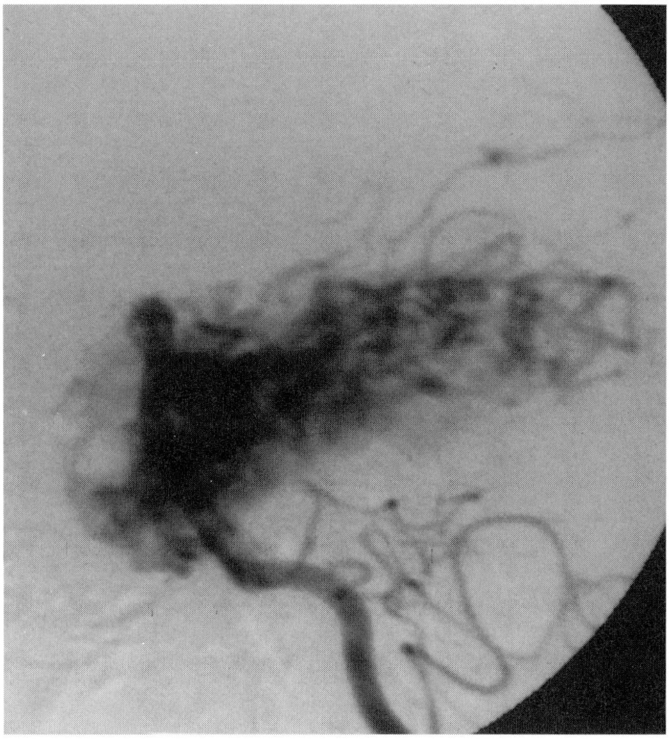

Figure 2C. Lateral projection from a left vertebral artery angiogram demonstrating the portion of the nidus supplied by the posterior cerebral artery. *Continued*

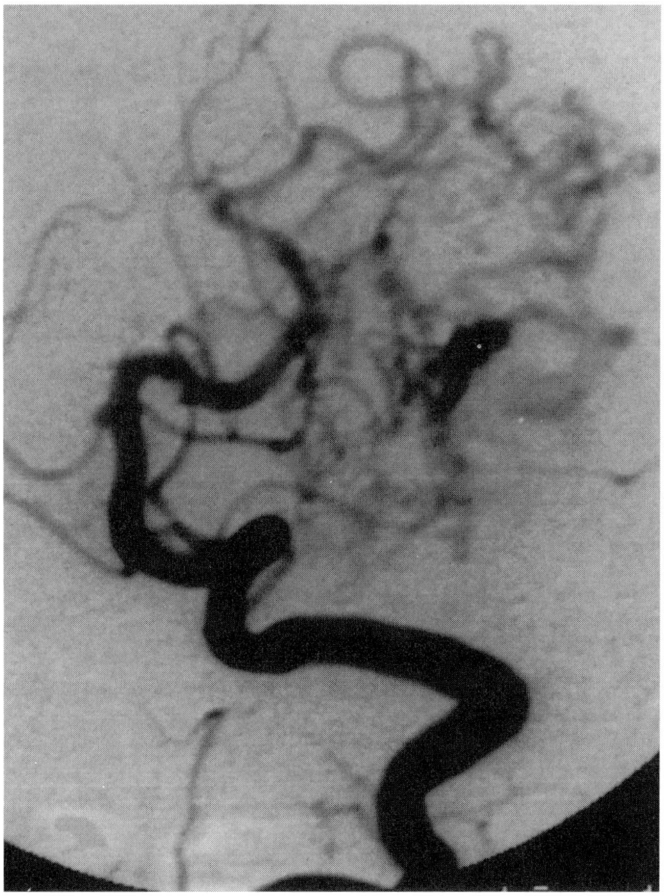

Figure 2D. AP projection from a left vertebral artery angiogram following embolization with cyanoacrylate showing significant reduction in AVM nidus volume; shunt flow has been achieved with embolization. *Continued*

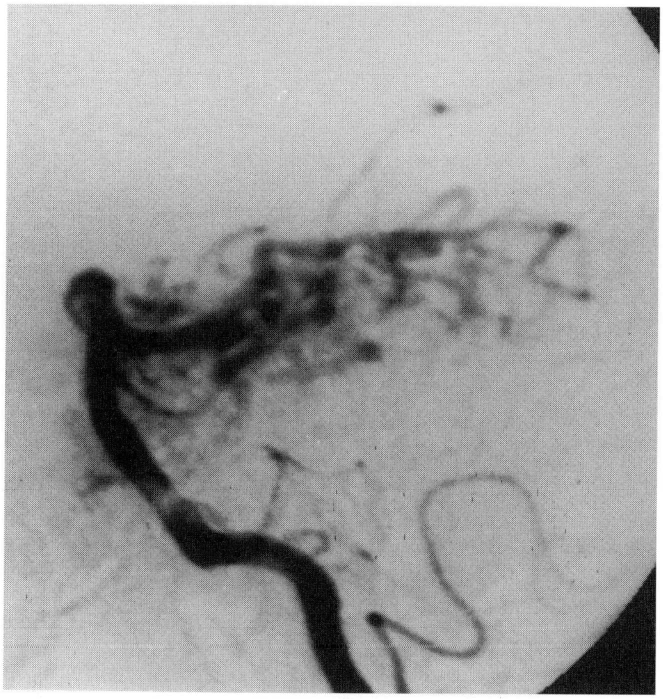

Figure 2E. Lateral projection from a left vertebral artery angiogram following embolization. *Continued*

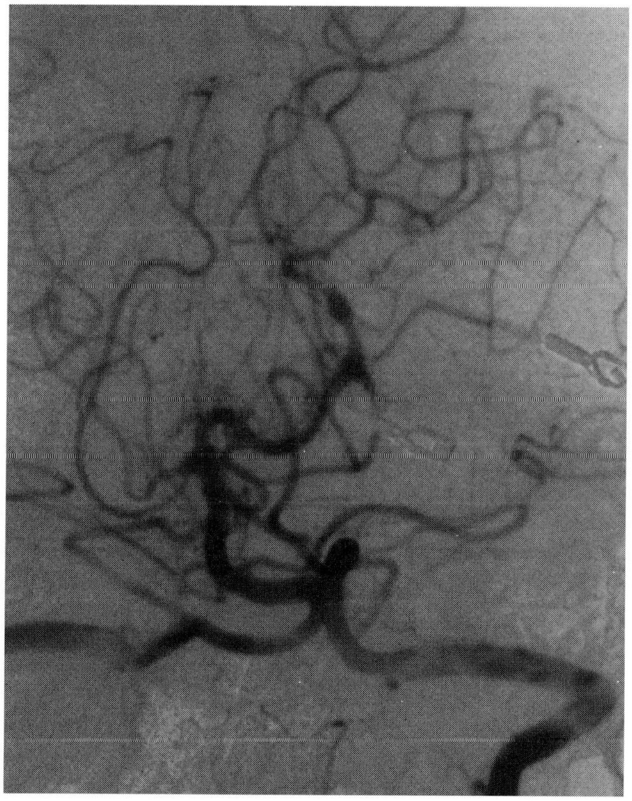

Figure 2F. AP projection following surgery in the same patient showing excision of the remaining arteriovenous shunt and obliteration of the AVM nidus. The patient had a mild expressive aphasia postoperatively that completely resolved after 3 months. Her seizures are completely controlled and she is neurologically normal. *Continued*

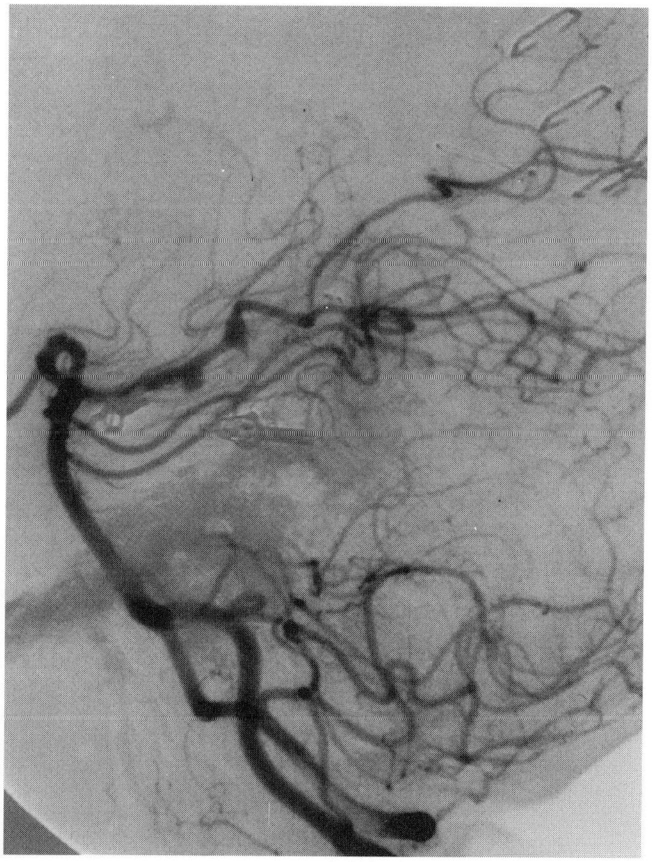

Figure 2G. Lateral projection following surgery showing excision of the remaining arteriovenous shunt and obliteration of the AVM nidus.

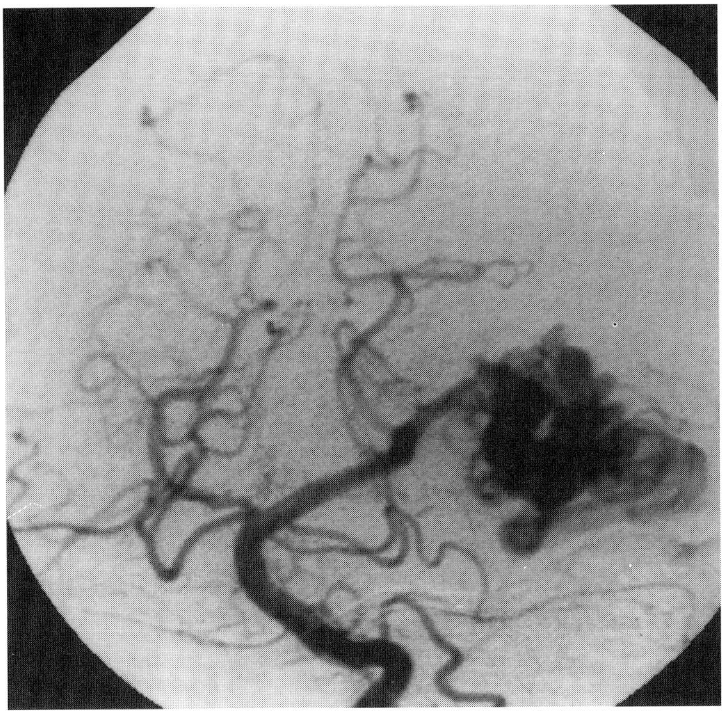

Figure 3. A 15-year-old boy who presented with an intraparenchymal hemorrhage and poorly controlled seizures from a left temporal AVM. He was previously treated by helium ion radiosurgery (35 GyE to 9000 mm^3). **A.** AP projection from a left vertebral artery angiogram showing the only supply to the AVM from the posterior cerebral artery. This angiogram was obtained 24 months following radiosurgery and demonstrated no change in the AVM nidus. *Continued*

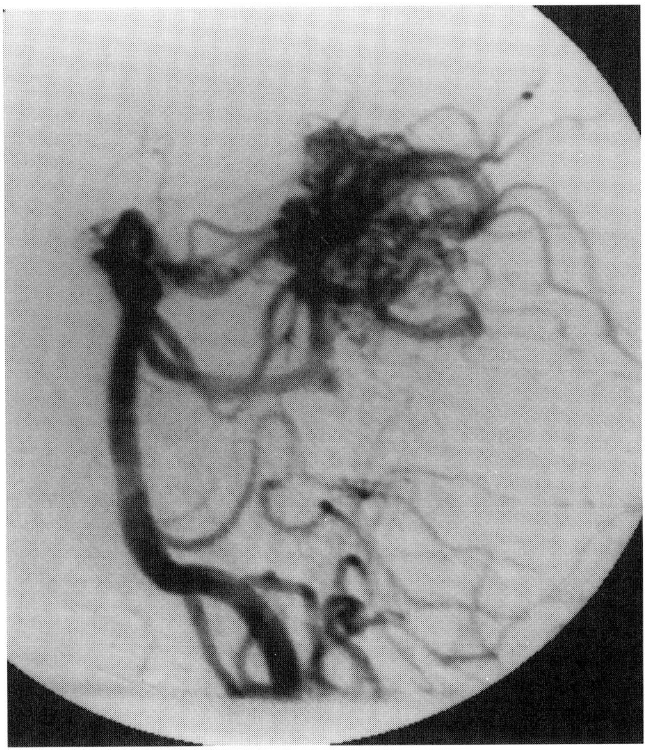

Figure 3B. Lateral projection of the same patient described in Figure 3A. *Continued*

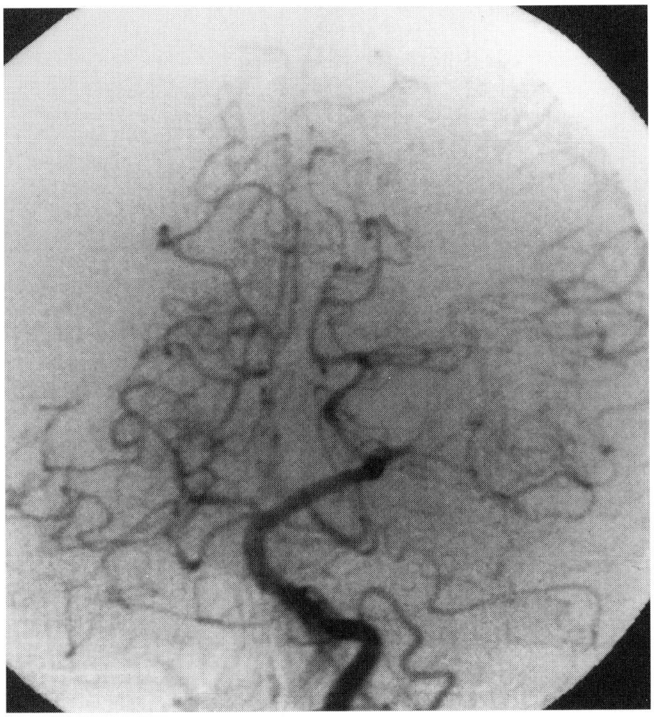

Figure 3C. AP projection from a left vertebral artery angiogram 2 years after embolization demonstrating no residual AVM or arteriovenous shunting. The patient has not had any further seizures and is neurologically normal. Used with permission from Marks MP, et al.[15] *Continued*

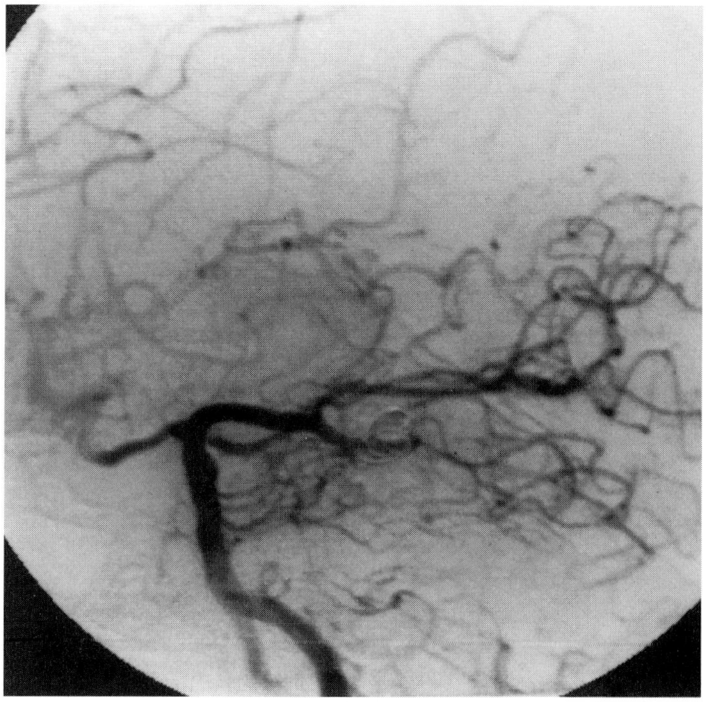

Figure 3D. Lateral projection, 2 years after embolization. Used with permission from Marks MP, et al.[15]

tion was curative in both of these patients, with excellent clinical results (Figure 3). Follow-up studies show the AVM remains angiographically obliterated 2 years later in one patient and 6 months later in the other patient.

Radiosurgery Followed by Microsurgery

In 17 patients whose AVMs did not obliterate completely within 3 years following radiosurgery, microsurgical resection of the residual AVM was performed. Prior to microsurgery, most of these patients showed no angiographic change in their AVM but a few showed partial angiographic obliteration. At surgery, the previously irradiated AVM was found to be markedly less vascular and easier to resect, compared with similar AVMs that had not been radiated. Pathological examination of the resected specimens disclosed extensive AVM thrombus involving small vessels of the AVM below the resolution of cerebral angiography. The surgery was curative in 15 of 17 cases, confirmed by postoperative angiography. Clinical outcome in these patients was generally excellent. Some patients suffered temporary, minor neurological deficits that resolved after 2–8 months. Most of the patients receiving this combination of therapy were neurologically normal or unchanged in long-term follow-up.[24,25]

Radiosurgery Followed by Embolization and Microsurgery

Seven patients who did not completely obliterate their AVM within 3 years of helium ion radiosurgery underwent subsequent endovascular embolization followed by microsurgical resection (Figure 4). Findings at surgery were similar to the group treated with helium ion irradiation and surgery, with the small vessel component of the AVM appearing to be largely obliterated in nonembolized areas. Pathology evaluation confirmed partial obliteration of the AVM that had not been appreciated angiographically. In 2 patients a subtotal resection was deliberately performed; 1 of these patients re-bled fatally. In the other 5 patients, angiography demonstrated complete resection of the AVM. Outcome was generally excellent. Some patients were temporarily worsened following this combination of treatments, but made a complete recovery within 3–6 months. One patient experienced radiation-induced necrosis with progressive hemiparesis and aphasia following radiosurgery. His deficits resolved completely 6 months after his AVM resection.[24,25]

Retreatment with Radiosurgery

Twenty patients whose AVMs were not obliterated 2–3 years after initial helium ion radiosurgery

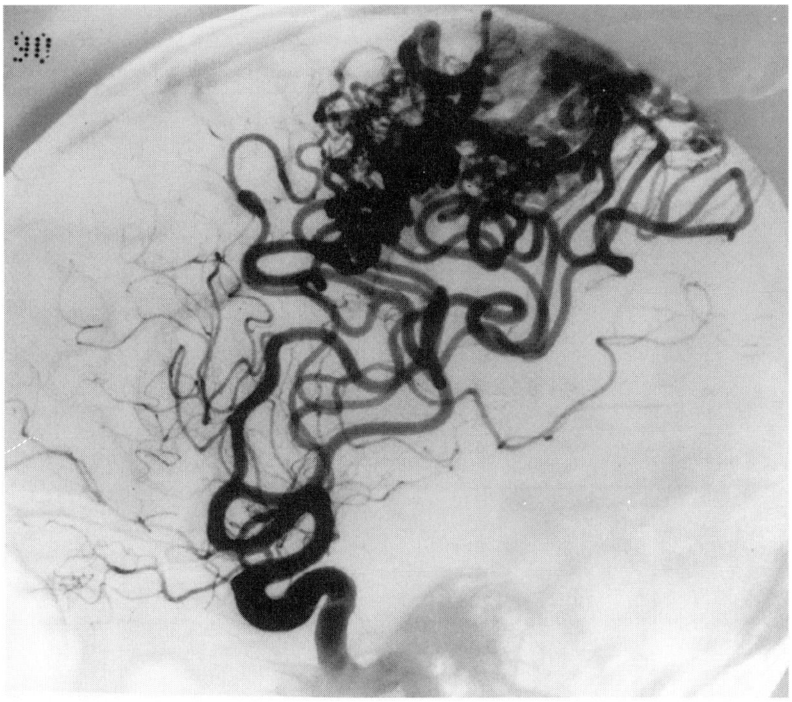

Figure 4. A 28-year-old male presenting with progressive neurological deficit and severe headaches from a left parietal AVM. The patient had previously received helium ion radiosurgery (18 GyE to 35,000 mm^3). **A.** Lateral projection from a left internal carotid artery angiogram demonstrating filling of the 5 cm AVM nidus overlying the region of the motor cortex. This angiogram was performed 34 months following radiosurgery and showed no change in the AVM. *Continued*

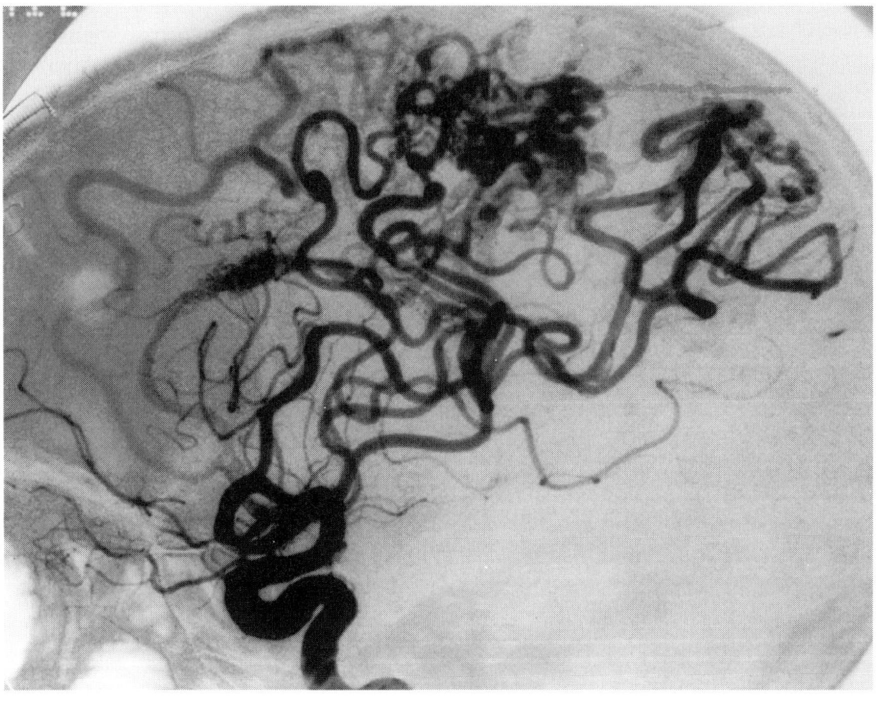

Figure 4B. Lateral projection from a left internal carotid artery angiogram following embolization showing reduction in the nidus size and occlusion of several middle cerebral artery opercular branches. *Continued*

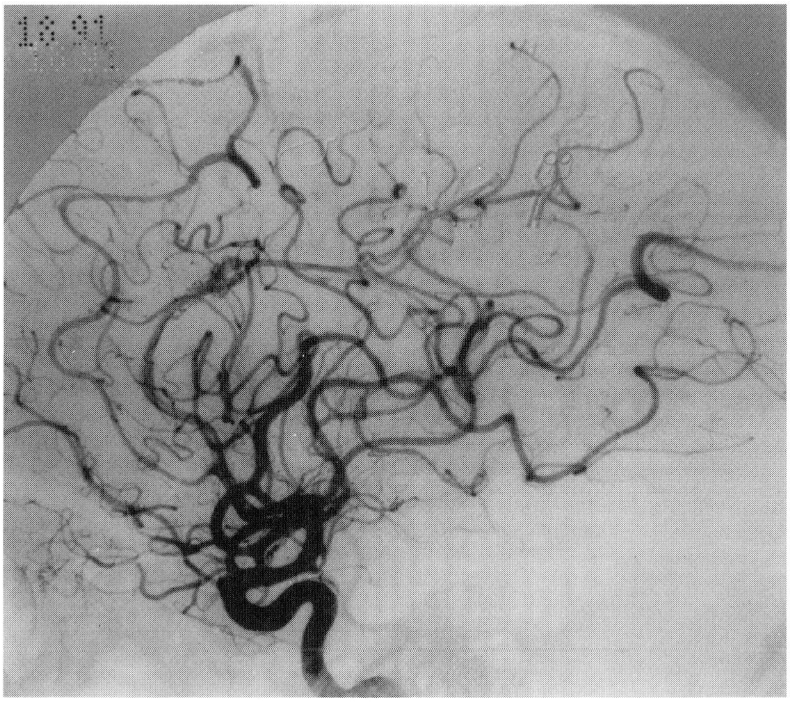

Figure 4C. Lateral projection of a left internal carotid artery angiogram following surgery demonstrating complete excision of the AVM without evidence of arteriovenous shunting. The patient had mild right leg weakness postoperatively that recovered fully over 2 months. He no longer has headaches. Used with permission from Marks MP, et al.[15]

received a second helium ion radiosurgical treatment. Follow-up is short on these patients, but 2 have gone on to complete angiographic obliteration and another patient 85% obliteration within 2 years after the second radiosurgery treatment. One patient developed radiation-induced white matter injury and transient hemiparesis after the second radiosurgery.

Angiographically Occult Vascular Malformations

Of the 47 patients with AOVMs treated using Bragg-peak helium ion radiosurgery, 8 (17%) experienced neurological deterioration due to recurrent hemorrhage from their AOVMs 2 months to 5 years following treatment. Five of these bleeds occurred within 13 months after treatment. Three of these patients had permanent worsening in their neurological status, while the remainder recovered to their previous neurological baseline. Fifteen percent of AOVM patients clinically worsened from probable radiation-induced injury, 3–12 months after treatment. One-third of this group recovered spontaneously, one-third had permanent worsening, and one-third recovered after microsurgical resection of the AOVM. A total of 7 patients with AOVMs underwent microsurgical resection of their malformations 6 months to 5 years following their helium ion treatment. At surgery, the AOVMs were found to be partially, but not completely, thrombosed. This was confirmed histologically.[20,21]

Because of our relatively poor success in treating AOVMs with stereotactic radiosurgery, several years ago we began using microsurgical resection for these vascular malformations in functional areas. The stereotactic approach using the CRW system has been particularly useful in localizing the AOVM through a small craniotomy and with minimal brain retraction. Our results using microsurgical resection for approximately 75 AOVMs in functional locations have been gratifying. Although there may be immediate postoperative neurological worsening, the vast majority of these patients made excellent recoveries over 1–6 months. For instance, of the 34 patients with brain stem, thalamic, or basal ganglia AOVMs that were microsurgically resected, the long-term results were generally excellent or good, with 56% of patients clinically improved, 32% unchanged, and only 12% worse. The AOVM was completely resected in 32 of 34 cases and no patients have subsequently deteriorated from re-bleeding.[23]

Discussion

Vascular malformations located in functional brain areas represent a challenge for neurosurgical treatment. The goal is to safely obliterate the vascular malformation completely, eliminating the potential for future hemorrhage, progressive neurological deficit, intractable seizures, or headaches refractory to medical therapy. To achieve this goal, we used various combinations of three modalities: endovascular embolization, open microsurgery, and stereotactic helium ion radiosurgery.

The particular treatment modality and order of treatment modalities is determined by our assessment of the relative risks of each treatment and each combination of therapies, in conjunction with our analysis of the natural history of the individual patient's AVM and the patient's preference (after the benefits and risks of each procedure have been explained).

The benefits of endovascular embolization include immediate reduction in AVM volume and decrease in AVM flow. This is usually performed with the patient awake during the procedure, obviating the need for general anesthesia, open craniotomy, or prolonged hospital stay. Occasionally, in the case of some very small AVMs, embolization alone is curative but, more commonly, it is to be used as an adjunct to open microsurgery, stereotactic radiosurgery, or both. In some cases we have used embolization following microsurgery and/or stereotactic radiosurgery, but generally it is used as a prelude to further microsurgery or radiosurgery. Disadvantages of embolization are the small risks of causing hemorrhage from residual AVM, dissections of cervical or intracranial arteries, infarcts from errant embolic material or excessive thrombosis in normal cerebral vessels, gluing of a catheter in cerebral vessels, and local minor complications at the femoral arterial cannulation site. In our experience, the risks of embolization can be minimized by meticulous attention to technical details, staging of embolization procedures (not obliterating too large a volume of AVM in any one session), close neurological clinical monitoring during the procedure, and the use of amytal provocative testing prior to permanent embolization. Monitoring of somatosensory evoked potentials (SSEPs) or brain stem auditory evoked potentials (BAEPs) has sometimes proved useful in assessing patients who require general anesthesia for embolization. We currently prefer glue embolization using NBCA because of its ease, versatility, and permanence. We have seen several cases of AVM recanalization after PVA embolization.

Microsurgical resection is the preferred mode of therapy for small AVMs in nonfunctional brain areas. For AVMs in functional cerebral regions, microsurgical resection still holds certain advantages: immediate and permanent cure of the lesion with elimination of future hemorrhage risk, and often improvement in other neurological symptoms and signs.[2,4,5,17–19,21] However, the risks of causing new neurological deficit with microsurgery can be significant when the AVM is situated in a critical brain area, especially if the AVM is larger than 3 cm diameter or has deep venous drainage.[2,4,5,17,18] Furthermore, open microsurgery requires general anesthesia and more prolonged hospitalization than either embolization or radiosurgery.

We have found a stereotactic approach, using the CRW system, to be extremely useful for microsurgically resecting deep-seated or small surface vascular malformations (AVMs and AOVMs).[23] This technique provides precise location of the vascular malformation (within a few millimeters) and allows for small craniotomy, limited dural opening, and minimal brain manipulation or unnecessary exposure. In our experience, it results in lower morbidity and shorter hospitalization compared with more conventional, larger craniotomies.

Intraoperative cortical mapping of functional areas (motor, sensory, language) with the patient asleep but nonparalyzed or the patient awake is also extremely valuable at the time of craniotomy. This procedure requires close collaboration with an epilepsy/neurophysiology team, and helps to determine if an AVM is situated within, rather than adjacent to, a critical functional region. Often an AVM will displace normal brain function to an atypical location.

Stereotactic, Bragg-peak helium ion radiosurgery has distinct advantages for the treatment of AVMs in functional brain areas, including a high obliteration rate (particularly with the small or moderate-sized AVMs, less than 3.7 cm diameter), low morbidity, and lack of need for general anesthesia or for hospitalization. It demonstrates a high rate of improvement in symptoms of headaches, seizures, and stabilization or improvement of progressive neurological deficit.[6,10,11,19,21]

The radiosurgery procedures have some disadvantages: there is a latency period of 1–2 years before complete obliteration of the AVM occurs, during which time the AVM can bleed, and there exists a small risk (1%–3%) of temporary or permanent delayed radiation complications (radiation-induced white matter changes or vasculopathy). Larger AVMs, greater than 3.7 cm diameters are more difficult to cure safely with stereotactic radiosurgery alone, since their complete obliteration is lower (42% at 2 years) and the risk of complications is higher than for smaller AVMs, even using the Bragg-peak helium ion technique.[6,10,11,19,21]

Approach to the Patient with an AVM in a Functional Brain Region

After reviewing the radiological studies (angiogram, MR, and CT), clinical presentation and age of each patient, our multidisciplinary AVM team assesses the natural history of the AVM in the particular patient under consideration (see the section describing methods). The relative risks of embolization, microsurgery, and stereotactic radiosurgery are estimated and discussed with the patient (and family) along with our assessment of the AVM's expected natural history. A decision regarding no treatment (except anticonvulsants or analgesics for symptomatic therapy) versus definitive treatment for the AVM is made between the members of the AVM team and the patient. In cases where the risks of treatment obviously outweigh the probable natural history of the AVM, a choice of no treatment is appropriate. For instance, a 20-year-old female we evaluated, with a 7 cm left temporo-occipital AVM, fed by anterior and posterior circulation and draining centrally, who suffered occasional migraine headaches, was advised to receive symptomatic treatment for her migraines and be followed clinically, but not receive other treatment for her AVM. Likewise, a 1.5 cm perimesencephalic cistern AVM that was discovered incidentally in a 77-year-old man was not treated.

Once a decision to treat a particular patient is made, our multidisciplinary team discusses the relative goals, benefits, and risks of each treatment modality separately and the additive benefits and risks of combined therapies. The overall aim of treatment in each patient is complete angiographic obliteration of the AVM, with elimination of future hemorrhage risk and improvement in neurological symptoms, with minimal risks of neurological complications.

For small AVMs (≤3.0 cm diameter), there are sometimes two good treatment choices: microsurgical resection, often using a stereotactic approach, or stereotactic radiosurgery (20–25 GyE). Occasionally, for the smallest AVMs (≤2.0 cm diameter), we will consider treatment with endovascular embolization aimed at complete AVM thrombosis and cure. If we conclude that endovascular embolization does not have a high potential for complete obliteration of small AVMs (≤3.0 cm diameter), it generally would not be used. The choice between recommending microsurgical resection or stereotactic radiosurgery depends on the precise AVM location, number of recent AVM hemorrhages, risk of future hemorrhage (based on angiographic risk factors), and the patient's current neurological symptoms and signs, general medical condition, age, and the patient's preferences after discussion of the relative risks and benefits. We tend to favor microsurgical resection if the small AVM presents to a pial or ependymal surface, or it can be approached safely, through "noneloquent" brain.

In our series, microsurgical resection of most small AVMs, 3 cm in diameter or less, even in functional areas, has been very successful in achieving complete AVM cure with low risk of permanent neurological deficits. This confirms the results of other reports.[4,8,18] It should be kept in mind that although some of these patients had immediate postoperative deficits, they recovered to normal over several weeks to months. We have found the use of a stereotactic technique with the CRW system to be extremely helpful in localizing and resecting some of these small AVMs.

For small AVMs in the motor/sensory cortex, coronal radiata, thalamic areas, internal capsule, or brain stem, we usually recommend radiosurgery (20–25 GyE) unless there is more urgency to obliterate the AVM sooner than 1–2 years (for instance, multiple recent bleeds). In our experience, open microsurgery for AVMs in these particular functional areas carries higher risk of causing neurological deficit than does radiosurgery. Radiosurgery is also often recommended for other small AVMs in functional areas, if the patient is considered a poor surgical risk (e.g., elderly or in poor medical condition) or the patient declines open surgery. Our previous publications document good results after helium ion radiosurgery for small AVMs, with a high rate of complete obliteration (94% at 2 years, 100% at 3 years), significant improvement in clinical symptoms and signs, and low risk of complications. However, there is still a latency period of 1–2 years for achieving complete obliteration, during which time bleeding can occur and neurological symptoms persist. Although most of our radiosurgery experience has been with the Bragg-peak helium ion method, gamma knife or LINAC radiosurgery appear to be comparable in terms of their success for smaller AVMs (≤3.0 cm).[3,7,9,26]

For AVMs in functional brain areas that are greater then 3.0 cm diameter, we usually recommend endovascular embolization prior to microsurgical resection or stereotactic radiosurgery (or both). The rationale underlying this approach is that larger volume AVMs carry higher risks of complications with either microsurgery or radiosurgery and have lower obliteration rates with radiosurgery than smaller AVMs. The goal of embolization is tailored to each case. If embolization is being used as a presurgical adjunct, our aims are to decrease AVM volume and flow as well as close deep AVM feeders that may be difficult to reach during the initial phase of surgery. We obliterate as much volume of AVM with embolization as is considered safely possible, but we will often use two or three different embolization sessions separated by at least 1 week to achieve this goal. We prefer to wait at least 1 week between embolization sessions and between the last embolization and surgery in order to allow hemodynamic stabilization of the AVM and surrounding vasculature. In our experience, this has substantially decreased the incidence of ischemic and hemorrhagic complications associated with both embolization and surgery. Typically, large AVM volumes are reduced 50%–85% by embolization. In selected cases of deep hemisphere or basal ganglia AVMs, we use intraoperative embolization (sometimes with temporary occlusion of normal arteries) to gain access to particular feeding vessels and inject large quantities of glue into inaccessible nidus.

Pre-radiosurgery embolization is designed to decrease the volume of AVM that will need to be treated with radiosurgery. We try to achieve residual AVM volumes of <25 cm^3 (<3.7 cm diameter) if possible, since our radiosurgery results are better for these small to moderate-sized AVMs.[6,10,11,19,21] Reduction of flow only, without AVM volume reduction, might theoretically increase the rate and extent of obliteration following radiosurgery. However, this approach is not of proven benefit, and treating the larger AVM volume would still carry some increased risk of complications unless a lower treatment dose were used. When AVM volume cannot be reduced below 25 cm^3, we will still often treat with stereotactic Bragg-peak radiosurgery (helium ions or protons), using a lower therapeutic dose (20 GyE).

In some cases we plan several stages of both endovascular embolization and microsurgery before using stereotactic radiosurgery for a particular AVM. This combined approach is used for especially large and complex AVMs in functional regions. One potential problem, in leaving some residual AVM after deliberate partial AVM resection, is bleeding. We take special precautions postoperatively, including induced hypotension and hypovolemia, for several days to avoid this complication. Since instituting this policy, we have experienced only two perioperative hemorrhages from residual AVM left deliberately. The incidence of delayed hemorrhage from residual AVM during the latency period after radiosurgery is also low, probably approximating the natural history of AVM bleeding.[6,10,11,19,21]

Approximately 15% of the AVMs we treated with radiosurgery alone did not obliterate completely after 3 years. These were mostly large AVMs and, in a few cases, AVMs treated with low doses (11–18 GyE) or incomplete nidus coverage. We have never observed an unobliterated AVM 3 years after radiosurgery that went on to complete obliteration in subsequent years. Also, there were no AVMs unchanged angiographically at 2 years following radiosurgery that obliterated completely in subsequent years. For these AVMs we usually recommend further treatment with embolization, microsurgery, or both modalities. We have successfully cured 22 of these previously radiated but unobliterated AVMs with: microsurgery alone (15), embolization alone (2), or combined embolization and microsurgery (5). Embolization of these lesions has suggested that these AVMs previously radiated have large shunts.[16]

Surgical observations and histopathology findings suggest that although radiosurgery did not alter the angiographic appearance of these large AVMs, many of the smaller vessels within the AVM were completely or partially thrombosed. In some cases, the radiosurgery appeared to obliterate the fine vessel AVM components, leaving larger AV fistulous elements. In many cases it was felt the radiosurgery transformed a high-risk, difficult resection into a straightforward, safe procedure with minimal blood loss and low morbidity.

There are also some large AVMs that have failed to obliterate after radiosurgery, where we still consider embolization or microsurgery too risky. We usually recommend a second course of stereotactic radiosurgery for these patients, recognizing that they may have a slightly higher risk of radiation-induced complications. This re-treatment with radiosurgery is usually reserved for symptomatic patients with complex, large AVMs in the corona radiata, basal ganglia, internal capsule, thalamus, or brain stem. Although follow-up is relatively short so far, it appears that some of these re-irradiated AVMs are obliterating without an excessively high complication rate.

The treatment of AOVMs in functional brain areas remains controversial. Our results with radiosurgical treatment of 47 AOVMs, mostly in the brain stem, thalamus, and basal ganglia, suggest that radiosurgery is not a good therapy for these lesions; it does not reliably lead to complete thrombosis of the AOVM (so there is continued risk of hemorrhage) and the complication rate is high. We have now resected about 75 AOVMs in functional regions, including brain stem, thalamus, corona radiata, or motor, sensory, visual, or language areas. Our results indicate that this direct microsurgical approach is curative and can yield excellent outcome, although some temporary morbidity should sometimes be expected.

Conclusion

Untreated vascular malformations in critical functional brain regions continue to cause significant morbidity and mortality. Their successful treatment remains a challenge. The use of individualized, multimodality therapy with different combinations of embolization, microsurgery, and radiosurgery has increased the chances for complete obliteration and improved clinical outcome in many of these patients. It is important to constantly review our patient selection criteria, radiological results, and clinical outcomes, and continually redesign our treatment strategies, in an effort to successfully treat patients with the largest and most complex vascular malformations located in these functional areas.

References

1. Abe M, Kjellberg RN, Adams RD. Clinical presentations of vascular malformations of the brain stem: Comparisons of angiographically positive and negative types. J Neurol Neurosurg Psychiatry 52:167–175, 1989.
2. Batjer H, Samson D. Arteriovenous malformations of the posterior fossa: Clinical presentation, diagnostic evaluation, and surgical treatment. J Neurosurg 64: 849–856, 1986.
3. Betti OO, Munari C, Rosler R. Stereotactic radiosurgery with the linear accelerator: Treatment of arteriovenous malformations. Neurosurgery 24:311–321, 1989.
4. Drake CG. Cerebral arteriovenous malformations: Considerations for and experience with surgical treatment in 166 cases. Clin Neurosurg 26:145–208, 1979.
5. Drake CG, Friedman AH, Peerless SJ. Posterior fossa arteriovenous malformations. J Neurosurg 64:1–10, 1986.
6. Fabrikant JI, Levy RP, Steinberg GK, et al. Charged-particle radiosurgery for intracranial vascular malformations. Neurosurg Clinic North Am 3:99–103, 1992.
7. Friedman WA, Bova FJ. LINAC radiosurgery for arteriovenous malformations. In Alexander E, Loeffler JS, Lunsford LD (eds): Stereotactic Radiosurgery. New York: McGraw-Hill, 1993, pp 147–155.
8. Heros RC, Korosue K, Diebold PM. Surgical excision of cerebral arteriovenous malformations: Late results. Neurosurgery 26:570–578, 1990.
9. Kondziolka D, Lunsford LD, Flickinger JC. Gamma knife stereotactic radiosurgery for cerebral vascular malformations. In Alexander E, Loeffler JS, Lunsford LD (eds): Stereotactic Radiosurgery. New York: McGraw-Hill, 1993, pp 136–146.
10. Levy RP, Fabrikant JI, Frankel KA, et al. Stereotactic heavy-charged particle Bragg-peak radiosurgery for the treatment of intracranial arteriovenous malformations in childhood and adolescence. Neurosurgery 24: 841–852, 1989.
11. Levy RP, Fabrikant JI, Frankel KA, et al. Charged-particle radiosurgery of the brain. Neurosurg Clin North Am 1:955–990, 1990.
12. Lobato RD, Rivas JJ, Gomez PA, et al. Comparison of the clinical presentation of symptomatic arteriovenous malformations (angiographically visualized) and occult vascular malformations. Neurosurgery 31: 391–397, 1992.
13. Marks MP, Bracci PM, Steinberg GK. The correlation of risk factors of hemorrhage with the natural history of brain arteriovenous malformations. Annual Meeting of Congress of Neurological Surgeons Program 43:95, 1993.
14. Marks MP, Lane B, Steinberg GK, et al. Hemorrhage in intracerebral arteriovenous malformations: Angiographic determinants. Radiology 176:807–813, 1990.
15. Marks MP, Lane B, Steinberg GK, et al. Vascular characteristics of intracerebral arteriovenous malformations in patients with clinical steal. AJNR 12:489–496, 1991.
16. Marks MP, Lane B, Steinberg GK, et al. Endovascular treatment of cerebral arteriovenous malformations following radiosurgery. AJNR 14:297–303, 1993.
17. Spetzler RM, Martin NA. A proposed grading system for arteriovenous malformations. J Neurosurg 65: 476–483, 1986.
18. Stein BM. Surgical decisions in vascular malformations of the brain. In Barnett HJM, Mohr JP, Stein BM, et al (eds): Stroke: Pathophysiology, Diagnosis, and Management. New York, Churchill-Livingstone, 1992, pp 1093–1133.
19. Steinberg GK, Fabrikant JI, Marks MP, et al. Stereotactic heavy-charged-particle Bragg-peak radiation for intracranial arteriovenous malformations. N Engl J Med 323:96–101, 1990.
20. Steinberg GK, Levy RP, Fabrikant JI, et al. Stereotactic helium ion Bragg-peak radiosurgery for angiographically occult intracranial vascular malformations. Stereotact Funct Neurosurg 57:64–71, 1991.
21. Steinberg GK, Levy RP, Marks MP, et al. Vascular malformations: Charged-particle radiosurgery. In Alexander E, Loeffler JS, Lunsford LD (eds): Stereotactic Radiosurgery. New York: McGraw-Hill, 1993, pp 122–135.
22. Steinberg GK, Marks MP, Shuer LM, et al. Occult vascular malformations of the optic chiasm: Magnetic resonance imaging diagnosis and surgical laser resection. Neurosurgery 27:466–470, 1990.
23. Steinberg GK, Vanefsky MA. Management of the patient with an angiographically occult vascular malformation. In Hadley MN (ed): Perspectives in Neurologi-

cal Surgery. St. Louis: Quality Medical Publishing, Inc., 1004 pp18–39.

24. Steinberg, GK, Chang SD, Levy RP, et al. Surgical resection of intracranial arteriovenous malformations following stereotactic radiosurgery. J Neurosurg 84: 920–928, 1996.
25. Chang SD, Steinberg GK. Other surgical options for stroke prevention. In Ginsberg M, Bougosslavsky J (eds): Cerebrovascular Disease: Pathophysiology, Diagnosis and Management. Volume II. Cambridge, MA: Blackwell Science, 1998, pp 1945–1963.
26. Steiner L. Radiosurgery in cerebral arteriovenous malformations. In Fein JM, Flamm ES (eds): Cerebrovascular Surgery, Vol.4. New York: Springer Verlag, 1985, pp 1161–1215.
27. Zimmerman RS, Spetzler RM, Lee KS, et al. Cavernous malformations of the brain stem. J Neurosurg 75:32–39, 1991.

Chapter 8

Stereotactic Radiosurgery for Arteriovenous Malformations of the Basal Ganglia and Thalamus

Ajay Niranjan, MCh, Douglas Kondziolka, MD, MSc, John C. Flickinger, MD, and L. Dade Lunsford, MD

Introduction

Thalamic and basal ganglia arteriovenous malformations (AVMs) are vascular disorders that present considerable management challenges to patients and their doctors. Patients are usually young at presentation and often present with an intracerebral hemorrhage that leads to temporary or permanent neurological deficits if not death. Hemorrhage is more common as the initial clinical event for a thalamic or basal ganglia AVM compared to a convexity AVM.[19] This is likely because diencephalic AVMs are rarely associated with seizures or headache. These AVMs may exhibit higher perfusion or venous pressures and a higher incidence of arterial or venous aneurysms. In one study, Sasaki et al. found a 13% re-bleeding rate for thalamic and basal ganglia AVMs in contrast to 2%–4% for other AVMs.[19] In a different study, Pollock et al. did not identify a higher rebleeding rate for deep AVMs compared to more superficial hemispheric AVMs.[16]

Anatomic Overview

An anatomic review of this region demonstrates the considerable and diverse clinical problems that may be manifest. The basal ganglia nuclei (caudate nucleus, putamen, globus pallidus, and subthalamus) surround the thalamus and are separated by fibers of the internal capsule. The corpus striatum is supplied mainly by the lateral striate arteries derived from the middle cerebral artery. The anteromedial part of the head of the caudate nucleus is supplied by the medial striate artery (of Heubner), while the tail of the caudate nucleus and the caudal part of the putamen are supplied by branches of the anterior choroidal artery. The lateral segment of the globus pallidus receives its supply from branches of both the lateral striate and the anterior choroidal arteries. The internal capsule is nourished mainly by the lateral striate arteries. The medial striate artery supplies the rostromedial part of the anterior limb of the internal capsule. The genu of the internal capsule receives some direct branches from the internal carotid artery while the ventral part of the posterior limb is supplied by branches of the anterior choroidal artery. The thalamus is supplied mainly from branches of the posterior cerebral artery (thalamoperforating and thalamogeniculate branches). Any damage to this region from manifestations of the AVM itself, or microsurgery, radiosurgery, or embolization may lead to profound contralateral weakness, sensory loss, visual deficits, or cognitive dysfunction. A knowledge of the neuroanatomic features of this region is important before recommending a specific management strategy (Figure 1).

Therapeutic Options

The three major therapeutic options include microsurgical resection, embolization, and radiosurgery. The fourth option, conservative management,

From Yamada S (ed): *Arteriovenous Malformations in Functional Areas of the Brain.* © Futura Publishing Co, Inc, Armonk, NY, 1999.

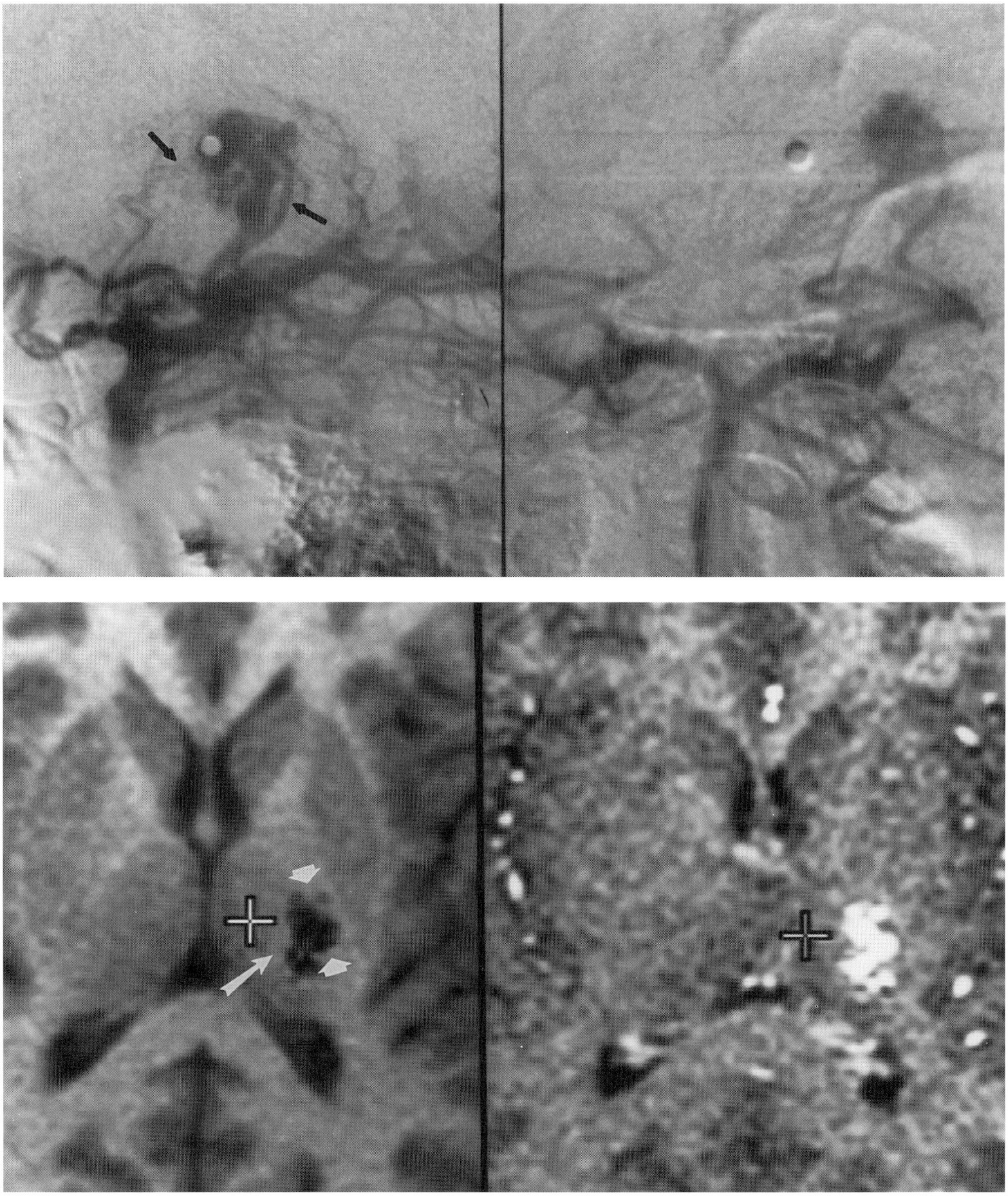

Figure 1. Lateral and anterior-posterior subtraction angiograms (top) showing a small internal capsule AVM supplied by thalamoperforating and choroidal arteries (black arrows). The MR images (bottom) show the AVM within the posterior limb of the internal capsule (small arrows) and lateral to the thalamus (large arrow). Two years after radiosurgery, complete obliteration was identified with no additional neurological deficits in this young woman.

always must be considered for patients with a malformation not deemed eradicable with acceptable risk. Embolization alone is useful only in a small number of patients, mainly as an adjunct to surgery or radiosurgery to reduce the volume of larger AVMs. The benefits of embolization with regard to improving the cure rate of radiosurgery are unknown.

Successful microsurgery offers immediate protection from hemorrhage if complete removal of the AVM is achieved. This approach is associated with a higher up-front mortality and morbidity risk. Unfortunately, many thalamic and basal ganglia AVMs are not suitable for resection due to their intimate relationship with critical brain structures. However, when the AVM presents to a pial or ependymal surface, resection may be possible.

Stereotactic radiosurgery is an effective and well-tolerated management modality for selected deep-seated AVMs and may be considered the treatment of choice for small intraparenchymal AVMs located within the parenchyma of the thalamus and basal ganglia. Its limitation in not providing immediate protection from hemorrhage is partly compensated for by the relatively low natural risk of bleeding, the acceptability by patients as a minimally invasive therapy, the lack of procedural mortality, and the low complication rate when carefully performed. Laboratory studies have shown that a single, large, focused dose of radiation produces localized endothelial proliferation. Complete luminal closure follows such endothelial cell proliferation, vascular wall thickening, and eventual malformation thrombosis.[23] These findings have been confirmed on histopathological examination of surgical or autopsy specimens after prior radiosurgery.[20]

Table 1
Patient Characteristics before AVM Radiosurgery

Age	Mean	27 yrs
	Range	2–65 yrs
Symptoms		
	Headache	43.7%
	Seizures	11.7%
	Prior embolization	14.6%
	Prior surgeries	12.6%
Volume (cm^3)		
	<1	24.3%
	1–10	72.8%
	>10	2.9%
Spetzler-Martin Grade		
	1	1.0%
	2	6.0%
	3	25.5%
	4	4.9%
	5	0%
	6	62.7%

Technique of Radiosurgery

Over a 7-year interval, 95 patients with angiographically identified thalamic and/or basal ganglia AVMs underwent stereotactic radiosurgery at our center and were suitable for follow-up beyond 2 years. The characteristics of the patients are listed in Table 1. Planned two-stage radiosurgery was performed for larger AVMs. Repeat radiosurgery of incompletely obliterated AVMs was generally recommended at 3 years. Relatively few AVMs were considered unsuitable for further irradiation due to their location or potential unacceptable morbidity. In this series 16 patients underwent staged radiosurgery.

Radiosurgery was performed using the 201 source cobalt-60 Gamma Knife (Elekta Instruments, Atlanta, GA). The treatment isodose plan, maximum dose, and dose to the margin were jointly decided by neurosurgeon, radiation oncologist, and medical physicist. All imaging and clinical patient data were reviewed at a multidisciplinary vascular malformation conference attended by neurosurgeons, radiation oncologists, and interventional neuroradiologists. If the AVM was considered suitable for treatment, this decision (along with the expected outcome) was communicated to the referring physician. The technique, rationale, risks, and benefits were discussed in detail with the patient and the family. A detailed informed consent with full explanation about possible complications and future treatment was obtained as an outpatient.

On the day of radiosurgery we begin with attachment of the stereotactic frame under buffered local anesthesia (5% marcaine and 1% xylocaine) supplemented by mild sedation when needed. In children under 13 years of age, general anesthesia is preferred. Since 1992 all eligible patients undergo MRI, which includes a sagittal scout sequence followed by a contrast-enhanced axial volume acquisition. On this spoiled grass gradient recombinant scan we use a low TE to enhance blood vessel definition. An MRA reconstruction is then obtained. The patient next undergoes conventional stereotactic angiography. Magnification subtraction images are transferred to the gamma knife workstation by ethernet (for MRI) or by scanner (for hard-copy angiograms).

Accurate definition of the AVM nidus is of the utmost importance in radiosurgery planning. It is important to carefully exclude draining veins, normal arterial vessels outside the nidus, and normal brain

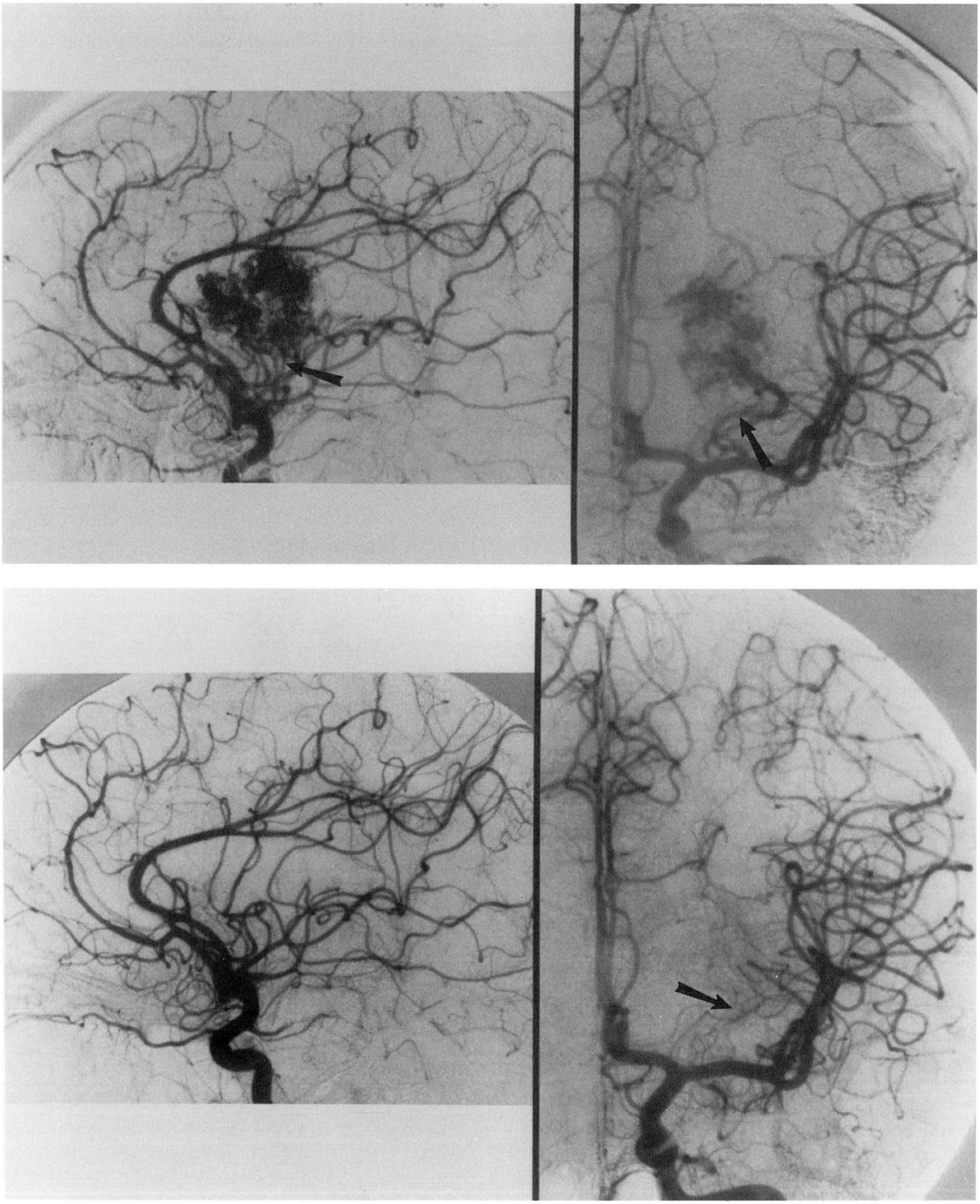

Figure 2. Angiograms at the time of radiosurgery (top) in a child with an anterior basal ganglia AVM. Two years later (bottom), complete obliteration was identified with preservation of the lateral striate arteries that had supplied the AVM (arrows).

tissue. We aim to construct a conformal radiosurgery volume that irradiates only the AVM nidus. Irradiation of the smallest target volume increases the success rate as a higher marginal dose can be delivered to a smaller target. Planning is first carried out on axial MR images assisted by coronal and sagittal reconstructions. A conformal plan is generally achieved using 1 to 12 isocenters of different diameters. After finalizing the plan on angiographic images, the integrated logistic formula for a 3% probability of permanent radiation-related complications is used. The expected obliteration rate based on margin dose also is checked.[3] The median dose to the AVM margin was 19.9 Gy (range 14–27 Gy). The mean AVM volume was 3.4 mL (range, 0.08–12.6 mL).

The patient then undergoes radiosurgery with the gamma knife. All patients receive a 40 mg dose of methylprednisolone at the conclusion of irradiation. After stereotactic frame removal, a light compression bandage is applied and then removed after a few hours. Patients are observed in the neurosurgical ward and discharged the next morning. Patients are followed with MRI scans at 6, 12, 24, and 36 months. Angiography is performed at 3 years if MRI suggests possible complete obliteration. In our experience, MRI accurately predicts obliteration and can be used as a guide to deciding the timing of final angiography.[18] We request post-radiosurgery angiography in all patients (Figure 2).

Results of Radiosurgery

Following radiosurgery, we obtained regular MRI scans in 80 patients and 3-year follow-up angiography in 55. Thirty six (65.5%) of these patients showed complete AVM obliteration. Evidence of a residual small nidus was seen in 19 (35.5%). The presence of a draining vein was initially assumed to represent incomplete obliteration and these patients were advised to undergo further angiography 1 year later. Three additional patients underwent angiography after the 3-year period and all showed complete obliteration. All 19 patients with subtotal obliteration (residual nidus) were recommended to receive second-stage radiosurgery. Five patients who underwent a second-stage radiosurgery procedure showed complete obliteration on follow-up angiography after 3 additional years. The rest have not reached the second 3-year period of follow-up. Thus, a total of 44 (76%) out of 58 patients followed angiographically eventually achieved complete obliteration. Two other patients had only an early draining vein, a feature heralding eventual complete obliteration. Of the 22 patients who were followed up with serial MRI scans, 19 showed MR evidence of complete AVM obliteration (no residual AVM flow-void when flow-void was seen before radiosurgery). If these 19 patients and the additional 2 patients with only an early draining vein (but no nidus) are included, then the obliteration rate for the entire series is 80% (Figure 3).

Table 2
Imaging Results after Radiosurgery for Thalamic or Basal Ganglia AVMs

Follow-up	*Total Patients*	*Complete Obliteration*
3 year angiogram	55	36 (65.45%)
5 year angiogram	58	39
2nd stage radiosurgery	14	5
Early draining vein	02	—
MRI obliteration	22	19
Total series	80	65 (80.3%)

The mean AVM volume in patients who achieved complete obliteration was 2.6 mL compared with 3.8 mL in the partial obliteration group. Both the mean margin (21.5 Gy) and maximum (37.4 Gy) doses were higher in the complete obliteration group than in the partial response group (19.2 Gy and 35 Gy, respectively), a feature related to dose reduction for larger AVMs.

Temporary complications reported by our patients included nausea and vomiting in the first few hours after radiosurgery (3.9%), transient motor or sensory symptoms related to cerebral edema (7.8%), and headache (1.9%). Ten patients (10%) showed improvement in their pre-radiosurgery neurological deficits and 12 (11.7%) noticed temporary deterioration. Eight percent of patients had a hemorrhage during follow-up and 3 patients died. Regrowth of an angiographically obliterated AVM was seen in one child.

Choice of Available Therapies

The management approaches toward basal ganglia and thalamic AVMs have evolved from observation to microsurgery as the predominant therapy to more multidisciplinary management that includes embolization and radiosurgery. Radiosurgery has emerged as the least invasive and potentially most effective and safest option. Although radiosurgery was originally advised for surgically high-risk AVMs (Spetzler-Martin[21] grade III or IV), increasingly patients and neurosurgeons have opted for it rather than microsurgery, even for the small or lower risk AVMs.[17] The overall results from a variety of centers have been consistent with complete obliteration rates

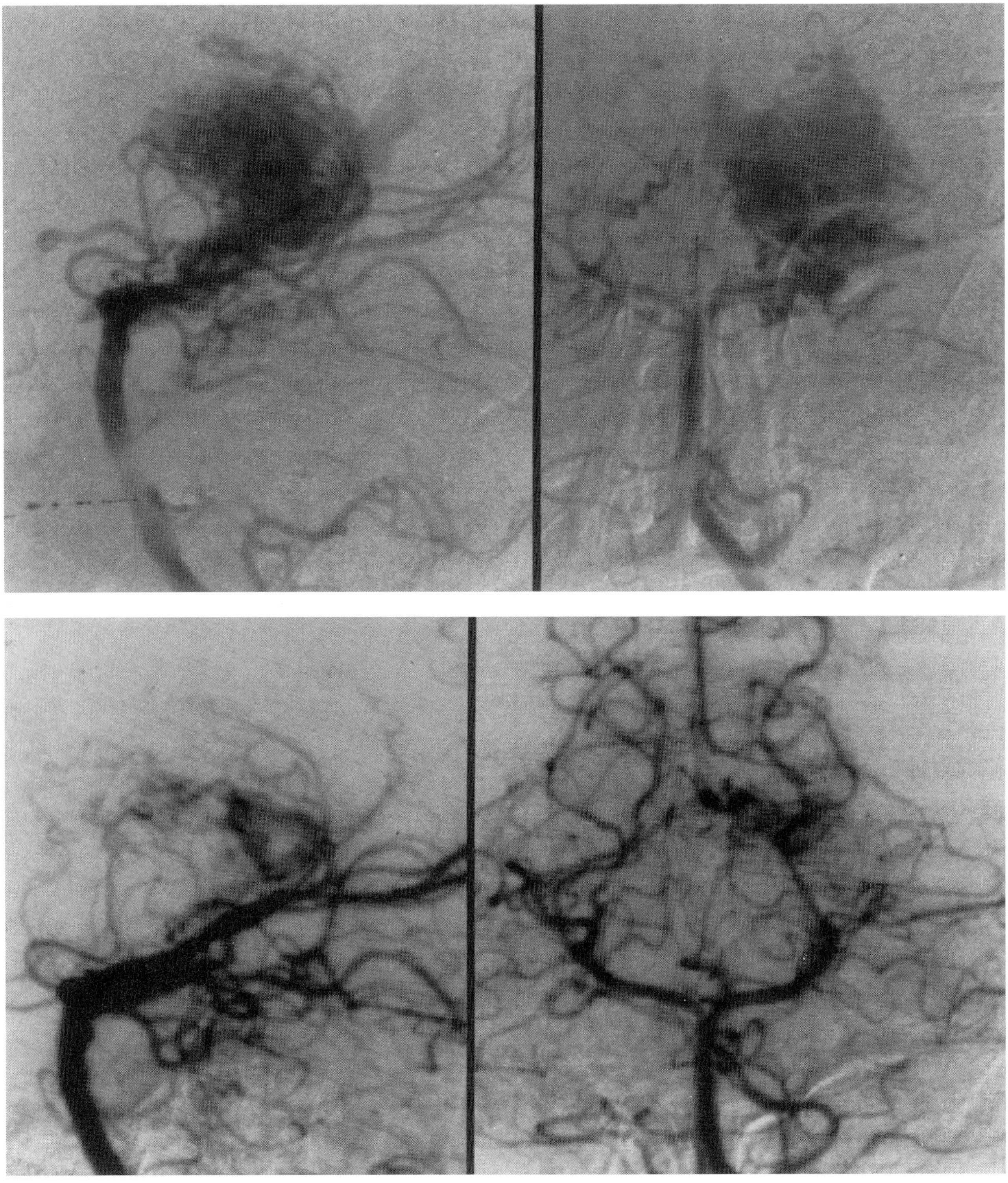

Figure 3. Angiograms at the time of radiosurgery (top) showing a thalamic AVM. Three years later (bottom), significant but subtotal obliteration was documented. She underwent a second radiosurgery procedure for the residual AVM nidus.

for AVMs that vary from 70% to 90%, depending on radiation dose and AVM volume.[14,17,19,22,24]

Although radiosurgery has been performed extensively for AVMs in all brain locations, there is no large series with long-term follow-up that addresses specifically thalamic and basal ganglia AVMs. Yamamoto et al. reported their long-term follow-up results in gamma knife radiosurgery for AVMs specifically focusing on complications occurring more than 5 years after irradiation.[24] Out of the 40 patients treated, only 9 had a thalamic or basal ganglia AVM. Complete angiographic obliteration was achieved in two-thirds of the cases over 5 years.[24] More recently, Kobayashi et al.[9] reported 71 patients with basal ganglia or thalamic AVMs treated with gamma knife radiosurgery and found an encouraging 92% 2-year complete obliteration rate in angiographically followed cases; however, only 55% of patients in their series underwent angiography. They found a higher obliteration rate in thalamic and basal ganglia AVMs when compared to other sites primarily because of their smaller average volume.[9]

Our results indicate that smaller AVMs have a higher rate of obliteration at 3 years. Apart from size, many other factors contributed to the obliteration of the nidus and these included: (1) the compactness of the nidus and the ease or difficulty of targeting, (2) the minimum dose prescribed to the margin, and (3) brain location. However, these factors are related to each other in several ways. The obliteration rate largely depends on the minimum dose delivered to the nidus, a dose that is limited by AVM volume and brain location. At the University of Pittsburgh, the criteria for dose prescription are based on an estimated 3% risk of delayed radiation-induced injury to the surrounding healthy brain.[3] The goal is to deliver the highest possible dose to the nidus margin, which has less than a 3% risk of probable complications. If the surrounding brain has already been damaged by hemorrhage or prior therapies, a higher risk may be taken by the surgeon and a higher (and potentially more effective) dose selected.

We previously found that the following factors were associated with incomplete obliteration: (1) large AVM volume in a critical area limiting minimum target dose, (2) a compressed AVM due to blood clot with the later reappearance of nidus not initially irradiated, (3) incomplete identification of the AVM on biplane angiography, (4) improper assessment of the AVM nidus shape despite the correct vessels being injected, and (5) recanalization of nidus after embolization. Finally, no definite cause (possible tissue resistance to radiation) was identified in some cases.[15]

In our experience, problems associated with definition of the nidus target were the greatest reason for failure to achieve obliteration. The conventional biplane two-dimensional angiogram fails to provide enough information about the true shape of the nidus to ensure inclusion of the entire nidus and exclude all normal tissue. Since 1992 we have used stereotactic MRI and MRA with angiography in all eligible patients. In our experience, high-resolution MRI provides excellent definition of the AVM to assist angiographic planning.[12] In many situations MRA can provide critical information on AVM shape that is not provided by the conventional angiogram alone.

At 3 years we generally recommend second-stage radiosurgery for incompletely obliterated AVMs. We consider re-treating the incompletely obliterated nidus at this time since few additional patients have further obliteration. Re-treatment is associated with a significant rate of further obliteration.[13] Five out of 14 re-treated AVMs have shown complete obliteration with additional follow-up pending. We now consider staged procedures for larger AVMs (volume staging) in patients who present with hemorrhage and are not found suitable for other procedures.

In our series one completely obliterated AVM showed regrowth 3 years after the documentation of complete obliteration by the 1-year follow-up angiogram. This young girl had a cerebral hemorrhage at the age of 6 and had radiosurgery. She probably represents one of the rare cases in children in whom further AVM formation is reported. Several authors have reported recurrence of an AVM after complete surgical excision and angiographic documentation of nidus absence. Many hypotheses have been put forward to explain this occurrence. Kondziolka et al., Sano et al., and Yasargil reported recurrences in surgically excised AVMs.[10–12] More recently Kader et al.[8] reported recurrence of AVMs in 5 children after complete excision. They hypothesized that AVM formation in children may be an active phenomenon in which synthesis of the abnormal vessels is induced by humoral factors such as vascular endothelial growth factor. Excision of these AVMs while they are still in the active phase of their growth may be associated with new growth from untreated cells responsible for the synthesis of angiogenic growth factors.[8] In our patient, consideration of other treatment options was found to be associated with too high a risk and this patient continues to have residual AVM.

Patients with large thalamic and basal ganglia AVMs have not fared as well. Out of 15 patients who underwent embolization prior to radiosurgery in our series, only one showed later complete obliteration. In a recent review of 1246 cases from the published literature involving many different centers, cure could be achieved only in 5% of patients using embolization alone. There was an 8% morbidity and 1% mortality rate.[6] Hurst et al. recently reported a 15% complete obliteration rate after embolization.[7] In 50% of cases the AVM was reduced in volume enough to permit radiosurgery. In cases of thalamic and basal ganglia AVMs, the complication rate was 14.3%.[7] Since recanalization of the nidus has been reported after embolization,[15] we use this technique only for patients with large AVMs where a definite and significant volume reduction is anticipated.

Radiosurgery has emerged as the treatment of choice for patients with small, high-risk thalamic or basal ganglia AVMs. The average diameter of these AVMs managed at our center was less than 25 mm. Encouraging and uniform long-term results have led to the expansion of inclusion criteria for radiosurgery. Staged radiosurgery, a concept similar to staged surgery, allows treatment of larger and surgically higher risk AVMs. With meticulous planning, the complication rate can be kept low. Multidisciplinary management strategies must be considered for patients with these difficult vascular lesions.

References

1. Colombo F, Pozza F, Chigeiro G, et al. Linear accelerator radiosurgery of cerebral arteriovenous malformation; an update. Neurosurgery 34:14–21, 1994.
2. Engenhart R, Wowra B, Debus J, et al. The role of high dose single-fraction irradiation in small and large intracranial arteriovenous malformation. Int J Radiat Oncol Biol Phys 30:521 529,1994.
3. Flickinger JC. An integrated formula for prediction of complication from radiosurgery. Int J Radiat Oncol Biol Phys 17:879–885, 1989.
4. Flickinger JC. Treatment planning for gamma knife radiosurgery with multiple isocenters. Int J Radiat Oncol Biol Phys 18:1495–1501, 1990.
5. Friedman WA, Bova FJ, Mendenhall WN. Linear accelerator radiosurgery of cerebral arteriovenous malformation: the relationship of size to outcome. J Neurosurg 82:180–189, 1995.
6. Frizzel RT, Fisher WS III. Cure, morbidity, and mortality associated with embolization of brain arteriovenous malformations: A review of 1246 patients in 32 series over a 35-year period. Neurosurgery 37:1031–1037, 1995.
7. Hurst RW, Berenstein A, Kupersmith MJ, et al. Deep central arteriovenous malformation of the brain: the role of endovascular treatment. J Neurosurg 82(2): 190–195, 1995.
8. Kader A, Goodrich JT, Sonstein WJ, et al. Recurrent cerebral arteriovenous malformations after negative postoperative angiograms. J Neurosurg 85:14–18, 1996.
9. Kobayashi T, Tanaka T, Omaya H, et al. Gamma knife treatment of the basal ganglia and thalamus AVMs. Brain Nerve 48(4):351–356, 1996.
10. Kondziolka D, Humphreys RP, Hoffman HJ, et al. Arteriovenous malformations of the brain in children: a forty-year experience. Can J Neurol Sci 19:40–45, 1992.
11. Kondziolka D, Dempsey PK, Lunsford LD, et al. A comparison between magnetic resonance imaging and computed tomography for stereotactic coordinate determination. Neurosurgery 30:402–407, 1992.
12. Kondziolka D, Lunsford LD, et al. Stereotactic magnetic resonance angiography imaging for targeting arteriovenous malformation in radiosurgery. Neurosurgery 35:585–591, 1994.
13. Lunsford LD. Stereotactic radiosurgery for arteriovenous malformation of the brain (editorial). Mayo Clinic Proc 70:305, 1995.
14. Lunsford LD, Kondziolka D, Flickinger JC, et al. Stereotactic radiosurgery for arteriovenous malformation of the brain. J Neurosurg 75:512–524, 1991.
15. Pollock BE, Kondziolka D, Lunsford LD, et al. Repeat stereotactic radiosurgery of arteriovenous malformation: Factors associated with incomplete obliteration. Neurosurgery 36:318– 324, 1996.
16. Pollock BE, Flickinger JC, Lunsford LD, et al. Hemorrhagic risk after stereotactic radiosurgery of arteriovenous malformations. Neurosurgery 38:651–652, 1996.
17. Pollock BE, Lunsford LD, Kondziolka D, et al. Patient outcomes after stereotactic radiosurgery for operable arteriovenous malformations. Neurosurgery 35:1–7, 1994.
18. Pollock BE, Kondziolka D, Patel AK, et al. Magnetic resonance imaging is an accurate method to evaluate arteriovenous malformations after stereotactic radiosurgery. J Neurosurg 85:1044–1049, 1996.
19. Sasaki T, Kurita H, Saito I, et al. Arteriovenous malformations in the basal ganglia and thalamus: management and results in 101 cases. J Neurosurg 88:285–292, 1998.
20. Schneider BF, Eberhard DA, Steiner LE. Histopathology of arteriovenous malformations after gamma knife radiosurgery. J Neurosurg 87:352–357, 1997.
21. Spetzler RF, Martin NA. A proposed grading system for arteriovenous malformations. J Neurosurg 65:476–483, 1986.
22. Steiner L, Lindquist C, Cail W, et al. Microsurgery and radiosurgery in brain arteriovenous malformations (editorial). J Neurosurg 79:647–652, 1993.
23. Yamaguchi N, Yamashima T, Yamashita J. A histopathological and flow cytometric study of dog brain endothelial cell injuries in delayed radiation necrosis. J Neurosurg 74:625–632, 1991.
24. Yamamato M, Jimbo M, Hara M, et al. Gamma knife radiosurgery for arteriovenous malformations: Long-term follow-up results focusing on complications occurring more than 5 years after irradiation. Neurosurgery 38:906–914, 1996.

Chapter 9

Hemodynamic Perturbations in Intracranial Arteriovenous Malformations:

Pathophysiology and Effects of Radiosurgery*

Eng H. Lo, PhD

Introduction

The management of intracranial arteriovenous malformations (AVMs) is one of the most difficult areas of vascular neurosurgery. Although the anatomic and angiographic architecture of these complex lesions have been the subject of many previous investigations,[23,27,60,66,74] the hemodynamic pathophysiology of these abnormal shunts is still not fully understood. It is important to recognize that the majority of AVM symptomatology is related to its abnormal hemodynamics. Regional alterations in cerebrovascular function result from the low-resistance, high-flow properties of the AVM shunts.[21,25,34,55–57,78] AVM hemodynamics may lead to vascular steal and chronic hypoperfusion of surrounding brain tissue that results in low-grade ischemia. In addition, the high-flow shunts are susceptible to hemorrhage. Neuronal damage due to ischemia or repeated hemorrhages may also provide a basis for seizures. Finally, AVM hemodynamics also impact on treatment outcomes; successful obliteration of the AVM should result in a reperfusion of areas previously subjected to steal,[55,56,59,78] but abrupt occlusion of shunts may also result in edema and hemorrhage. This latter phenomenon was first described by Spetzler in 1978 and was termed "perfusion pressure breakthrough."[67] These hyperemic events have been observed in clinical patients and represent a serious complication in AVM therapy, especially when the AVM resides in or close to functional brain areas.[2–4,76,78]

Advances in microsurgical techniques have allowed the excision of AVMs in functionally critical brain areas[76,77] and embolization techniques have been used with and without surgery to treat large AVMs.[19,32,72] Additionally, stereotactic radiosurgery with charged particles, modified linear accelerators, and the gamma knife have been used to alter AVM flow noninvasively.[7,8,13,28,38,43,45,58,69] More recently, multimodality treatments that combine surgery, embolization, and/or radiosurgery are beginning to yield results.[12,15,48,68] The efficacy of these various approaches is dependent on the successful conversion of abnormal hemodynamics into flow patterns consistent with normal brain function. It is thus important to examine AVM hemodynamics in order to understand its pathophysiology as well as its response to treatment.

In this chapter, a biomathematical analysis of hemodynamic alterations in AVMs and the adjacent vasculature is presented. Alterations in blood flow,

From Yamada S (ed): *Arteriovenous Malformations in Functional Areas of the Brain.*

* Dedicated to the memory of Professor Jacob I. Fabrikant (1928–1993), one of the pioneers in the applications of radiosurgery for the treatment of intracranial vascular malformations.

Research supported in part by NS32806, and NS37074 and a Grant-in-Aid from the American Heart Association.

pressure gradients, and hemodynamic resistance are calculated based on a model of Poiseillean flow dynamics. The model will also examine the biomechanical response to radiosurgery. Intramural stress in the shunt walls is calculated based on radiosurgically induced luminal narrowing and obliteration. Finally, biological consequences of AVM radiosurgery are discussed as they may relate to the hemodynamic perturbations before and after treatment.

Hemodynamic Analysis

Derivation of Biomathematical Model

The precise analysis of cerebral hemodynamics using fluid dynamic mathematics is quite complex. The pulsatile nature of flow coupled with the intricately branched and tapered structure of the cerebrovascular tree requires Navier-Stokes formulations and impedance calculations to account for multiple wave reflections.[49] In order to simplify the analysis, we assume first-order nonpulsatile flow through the AVM and surrounding vasculature.[20,35,36,39,52,53] The AVM is represented as a parallel set of multiple flow compartments, itself in parallel with a normal vessel compartment (Figure 1). This formulation allows the representation of any AVM as an arbitrary distribution of different sized shunts. Blood viscosity is υ.

The total cerebral blood flow (F_{tot}) to the region-of-analysis is thus comprised of AVM flow (F_{avm}) and blood flow to surrounding normal brain (F_{br}):

$$F_{tot} = F_{br} + F_{avm} \tag{1}$$

R_{avm} is comprised of multiple resistances of its various parallel compartments R_i, where N_i is the num-

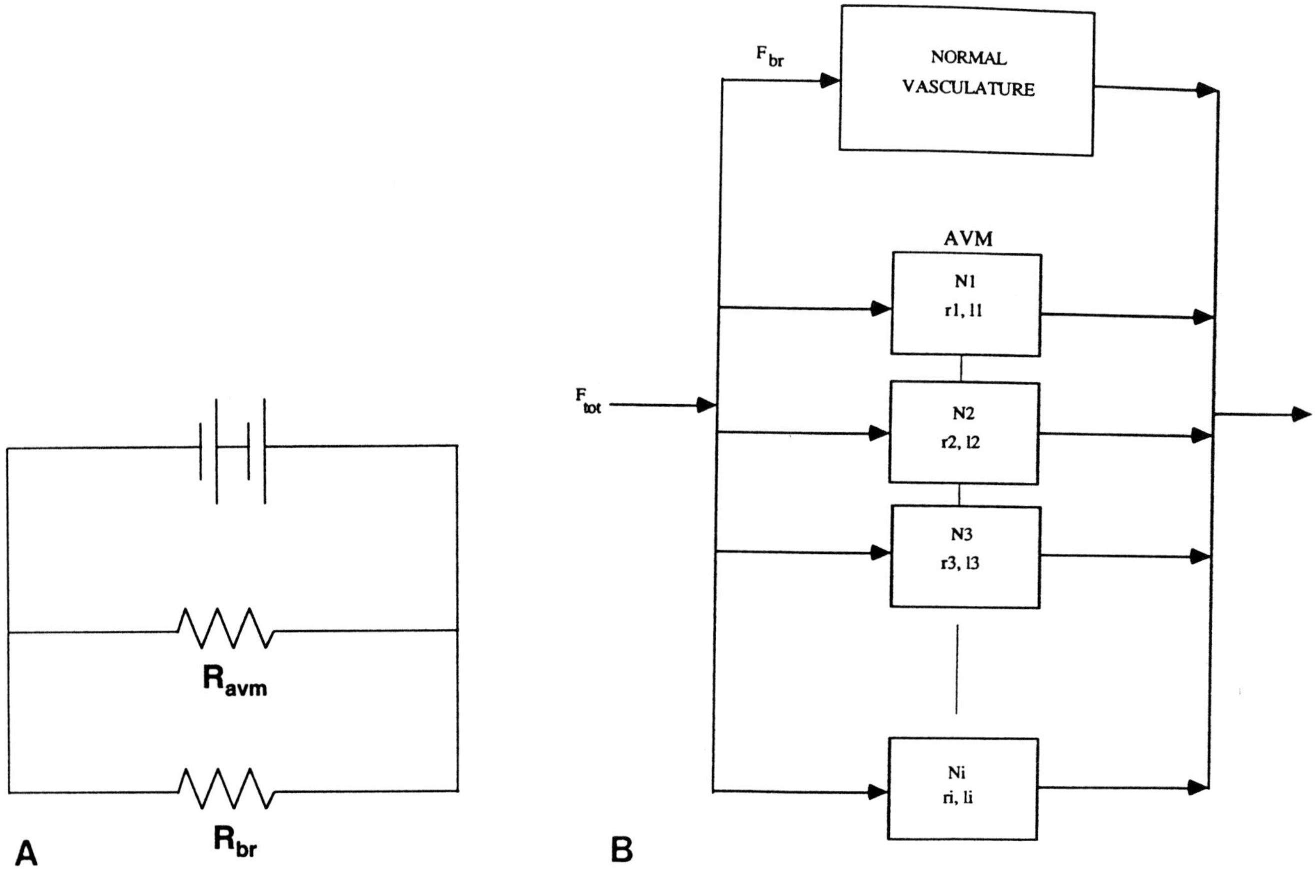

Figure 1A. The AVM flow compartment model can be thought of as being analogous to an electrical circuit where the AVM "resistor" (R_{avm}) lies in parallel with another resistor representing normal vasculature in adjacent brain (R_{br}). The electrical current flowing through the circuit is the blood flow and the battery provides the voltage or the cerebral perfusion pressure. Adapted and used with permission from Lo EH.[35] **B.** A more detailed schematic representation of the flow compartments used to model AVM hemodynamics. Normal adjacent vasculature is represented as a flow compartment placed in parallel with the AVM. The AVM itself is comprised of multiple flow compartments with an arbitrary distribution of shunt lengths and radii.

ber of shunts in that compartment and l_i is the length of these shunts,

$$R_{avm} = 1/(\Sigma 1/R_i) \quad (2)$$

$$R_i = 8\upsilon l_i/N_i \pi r_i^4 \quad (3)$$

Cerebral perfusion pressure (CPP) is defined as the blood pressure gradient across this region-of-analysis. The total hemodynamic resistance is R_{tot} (R_{br} in parallel with R_{avm}) so that,

$$CPP = F_{tot}R_{tot} = F_{tot}R_{br}R_{avm}/(R_{br} + R_{avm}) \quad (4)$$

Blood flow through the AVM is:

$$F_{avm} = CPP/R_{avm} \quad (5)$$

and flow through the surrounding normal brain is:

$$F_{br} = CPP/R_{br} \quad (6)$$

Based on these equations, the various hemodynamic perturbations associated with AVMs may be examined, including vascular steal, hemorrhage, reperfusion, and the response to treatment.

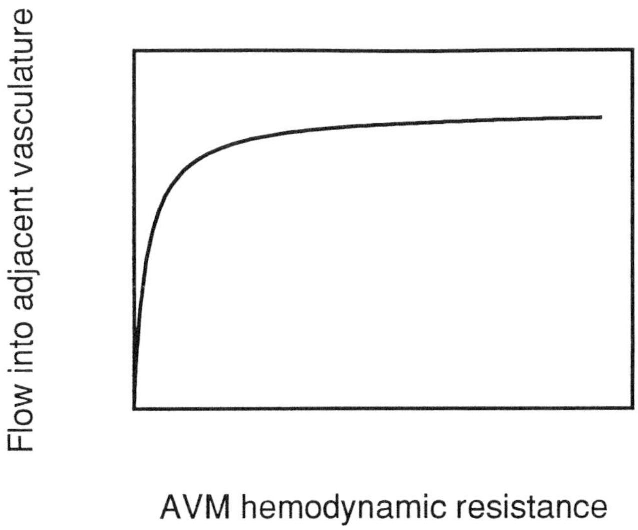

Figure 2. A schematic showing that the amount of blood flow remaining in adjacent vasculature is subject to steal from the high flow AVM. Flow into surrounding areas is dependent on the hemodynamic resistance of the AVM. The lower the AVM resistance, the lower the level of flow into normal vessel compartments. After radiosurgery, as the AVM is slowly obliterated, the hemodynamic resistance increases and flow is restored into adjacent vasculature. Adapted and used with permission from Lo EH.[35]

Vascular Steal

The degree of blood flow redirected through the AVM is related to the relative hemodynamic resistances of the AVM versus the surrounding vasculature.[34,35,46,52,53,55,56,64] A direct relationship between these flow values will be present if the total blood flow (F_{tot}) to that region is constant. Therefore, the remaining flow to normal brain would be total flow less that shunted through the AVM (Figure 2).

$$F_{br} = F_{tot} - F_{avm} = F_{tot} - (CPP/R_{avm}) \quad (7)$$

$$F_{br} = F_{tot}[1 - R_{br}/(R_{avm} + R_{br})] \quad (8)$$

Intracranial Hemorrhage

The risks of hemorrhage are likely to be related to the biomechanical stress across the AVM vessel walls. Therefore, by calculating the changes in stress within the AVM shunt walls, one may be able to estimate the changes in hemorrhage probabilities. Stress in the circumferential direction for thin-walled cylindrical tubes may be expressed as:

$$S\vartheta = Pr/h \quad (9)$$

where P is transmural pressure, r is the radius of the tube, and h is the vessel wall thickness. The summation of circumferential stress across all AVM shunts is:

$$\Sigma S\vartheta \sim \Sigma(N_i P_i r_i/h_i) \quad (10)$$

Assuming that the venous pressure is equivalent to the intracranial pressure outside the vessels, the parallel arrangement of the AVM shunts imply that, on average, $P_i = CPP$. Therefore,

$$\Sigma S\vartheta \sim \Sigma(N_i CPP r_i/h_i) = CPP\Sigma(N_i r_i/h_i) \quad (11)$$

Equation (11) implies that the probability of hemorrhage is proportional to the pressure gradient CPP across the AVM, which is not surprising. These results also suggest that AVMs with large (high value for r_i) and thin-walled (small value for h_i) shunts may be more susceptible to hemorrhage. Although the intramural stress within the AVM shunt walls is not directly predictive of hemorrhage, it may represent a useful index for risk. The relationship between anatomic factors and the stress index proposed in this section is unclear. However, until a more direct clinical parameter is identified, the use of biomechanical stress appears to be a reasonable parameter for our theoretical model. The use of shunt wall stress as an index for biomechanical changes in the AVM after radiosurgery will be examined in a separate section below.

Some studies have attempted to correlate the angiographic pattern of feeders and the AVM nidus with hemorrhage risks.[47,60] Other groups have suggested that venous drainage may be more important than arterial compartments in terms of hemorrhage.[1,16,50] Additionally, some data also suggest that AVM size (which may in turn affect pressure and shunt wall stress) might influence hemorrhage risks as well.[26,65] More recently, sophisticated approaches based on logistic and multivariate analysis have been proposed in an attempt to assess the risks of AVM hemorrhage and predict results and overall complication rates, especially after radiosurgical treatment.[9,61,73]

Reperfusion After AVM Obliteration

Upon obliteration (partial or complete) of the AVM, blood flow should be redirected back into normal flow patterns.[4,20,35,39,55,56,59,78] From a theoretical standpoint, there are two limiting cases. In the first case, when CPP remains constant, there is no redirection of flow into normal vasculature. In this scenario, total blood flow to the brain is reduced. In the other limiting case, F_{tot} remains constant and the degree of reperfusion is a function of the ratio of hemodynamic resistance of surrounding vessels to the resistance of any residual AVM shunts (equation 8, Figure 2).

The occurrence of hyperemic complications following treatment may be related to the sudden surge of pressure into previously low-flow regions of adjacent brain. Large relative increases in pressure may induce hemorrhage and/or edema. In the event that complete AVM obliteration has occurred, all the flow through the AVM is now redirected into the surrounding normal vessels:

$$F_{br} = F_{tot} = CPP/R_{br} + CPP/R_{avm} \qquad (12)$$

The new pressure gradient across the normal vasculature is now P_{br} so that:

$$F_{br} = P_{br}/R_{br} \qquad (13)$$

Equating 12 and 13 reveals that the relative increase in pressure is:

$$\begin{aligned}(P_{br} - CPP)/CPP &= R_{br}/R_{avm}CPP \\ &= F_{avm}/F_{br}CPP\end{aligned} \qquad (14)$$

Equation 14 implies that the degree of reperfusion pressure is related to the ratio of original AVM flow versus normal flow, i.e., the degree of vascular steal present. In addition, the results paradoxically suggest that AVMs in brain regions with high perfusion pressures to begin with, may be less susceptible to hyperemic reperfusion and "perfusion pressure breakthrough" complications.

Biomechanical Consequences of Radiosurgery

Stereotactic radiosurgery is being increasingly used to treat intracranial AVMs. However successful radiosurgery may involve latent periods of 1–2 years prior to complete obliteration.[7,28,38,43,58,69] This latent period includes states of altered hemodynamics that may influence hemorrhage probabilities. Transient increases in intra-AVM pressure could increase hemorrhage risks. Alternatively, radiosurgery is believed to induce progressive shunt wall thickening leading to luminal closure. Thus, it is conceivable that even prior to complete obliteration, the radiosurgically thickened shunt walls may reduce transmural stress and decrease hemorrhage risks.

The compartmental model described above was used to examine the changes in biomechanical stress after radiosurgery. Based on equations 1–7, parameters were selected (Table 1) to duplicate typical AVM flow rates and pressure gradients obtained by various groups using both intraoperative and noninvasive measurements.[17,34–36,41] A Poisson function was used to represent AVM shunt distributions. The resistance of the AVM was approximately 15,000 dynes-sec/cm^2 and F_{avm} was calculated to be about 140 mL/min. Perfusion to adjacent brain was, therefore, compromised due to steal. It was assumed that the AVM would affect approximately 500 cm^3 of

Table 1
Arteriovenous Malformation Model Parameters, Hemodynamic Values, and Biomechanical Stresses

Total number of shunts	18
Shunt radii	0.01–0.07 cm
Shunt lengths	10 cm
R_{avm}	16,681 dynes-sec/cm^2
rCPP	27.9 mm Hg
F_{avm}	134 mL/min
F_{br}	116 mL/min
$S\epsilon$	6.72 × 10^6 dynes/cm^2
$S\epsilon\epsilon$	2.16 × 10^7 dynes/cm^2

rCPP = cerebral perfusion pressure; R_{avm} = AVM resistance; F_{br} = blood flow to normal brain; F_{avm} = AVM flow.

brain tissue. Hence, F_{tot} was 250 mL/min and F_{br} was calculated to be 110 mL/min, resulting in average perfusion rates of approximately 22 mL/100 g/min for the surrounding brain tissue affected by the AVM. Note that normal perfusion levels for human brain is considered to be in the 50–80 mL/100 g/min range.

The stresses in an isotropic thick-walled elastic tube can be resolved into three components in the radial, longitudinal, and circumferential directions.[49] The greatest stress is circumferential and would occur at the inner wall of the tube. For thin-walled tubes, circumferential stress can be expressed as equation 9. For cases where the thin-wall approximation is not valid, the stress is:

$$S\vartheta\vartheta = P(r_i^2 + r_o^2)/(r_o^2 - r_i^2) \qquad (15)$$

where r_i and r_o represent inner and outer radii, respectively. In this analysis, the total biomechanical stress in dynes/cm^2 was calculated based on the distributions of shunt radii and a constant shunt wall thickness of 0.001 cm. As shunts were progressively obliterated over the course of the latent period post-radiosurgery, the change in biomechanical stress was expressed as a percent change from pre-treatment baseline values. Two different obliteration models[36] were used to simulate the latent period after radiosurgery during which the AVM shunts are slowly obliterated: Model I where the distribution of AVM shunts was subjected to a step-function elimination process, i.e., at selected time points, shunts were instantaneously eliminated; and Model II where the shunt walls are slowly thickened to simulate progressive luminal narrowing.

For Model I, since no luminal narrowing was involved, the thin-wall approximation for circumferential stress (equation 8) was used. As predicted by equations 1–7, a progressive reduction in F_{avm} resulted in an accompanying increase in F_{br}. Regional pressure gradients (rCPP) returned to normal levels when the AVM was completely obliterated. Biomechanical changes were significantly dependent on the selection of shunts that were being obliterated. Random series of shunt selection generated from a spreadsheet demonstrated that there may be transient increases in biomechanical stress prior to complete obliteration (Figure 3). Although a general trend of reduced biomechanical stress was obtained, there existed a finite probability that transient increases in stress within the AVM shunts would occur prior to complete AVM obliteration.

In Model II, changes in F_{avm}, F_{br}, and rCPP were, in general, similar to those found in Model I. However, the biomechanical stress for this model was computed based on slowly thickening shunt walls subjected to radiation-induced luminal narrowing (equation 9). If all shunts were simultaneously narrowed in a uniform manner, the change in circumferential stress in the inner shunt walls demonstrated a rapid decrease to zero. However, uniform luminal narrowing may not be a biologically realistic situation; therefore, a random shunt selection process was

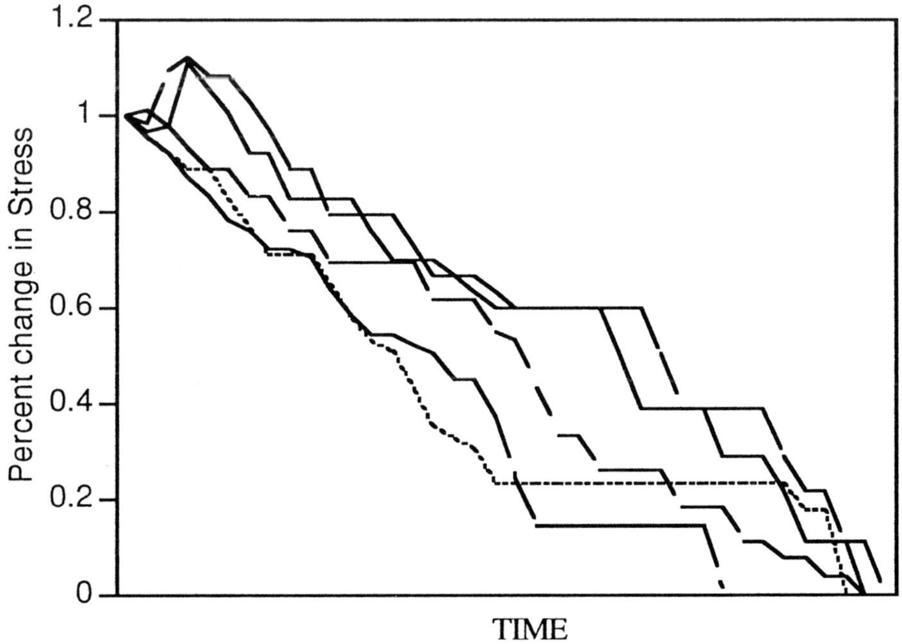

Figure 3. Changes in biomechanical stress in a Poisson distribution of AVM shunts subjected to a random obliteration process. Five random series are represented to demonstrate that, following radiosurgery, it is theoretically possible for transient increases in stress to occur prior to complete obliteration. Adapted and used with permission from Lo EH.[36]

also examined where the latent period for the induction of luminal narrowing was dependent on shunt radii. In this scenario, the initial period of luminal narrowing was associated with large variations in stress. When changes in F_{avm} were compared with alteration in stress, the upper and lower bounds encompassed regions where relatively large decreases in AVM flow resulted in only minimal reductions in stress. This characteristic was similar to that observed in Model I, and again demonstrated that, although radiosurgically induced luminal narrowing with concomitant wall thickening would generally result in decreased stress, there remained the possibility that no significant reduction in stress will occur until the AVM was almost completely obliterated. This suggests that protection may not be assured until complete angiographic obliteration of all AVM shunts has been demonstrated. This is an important point and appears to be in agreement with emerging clinical findings.[7,14,62]

Hemodynamic Consequences of Partial Obliteration

One of the limiting factors in AVM radiosurgery is the dose to surrounding brain. Due to profound dose-volume effects of brain irradiation,[10,38,43,44,69] there has been some effort to limit the full radiosurgical dose to the nidus of the AVM. This strategy is based on the assumption that obliteration of the nidus would eliminate all flow through the AVM. It is often difficult to identify the true nidus of an AVM based on angiographic and MRI data. From the point of blood flow dynamics, the nidus is the hemodynamic or physiological center of the AVM through which all AVM shunt flow must pass. The nidus of the AVM is not necessarily its anatomic core. Therefore, limiting the radiosurgical target volume to the central anatomic portions of the AVM may not lead to complete obliteration if true physiological nidus has not been properly identified.

In order to examine the hemodynamic response to incomplete radiosurgery, we apply the compartmental model described above to calculate changes in flow and pressure gradient.[36] The model is further refined to include separate compartments for the various portions of the AVM, feeding arteries, shunting arterioles, and core vessels (Figure 4), based on the classification derived by Yamada.[78] Reduction of flow and pressure gradients within the various AVM compartments occurred, as expected (Figure 5). However, the model suggested that transient pressure increases in the shunting arterioles may occur before the AVM is completely obliterated. For partial volume radiosurgery, incomplete obliteration was achieved (Figure 6). AVM shunt flow was reduced but did not go to zero, and pressure gradients may be permanently increased in certain compartments. This result agrees with clinical data demonstrating that uniform irradiation of the entire arterial phase of the AVM is necessary for complete obliteration.[7,38,43] However, it is not currently possible to confirm the predicted pressure changes in the individual compartments.

Higher Order Models

The model described above provides the first order fundamentals for a theoretical analysis of AVM hemodynamics and biomechanics. Although unequivocal validation of model predictions may remain unattainable because of the difficulty of obtaining robust clinical parameters of flow, pressure, and stress, the model yields a useful framework for further investigations into AVM pathophysiology.

More recently, higher order models have been

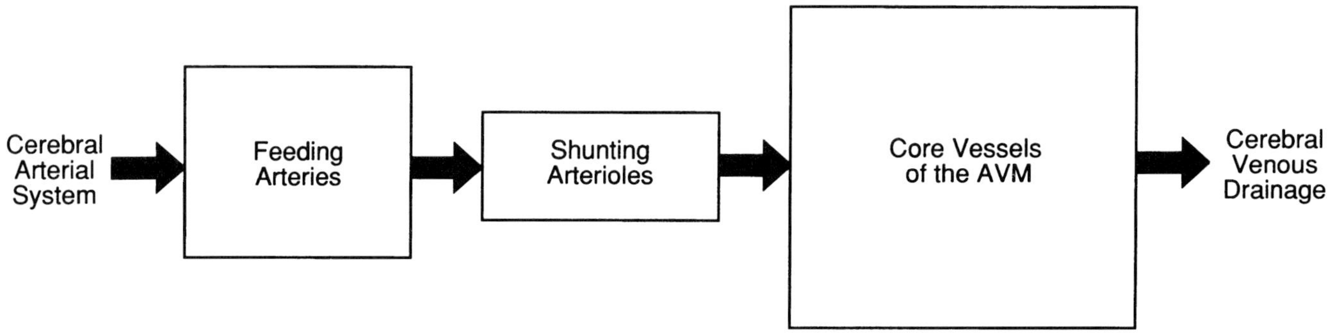

Figure 4. The intracranial AVM is modeled as a series of linked flow compartments based on the hemodynamic anatomy proposed by Yamada. Each flow compartment is comprised of parallel shunts with a selected distribution of shunt radii and lengths. The relative size of each compartment in this schematic is indicative of the relative blood volumes present in the various flow compartments of the AVM. Used with permission from Lo EH, et al.[39]

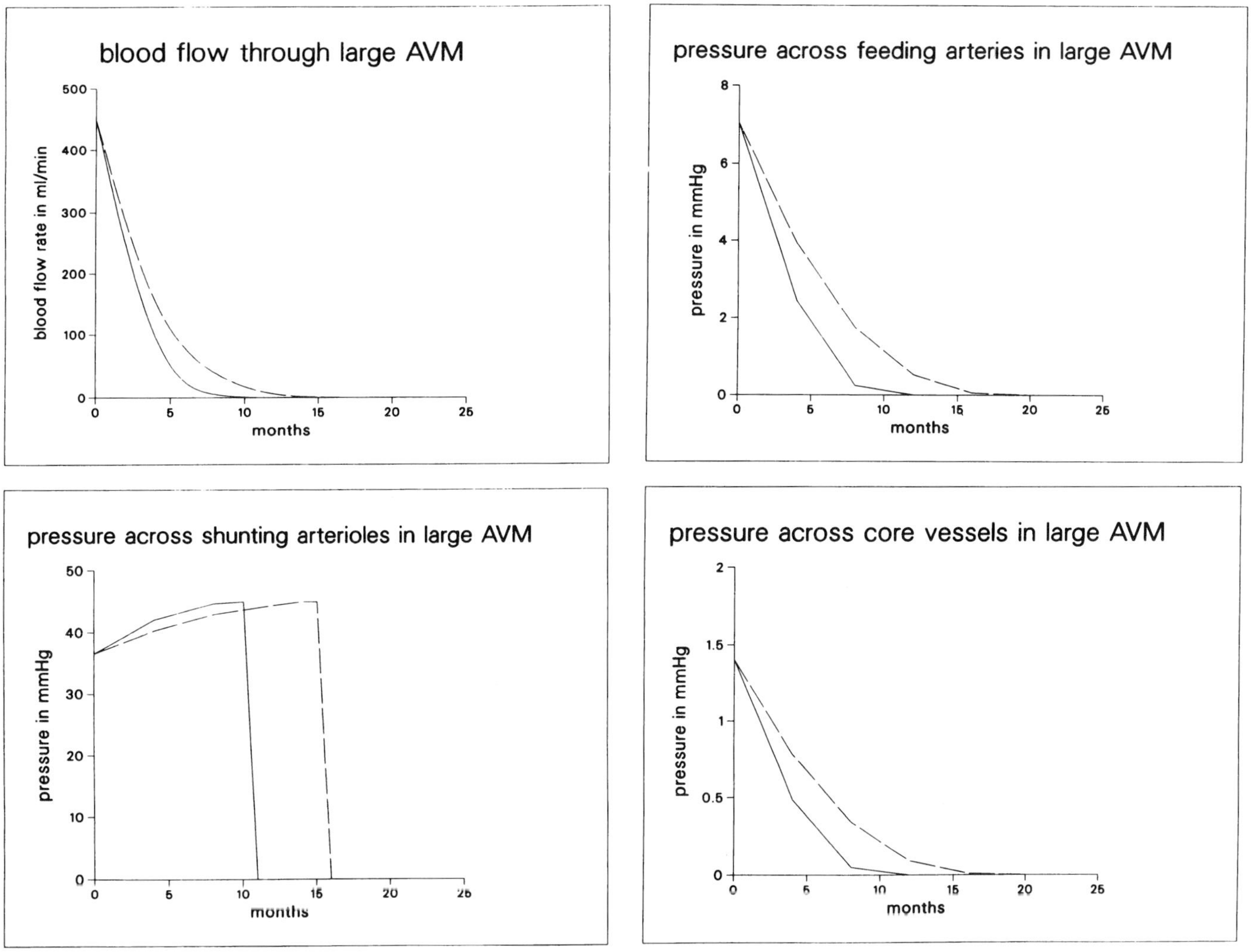

Figure 5. AVM blood flow rates and pressure gradients in the different compartments after complete volume radiosurgery. Shunt radii are reduced to simulate the effects of radiosurgery in a large high-flow (440 mL/min) AVM. Variable latent periods may be present after radiosurgery. Therefore, the plots only demonstrate the hemodynamic changes that occur after the latent period. Two different luminal narrowing processes are shown: a radius independent rate of 0.025 mm/month and a progressive radius dependent process where large shunts (greater than 0.2 mm) narrow at 0.025 mm/month and small shunts (smaller than 0.2 mm) narrow at 0.05 mm/month. Used with permission from Lo EH, et al.[39]

proposed that incorporate the more complex characteristics of cerebral hemodynamics including autoregulation, the pulsatile nature of blood flow, the elastic modulus of blood vessels, and multiple flow networks that extend beyond the immediate periphery of the AVM itself. In particular, two models may be especially promising. The first utilizes electrical network analysis to simulate the complicated branching relationships of the multi-shunt AVM and related arterial trees.[17] This approach has been successfully applied to examine the outcomes of AVM venous drainage occlusions.[16] The second model utilizes a combination of electrical network analysis and hydrodynamics to simulate the effects of AVMs on the whole brain.[11] This model has been used to show that hyperemic events after AVM removal may be related to more than simple hemodynamic readjustments alone. Sophisticated approaches such as these will surely lead to a better theoretical understanding of the complex hemodynamic behavior of cerebral AVMs.

Effects of Radiosurgery

Cerebrovascular Effects

Cerebrovascular effects after brain irradiation are usually comprised of hemodynamic alterations and

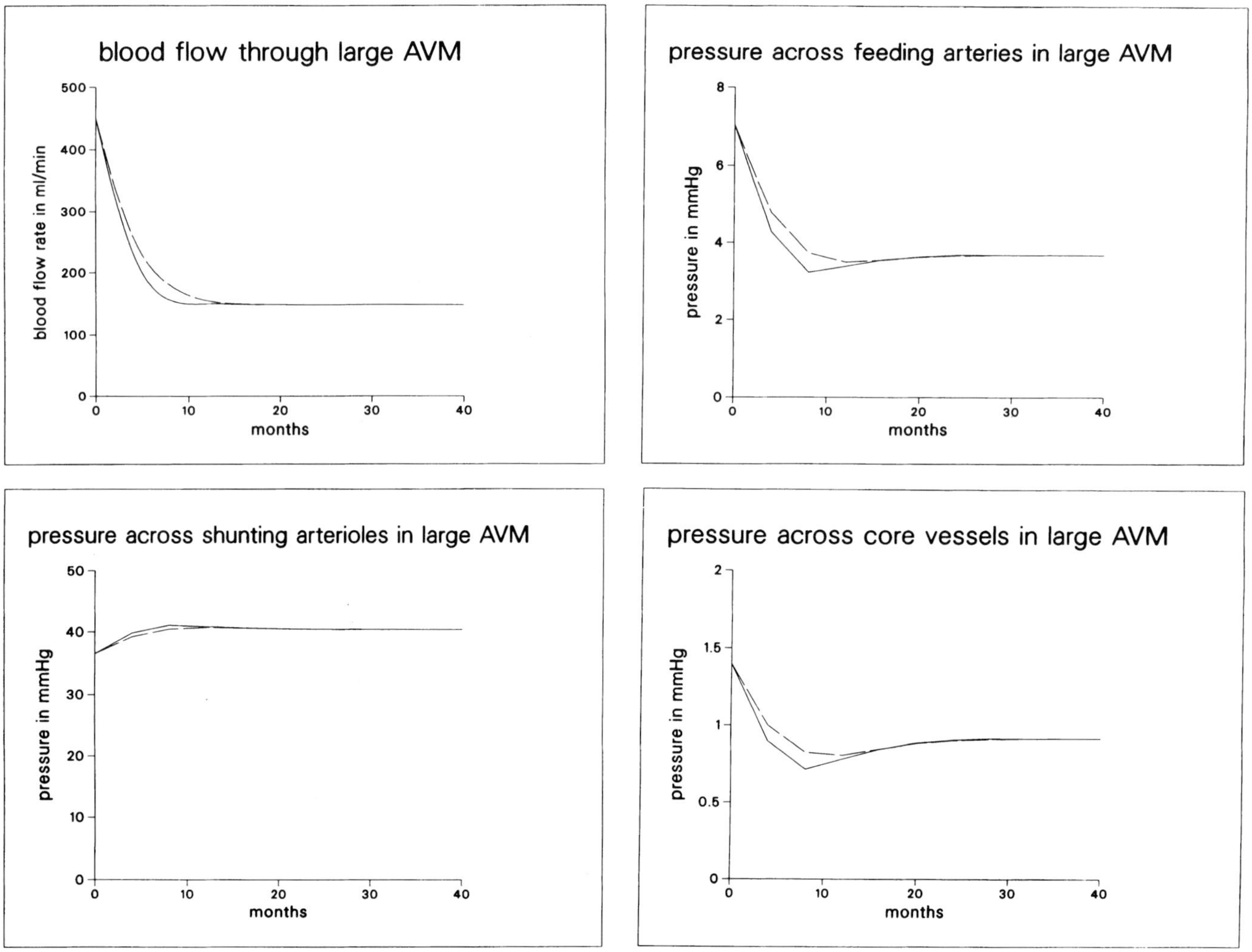

Figure 6. Alterations in AVM shunt flow and pressure gradients after partial volume radiosurgery where only 50% of shunts in all three compartments were treated. Blood flow does not reduce to zero and persistent alterations in pressure gradients remain in the various compartments. Used with permission from Lo EH, et al.[39]

blood-brain barrier (BBB) changes. In AVM radiosurgery, hemodynamic alterations are best demonstrated on follow-up cerebral angiography. Successful obliteration of abnormal shunts in high-flow AVMs often results in a dramatic reversal of steal and restoration of normal cerebral perfusion patterns (Figure 7). The biomathematical analysis described above showed that the degree of reperfusion is proportional to the hemodynamic resistance of the remaining shunts and restoration of regional perfusion pressure is related to the ratio of AVM versus normal flow. However, based on the current inability to measure the necessary parameters such as shunt resistance, it is not possible to quantitatively predict the degree of hemodynamic changes after AVM radiosurgery.

BBB disruptions are more difficult to assess. Radiosurgery may alter BBB function in both normal and abnormal vessels within and around the target volume. GdDTPA-enhanced MRI is usually used to detect changes in barrier permeability, but pretreatment scans of AVMs will often demonstrate variable degrees of contrast enhancement, thus making it difficult to distinguish radiosurgical effects from AVM enhancement.[38,43,71] Barrier disruption may be related to the most common radiological sequelae from radiosurgery, i.e., the observation of changes compatible with radiation edema in deep white matter areas adjacent to the radiosurgical target volume. Approximately 20%–30% of all patients will demonstrate either high-intensity signal on T2-weighted MRI or hypodensity on CT scans.[58] These changes usually develop 1–2 years after treatment and may resolve over several months or years. These sequalae may

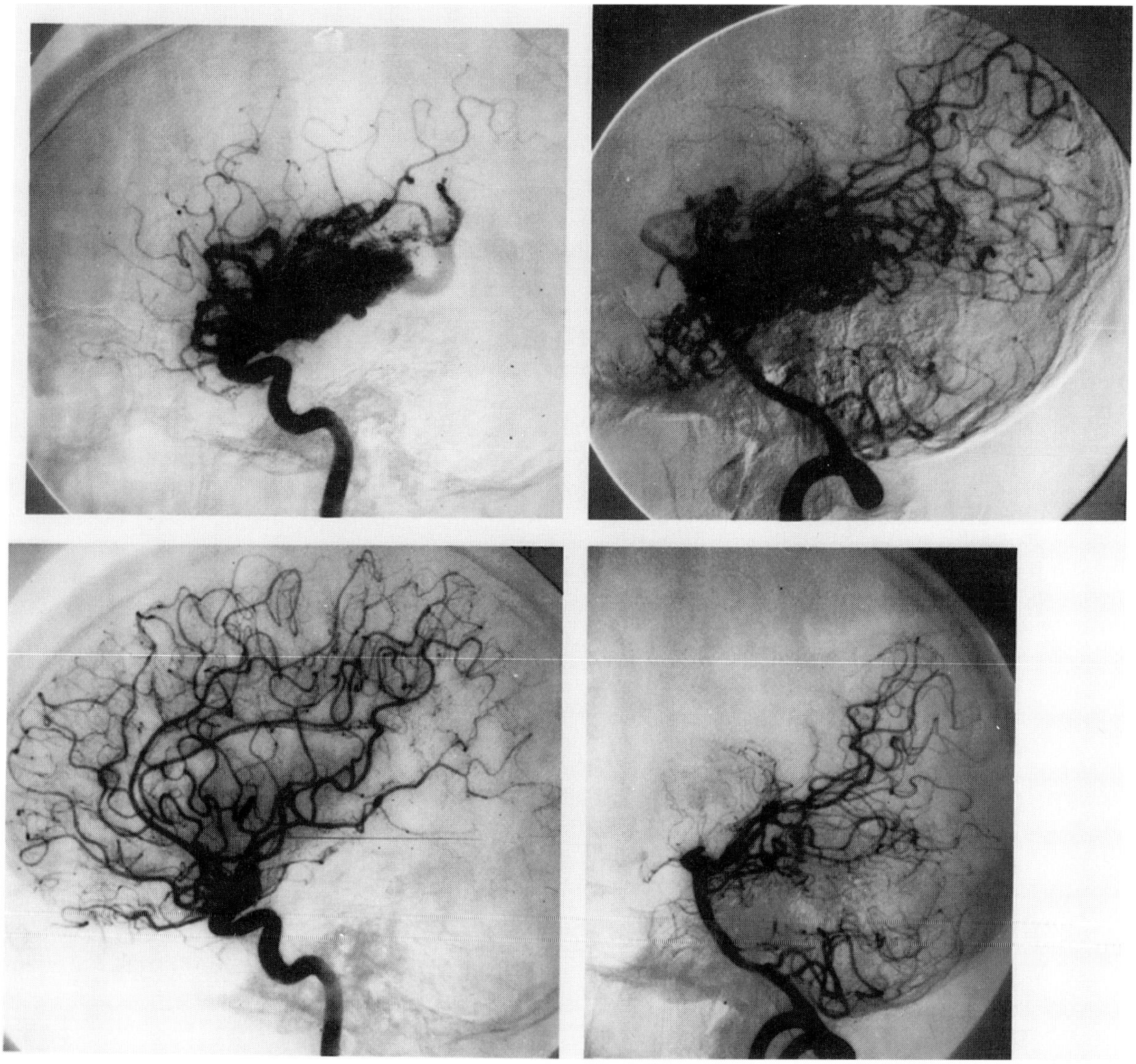

Figure 7. Hemodynamic alterations after successful radiosurgery (1 year after 27 Gy Bragg-peak 230 MeV/U helium ions). Complete obliteration of a large temporal lobe AVM is clearly accompanied by reversal of vascular steal and restoration of normal cerebral perfusion patterns. Used with permission from Lo EH, et al.[38]

be symptomatic or asymptomatic depending on the lesion location. Although direct evidence is still lacking, it is likely that these effects are due to radiation-induced changes in BBB permeability that lead to spreading edema.

Metabolic Effects

Approximately 10%–15% of patients will develop reversible and irreversible neurological dysfunction following radiosurgery.[38,43,44,69] For AVMs located in functional areas, this becomes a crucial consideration. This subset appears to be primarily composed of patients exposed to high doses in large brain volumes.[43] Widespread changes detected on MRI may be correlated to metabolic suppression as measured using fluorodeoxyglucose positron emission tomography (PET).[38,71] Extensive decreases in glucose metabolism may be observed in the associated cortical and subcortical regions. HIPDM tracer flow studies show that decreased blood flow often accompanies these metabolic suppressions.[71] This suggests that the metabolic suppression is not related to the redistribution of flow following hemodynamic obliteration of the AVM, but rather, may be indicative of radiation necrosis of normal brain. The temporal progression of clinical symptoms is usually well correlated with the pattern of PET metabolic activity over time. Spatial alterations in metabolic profile appear to be related to spreading edema, and the subsequent suppression of cerebral glucose metabolism corresponds with progressive neurological dysfunction.

Experimental Models

In spite of the increasingly widespread use of radiosurgery, the effects of large single-dose brain irradiation are not fully defined. These include latent periods, temporal progression, dose-volume effects, functional reactions, and other modifying factors.[33] In part, these issues may be addressed by experimental studies in various animal models.

The reaction to radiosurgery in the brain involves both early and delayed cerebrovascular and metabolic alterations. Stereotactic gamma irradiation of the cat basilar artery with 300 Gy induced endothelial swelling and laminar and smooth muscle degeneration as early as 1 week post-irradiation,[54] but these doses are much higher than clinical radiosurgical levels. Whole-brain irradiation in rats with 20 Gy resulted in transient decreases in iodoantipyrine extraction at 3 months followed by delayed increases at 9–12 months.[51] When a lower dose of 15 Gy was used, glucose metabolism was suppressed in 1 month.[24] Hemibrain irradiation of the rabbit brain with 60 Gy of 225 keV x-rays resulted in perturbed BBB and blood flow primarily in the hippocampal regions after only 2–3 months.[40] These changes were associated with histologic evidence of radiation-induced telangiectasia. These studies, however, involved larger brain volumes than the focal target volumes typically used in radiosurgery.

Focal brain irradiation in animal models also shows dramatic alterations in brain function. Histologic results, in general, demonstrate that focal lesions can be induced in the brain with minimal injury to adjacent structures, thus validating the radiosurgical approach. In the rabbit brain, focal irradiation with 20 Gy of neon particles induced a mild sclerosis of blood vessels and some fragmentation of myelin with 6 months.[75] Higher doses (40–80 Gy) induced cystic necrosis and cavitation. All border zones showed a sharp transition between the irradiated areas and normal brain spanning only 0.5–1.0 mm. High doses (150 Gy) from a gamma knife induced well-circumscribed lesions in the baboon brain detected with in vivo CT and MRI that were confirmed with histology.[42] Focal irradiation with 30 Gy from the Bragg-peak of a radiosurgical helium beam induced discrete regions of BBB disruption and necrosis in the deep perithalamic areas of the rabbit brain within 10 months.[37,41] However, extensive cortical metabolic suppression was detected with FDG-PET scanning, suggesting that focal injury may also induce secondary and more widespread functional effects.

It is likely that vascular responses may predominate at the dose levels used in radiosurgery. Dose response studies in the hemibrain-irradiated rat demonstrated that demyelination preceded vascular damage only at doses higher than 30–40 Gy.[22] Irradiation of the rat brain with a 3 mm proton beam showed that capillary impairment precedes parenchymal necrosis,[31] and focal irradiation of the monkey occipital lobe with a single dose of 35 Gy x-rays induced a reduction in cerebral blood flow subsequent to severe edema.[70]

The temporal progression of radiosurgical changes appears to be significantly dependent on dose and volume. Irradiation of a 0.5 mL volume in the rat brain with focused helium ions showed an inverse relationship between dose (20–60 Gy) and latent period for BBB damage (7-3 months).[63] Studies at the early phase (3 months) after a gamma knife treatment using a 4 mm port showed that increasing dose (30–150 Gy) led to increasing damage (from no changes to gross cystic necrosis) in the rat cortex.[29] A comprehensive study that examined the volume response in rabbit brain using "slit" irradiations from 2% to 100% of one hemisphere demonstrated that the frequency of various histologic alterations (vascular lesions, hemorrhage, demyelination, and necrosis) was significantly dependent on the volume of irradiated brain.[5]

The induction of delayed radiation injury in the brain is a complex process and it is difficult to separate primary from secondary effects. The aim of AVM radiosurgery is the elimination of abnormal high-flow shunts. Thus, the cellular target for radiosurgery appears to be the endothelial cell and/or smooth muscle lamina of the AVM. It is, however, inevitable that other cellular elements will also be present in the target volume, including glial and neuronal cells. There may be considerable interaction between these various elements during the latent period prior to successful AVM obliteration (Figure 8). Parenchymal cells cannot exist without an adequate vascular supply and conversely, cerebrovascular function is dependent on the metabolic demands of the parenchyma. Thus, injury to one component will lead to altered function in the other. The differential responses between vascular versus neuronal and glial elements may profoundly impact on radiosurgical outcomes, especially for large treatment volumes. Indeed, radiobiological principles based on the dose

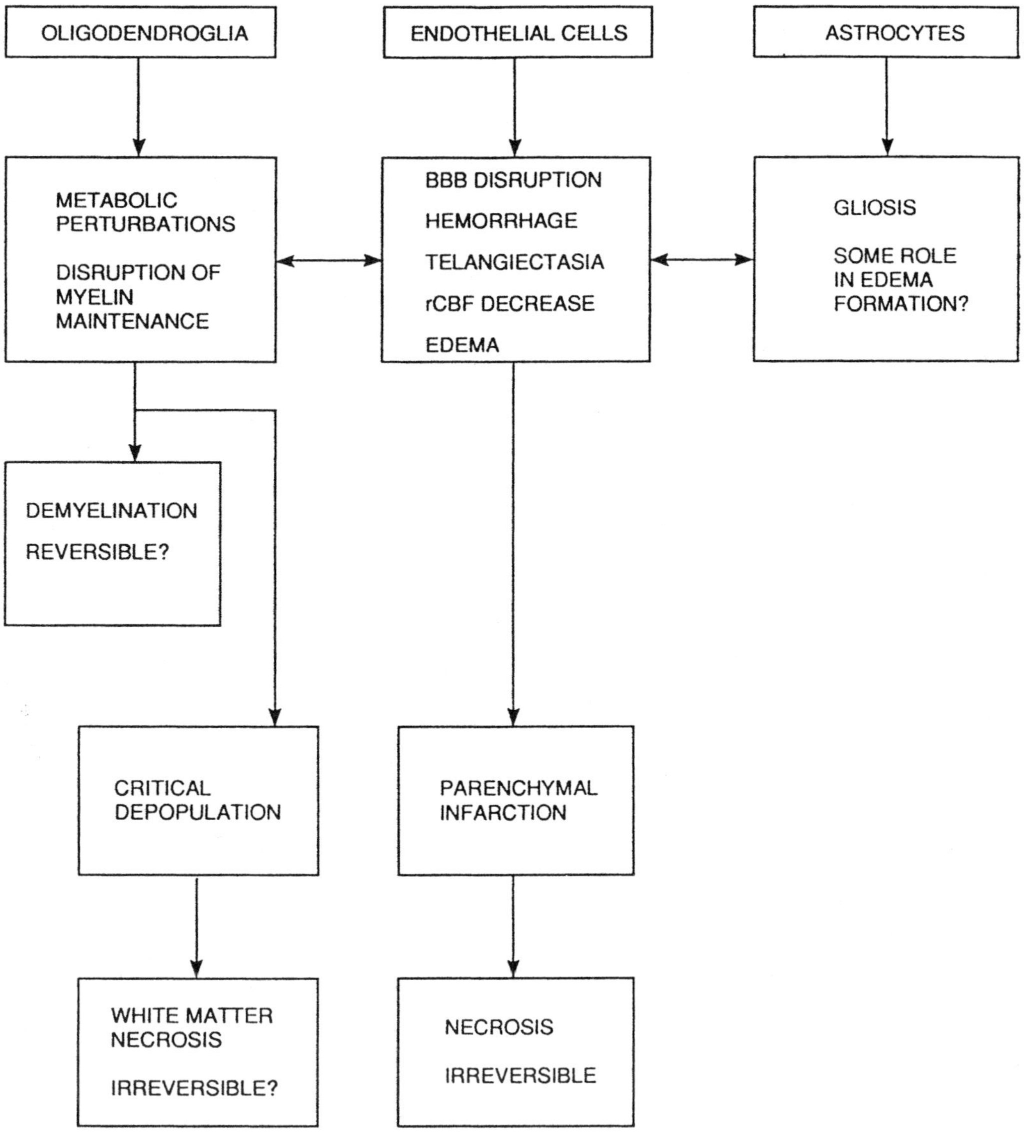
OLIGODENDROGLIA
ENDOTHELIAL CELLS
ASTROCYTES
METABOLIC PERTURBATIONS
DISRUPTION OF MYELIN MAINTENANCE
BBB DISRUPTION
HEMORRHAGE
TELANGIECTASIA
rCBF DECREASE
EDEMA
GLIOSIS
SOME ROLE IN EDEMA FORMATION?
DEMYELINATION
REVERSIBLE?
CRITICAL DEPOPULATION
PARENCHYMAL INFARCTION
WHITE MATTER NECROSIS
IRREVERSIBLE?
NECROSIS
IRREVERSIBLE

Figure 8. A schematic showing the possible interactions between various target cells in the development of delayed radiation injury following radiosurgery. BBB = blood-brain barrier; rCBF = regional cerebral blood flow. Used with permission from Lo EH, et al.[38]

response of early versus late responding tissues dictate the proper design of radiosurgery for vascular malformations as opposed to malignancies.[18] More recently, novel approaches have been investigated that combine pharmaceutical neuroprotectants with radiosurgery in an attempt to maximize vascular response and minimize parenchymal damage.[6,30]

Summary and Conclusions

The analysis presented in this chapter has demonstrated that complex hemodynamic alterations are central to the pathophysiology of the intracranial AVM. High shunt flow, steal, abnormal perfusion pressure gradients, and elevated risks of hemorrhage may be modeled by a set of biomathematical equations that link blood flow to the hemodynamic resistance of the AVM and its adjacent vasculature. The main limitation of this and other higher order models is the inability to obtain reliable quantitative parameters from clinical data, thereby precluding direct empirical testing of the model and its predictions. In general, however, the theoretical results agree well with current clinical impressions, thus validating the approach.

At present, the variables for radiosurgery continue to be defined. For the purposes of AVM treatment, it is clear that hemodynamic factors will predominate. However, as described in this chapter, other reactions to radiosurgery including BBB and metabolic events may also significantly influence outcomes and complications, especially for AVMs located in functional brain areas. Furthermore, as the role of radiosurgery is expanded to include other intracranial disorders including primary tumors and metastases, it becomes critical that these functional and cellular responses are carefully characterized. Although experimental studies can reveal useful information regarding the mechanisms of radiosurgery, the optimal parameters will ultimately have to be determined from a careful multi-institutional analysis of clinical experience and data.

References

1. al-Rodhan N, Sundt T, Piepgras D, et al. Occlusive hyperemia: a theory for the hemodynamic complications following resection of intracerebral arteriovenous malformations. J Neurosurg 78:167–175, 1993.
2. Auger R, Wiebers D, et al. Management of unruptured intracranial arteriovenous malformations: a decision analysis. Neurosurgery 30:561–569, 1992.
3. Batjer HH, Devous MD, Meyer YJ, et al. Cerebrovascular hemodynamics in arteriovenous malformation complicated by normal prefusion presure breakthrough. Neurosurgery 22:503–509, 1988.
4. Batjer HH, Purdy PD, Giller CA, et al. Evidence for redistribution of cerebral blood flow during treatment for an intracranial arteriovenous malformation. Neurosurgery 25:599–605, 1989.
5. Berg N, Lindgren M. Relationship between filed size and tolerance of rabbit brain to roentgen irradiation via a slit field. Acta Radiol 1:147–152, 1963.
6. Buatti J, Friedman W, Theele D, et al. The lazaroid U74389G protects normal brain from stereotactic radiosurgery induced radiation injury. Int J Radiat Oncol Biol Phys 34:591–597, 1996.
7. Colombo F, Pozza F, Chierego G, et al. Linear accelerator radiosurgery of cerebral arteriovenous malformations: an update. Neurosurgery 34:14–21, 1994.
8. Columbo F, Benedetti A, Pozza A. Linear accelerator radiosurgery of cerebral arteriovenous malformations. Neurosurgery 24:833–840, 1989.
9. Flickinger J, Kondziolka D, Pollock B, et al. Complications from arteriovenous malformation radiosurgery: multivariate analysis and modeling. Int J Radiat Oncol Biol Phys 38:485–490, 1997.
10. Flickinger J, Pollock B, Kondziolka D, et al. A dose response analysis of arteriovenous malformation obliteration after radiosurgery. Int J Radiat Oncol Biol Phys 36:373–379, 1996.
11. Gao E, Young W, Ornstein E, et al. A theoretical model of cerebral hemodynamics: application to the study of arteriovenous malformations. J Cereb Blood Flow Metab 17:905–918, 1997.
12. Gobin Y, Laurent A, Merienne L, et al. Treatment of brain arteriovenous malformations by embolization and radiosurgery. J Neurosurg 85:19–28, 1997.
13. Guo W. Radiological aspects of gamma knife radiosurgery for arteriovenous malformations. Acta Radiol 388: 1–34, 1993.
14. Guo W, Karlsson B, Ericson K, et al. Even the smallest remnant of AVM constitutes a risk of further bleeding (case report). Acta Neurochir 121:212–215, 1993.
15. Guo W, Wikholm G, Karlsson B, et al. Combined embolization and gamma knife radiosurgery for cerebral arteriovenous malformations. Acta Radiol 34:600–606, 1993.
16. Hademenos G, Massoud T. Risk of intracranial arteriovenous malformation rupture due to venous drainage impairment: a theoretical analysis. Stroke 27: 1072–1083, 1996.
17. Hademenos G, Massoud T, Vinuela F. A biomathematical model of intracranial arteriovenous malformations based on electrical network analysis: theory and hemodynamics. Neurosurgery 38:1005–1015, 1996.
18. Hall E, Brenner D. The radiobiology of radiosurgery: rationale for different treatment regimes for AVMs and malignancies. Int J Radiat Oncol Biol Phys 25:381–385, 1993.
19. Harders A, Bien S, Eggergt H, et al. Hemodynamic changes in arteriovenous malformations induced by superselective embolization. Neurol Res 10:239–245, 1988.
20. Hecht ST, Horton JA, Kerber CW, et al. Hemodynamics of the central nervous system arteriovenous malformation nidus during particulate embolization: a computer model. Neuroradiology 33:62–64, 1991.
21. Homan R, Devous M, Stokely E, et al. Quantification of intracerebral steal in patients with arteriovenous malformations. Arch Neurol 43:779–785, 1986.
22. Hopewell J, Campling D, Calvo W, et al. Vascular irradiation damage: its cellular basis and likely consequences. Br J Cancer 53:181–191, 1986.
23. Inoue H, Kohga H, Kurihara H, et al. Classification of arteriovenous malformations for radiosurgery: neuroimaging, histopathology and radiobiologic effects. Stereotact Funct Neurosurg 64(Suppl 1):110–117, 1995.
24. Ito M, Patronas N, DiChiro G, et al. Effect of moderate level x-irradiation to brain on cerebral glucose metabolism. J Compt Tomogr 10:584–588, 1986.
25. Kader A, Young W. The effects of intracranial arteriovenous malformations on cerebral hemodynamics. Neurosurg Clin 7:767–781, 1996.
26. Kader A, Young W, Pile-Spellman J, et al. The influence of hemodynamic and anatomic factors on hemorrhage from cerebral arteriovenous malformations. Neurosurgery 34:801–807, 1994.
27. Kaplan H, Aronsen S, Browder E. Vascular malformations of the brain, an anatomical study. J Neurosurg 18:630–635, 1961.
28. Kjellberg R, Hanamura T, Davis K, et al. Bragg peak

proton beam therapy for arteriovenous malformations of the brain. N Engl J Med 309:269–274, 1983.
29. Kondziolka D, Lundsford L, Claasen D, et al. Radiobiology of radiosurgery: the normal rat brain. Neurosurgery 31:271–279, 1992.
30. Kondziolka D, Somaza S, Martinez A, et al. Radioprotective effects of the 21-aminoateroid U-74389G for stereotactic radiosurgery. Neurosurgery 41:203–208, 1997.
31. Larsson B. Blood vessel changes following local irradiation of the brain with high energy protons. Acta Soc Med Uppsala 65:65–71, 1960.
32. Lasjaunis P, Manelfe C, Terbrugge K, et al. Endovascular treatment of cerebral arteriovenous malformations. Neurosurg Rev 9:265–275, 1986.
33. Levy R, Lo EH, Fabrikant JI. Biologic basis for stereotactic radiosurgery. In Phillips M: Physical Aspects of Stereotactic Radiosurgery. New York: Plenum Medical Book Co, 1993, pp 189–238.
34. Lindegaard K, Gromilund P, Aaslid R, et al. Evaluation of cerebral AVMs using transcranial Doppler ultrasound. J Neurosurg 65:335–344, 1986.
35. Lo EH. A hemodynamic analysis of intracranial arteriovenous malformations. Neurol Res 15:51–55, 1993.
36. Lo EH. A theoretical analysis of hemodynamic and biomechanical alterations in intracranial AVMs after radiosurgery. Int J Radiat Oncol Biol Phys 27:353–361, 1993.
37. Lo EH, DeLapaz RL, Frankel KA, et al. MRI and PET of delayed heavy-ion radiation injury in the rabbit brain. Int J Radiat Oncol Biol Phys 20:689–698, 1991.
38. Lo EH, Fabrikant JI. Delayed biologic reactions to stereotactic charged particle radiosurgery in the human brain. Sterotact Funct Neurosurg 56:197–211, 1991.
39. Lo EH, Fabrikant JI, Levy RP, et al. An experimental compartmental flow model for assessing the hemodynamic response of intracranial arteriovenous malformations to stereotactic radiosurgery. Neurosurgery 28: 251–261, 1991.
40. Lo EH, Franjek KA, Steinberg GK, et al. High dose single fraction brain irradiation: MRI, cerebral blood flow, electrophysiological, and histological studies. Int J Radiat Oncol Biol Phys 22:47–55, 1992.
41. Lo EH, Frankel KA, DeLapaz RL, et al. Cerebrovascular and metabolic perturbations in delayed heavy charged particle radiation injury. Brain Res 504:168–172, 1989.
42. Lunsford L, Altschuler E, Flickinger J, et al. In vivo biological effects of stereotactic radiosurgery: a primate model. Neurosurgery 27:373–382, 1990.
43. Lunsford L, Kondziolka D, Flickinger J, et al. Stereotactic radiosurgery for arteriovenous malformations of the brain. J Neurosurg 75:512–524, 1991.
44. Marks M, DeLapaz R, Fabrikant J, et al. Intracranial vascular malformations: imaging of charged particle radiosurgery. Part 2. Complications. Radiology 168: 457–462, 1988.
45. Marks M, DeLapaz RL, Fabrikant J, et al. Intracranial vascular malformations: imaging of charged particle radiosurgery. Part I: Results of therapy. Radiology 168: 447–455, 1988.
46. Marks M, Lane B, Steinberg G, et al. Vascular characteristics of intracerebral arteriovenous malformations in patients with clinical steal. Am J Neuroradiol 12: 489–496, 1991.
47. Marks M, Lane B, Steinberg G, et al. Hemorrhage in intracranial arteriovenous malformations: angiographic determinants. Radiology 176:807–813, 1990.
48. Mathis J, Barr J, Horton J, et al. The efficacy of particulate embolization combined with stereotactic radiosurgery for treatment of large arteriovenous malformations of the brain. Am J Neuroradiol 16:299–306, 1995.
49. Milnor W. Hemodynamics. Baltimore: Williams and Wilkins, 1989.
50. Miyasaka Y, Yada K, Ohwada T, et al. An analysis of the venous drainage system as a factor in hemorrhage from arteriovenous malformations. J Neurosurg 76: 239–243, 1992.
51. Moustafa H, Hopewell J. Late functional changes in vasculature of the rat brain after local x-irradiation. Br J Radiol 53:21–25, 1980.
52. Nagasawa S, Kawanishi M, Kondoh S, et al. Hemodynamic simulation study of cerebral arteriovenous malformations: effects of impaired autoregulation. J Cereb Blood Flow Metab 16:162–169, 1996.
53. Nagasawa S, Kawanishi M, Tanaka H, et al. Hemodynamic study of arteriovenous malformations using a hydraulic model. Neurol Res 15:409–412, 1993.
54. Nilsson A, Wennerstrand J, Leksell D, et al. Stereotactic basilar artery irradiation in cat. Acta Radiol Oncol 17: 150–160, 1978.
55. Nornes H. Quantitation of altered hemodynamics. In Wilson C, Stein B (eds): Intracranial Arteriovenous Malformations. Baltimore: Williams & Wilkins, 1984, pp 32–43.
56. Nornes H, Grip A. Hemodynamic aspects of cerebral arteriovenous malformations. J Neurosurg 53:456–464, 1980.
57. Nornes H, Grip A, Wikeby P. Intraoperative evaluation of cerebral hemodynamics using directional Doppler. J Neurosurg 50:145–151, 1979.
58. Ogilvy CS. Radiation therapy for arteriovenous malformations: a review. Neurosurgery 76:725–735, 1990.
59. Okabe T, Meyer J, Okayasu H, et al. Xenon-enhanced CT CBF measurements in cerebral AVMs before and after excision. J Neurosurg 59:21–31, 1983.
60. Pasqualin A, Barone G, Cioffi F, et al. The relevance of anatomic and hemodynamic factors to a classification of cerebral arteriovenous malformations. Neurosurgery 28:370–379, 1991.
61. Pollock B, Flickinger J, Lunsford L, et al. Factors that predict the bleeding risk of cerebral arteriovenous malformations. Stroke 27:1–6, 1996.
62. Pollock B, Flickinger J, Lunsford L, et al. Hemorrhage risk after stereotactic radiosurgery of arteriovenous malformations. Neurosurgery 38:652–659, 1996.
63. Remler M, Marcussen W, Tiller-Borsisch J, et al. The late effects of radiation on the blood-brain barrier. Int J Radiat Oncol Biol Phys 12:1965–1969, 1986.
64. Rosenblum B, Bonner R, Oldfield E. Intraoperative measurement of cortical blood flow adjacent to cerebral AVMs using laser Doppler velocimetry. J Neurosurg 66:396–399, 1987.
65. Spetzler RF, Hargraves RW, McCormick PW, et al. Relationship of perfusion pressure and size to risk of hemorrhage from arteriovenous malformations. J Neurosurg 76:918–923, 1992.
66. Spetzler R, Martin N. A proposed grading system for

arteriovenous malformations. J Neurosurg 65:476–483, 1986.

67. Spetzler R, Wilson C, Weinstein B, et al. Normal perfusion pressure breakthrough theory. Clin Neurosurg 25: 651–672, 1978.
68. Steinberg G, Chang S, Levy R, et al. Surgical resection of large incompletely treated intracranial arteriovenous malformations following stereotactic radiosurgery. J Neurosurg 84:920–928, 1996.
69. Steinberg G, Fabrikant J, Marks M, et al. Stereotactic heavy charged particle Bragg peak radiation for intracranial arteriovenous malformations. N Engl J Med 323:96–101, 1990.
70. Tanaka A, Ueno H, Yamashita Y, et al. Regional cerebral blood flow in delayed brain swelling following x-irradiation of the occipital lobe in the monkey. Brain Res 96:233–246, 1975.
71. Valk P, Dillon W. Radiation injury of the brain. Am J Neuroradiol 12:45–62, 1991.
72. Van Alphen H. Intraoperative embolization of cerebral arteriovenous malformations. Neurosurg Rev 9:77–86, 1986.
73. Voges J, Treuer H, Sturm V, et al. Risk analysis of linear accelerator radiosurgery. Int J Radiat Oncol Biol Phys 36:1055–1063, 1996.
74. Waltimo O. The relationship of size, density, and localization of intracranial arteriovenous malformations to type of initial symptoms. J Neurol Sci 19:13–19, 1973.
75. Woodruff K, Lyman J, Fabrikant J. Heavy charged particle induced lesions in rabbit cerebral cortex. Int J Radiat Oncol Biol Phys 14:301–307, 1987.
76. Yamada S. Arteriovenous malformations in the functional area: surgical treatment and regional cerebral blood flow. Neurol Res 4:283–322, 1982.
77. Yamada S, Brauer F, Knierim D. Direct approach to arteriovenous malformations in functional areas of the cerebral hemisphere. J Neurosurg 72:418–425, 1990.
78. Yamada S, Cojocaru T. Arteriovenous malformations. In Wood J: Cerebral Blood Flow: Physiologic and Clinical Aspects. New York: McGraw Hill, 1987, pp 580–592.

Chapter 10

Ancillary Studies for Arteriovenous Malformation Surgery in Functional Areas of the Brain:

Evoked Potentials, Magnetic Source Imaging, Color Doppler Ultrasonography, and Endoscopy

Introduction

Technological advances in recent years have elevated the surgeon's capability of performing procedures of increasing complexity with relative safety. Such is the case for arteriovenous malformation (AVM) surgery in functional areas of the brain. Somatosensory evoked potentials (SSEPs), magnetic source imaging, color Doppler ultrasonography, and endoscopy are the supportive studies used by the authors in pinpointing delicate functional structures for preoperative decision-making as well as the enhancement of surgical precision. This chapter focuses on these studies and their usefulness for this purpose.

From Yamada S (ed): *Arteriovenous Malformations in Functional Areas of the Brain.* © Futura Publishing Co, Inc, Armonk, NY, 1999.

Section 1

Somatosensory Evoked Potentials and Controlled Hypotension

Shokei Yamada, MD, PhD, David S. Knierim, MD, and Shoko M. Yamada, MD, PhD

Hypoxemia, ischemia, degree of impairment in oxidative metabolism, and electrophysiological activity of the brain are all closely interrelated. The balance between energy production and consumption is another factor in the control of cerebral metabolism and function. During surgical removal of AVMs, an unexpectedly large amount of bleeding may occur from abnormal vessels and consequent ischemia can interfere with cerebral function and further lead to irreversible brain damage or even fatality.[14,24] The use of controlled hypotension can ameliorate the risk,[8,14,34,35] but in its own right may lead to serious ischemia of the brain, first at the penumbral level and later at the stroke level. This section introduces the value of SSEPs, which are intimately correlated with oxidative metabolism, as an important indicator of the safety level of cerebral function. Conversely, surgical, anesthetic, or any insult to the sensory cortex and its pathways in the brain is predictable. The following is based on a previously published report[36] about modified surgical management of AVMs in functional areas.

For an individual patient, what is the safe level of controlled hypotension? Various methods[28] have been proposed for monitoring cerebral circulation, oxygenation,[2] and energy status[15,26,30] during diagnostic and surgical procedures. Do these methods actually provide an early warning signal of brain dysfunction? Decreased cerebral blood flow (CBF)[3,16,29,33,41] can be partially compensated by an increase in oxygen extraction factor[22] and partly by a decrease in oxygen and energy consumption.[38] Therefore, CBF changes may not be definite indicators of brain dysfunction. Positron emission tomography (PET),[25] magnetic resonance spectroscopy (MRS),[12] and optical techniques[2,9,18,20,27] can all be useful tools to determine metabolic status of the brain; however, these procedures are difficult to apply clinically in the operating room. What may be useful during neurosurgical procedures is identification of one or more signals that would take into account the dynamics between energy conservation and use. The goal of such monitoring would be to warn of a metabolic trend, indicating that the brain may be entering a silent state from which recovery becomes questionable. Steps toward this goal are offered in this section, which describes the simultaneous monitoring of: (1) the reduction/oxidation (redox) ratio of cytochrome a,a_3 by reflection spectrophotometry; and (2) SSEPs.

The authors' study indicated that SSEP changes correlate with redox shifts in animal and human brains during and after controlled hypotension and that SSEP monitoring is a valuable and practical means to determine the safety level of controlled hypotension.

Materials and Methods

Controlled Hypotension in Humans

One hundred thirty-five patients underwent AVM resection under general anesthesia with nitrous oxide or isofluorane, and analgesics. Some degree of hypotension was induced in all patients. One hundred twenty patients had SSEP recordings and 30 patients had measurement of redox of cyctochrome a,a_3 by reflection spectrophotometry. The mean arterial pressure (MAP) was maintained routinely between 40 and 60 mm Hg by intravenous infusion of nitroprusside. At this level, pulsation of the AVM core diminished to a barely noticeable degree. The MAP was lowered to below 60 mm Hg, even as low as 40 mm Hg, when bleeding control was difficult.

The median or ulnar nerve was stimulated with a bipolar electrode (30 sec square wave pulse trains, 0.3 ms pulses at 4.1 Hz, 3–5 mA). Recording electrodes were placed in both the left and the right sensory areas. A negative electrode was placed at the glabella. A monopolar recording electrode was inserted percutaneously to the second cervical spinous process to monitor central conduction time. Evoked potentials were recorded and redox activity of cytochrome a,a_3 was measured in the manner described previously.

Results

At a MAP of 40–60 mm Hg, cerebral cytochrome a,a_3 was reduced (Figure 1) although SSEPs were unchanged (Figure 2A). When the MAP fell unintentionally below 40 mm Hg due to blood loss, the cyto-

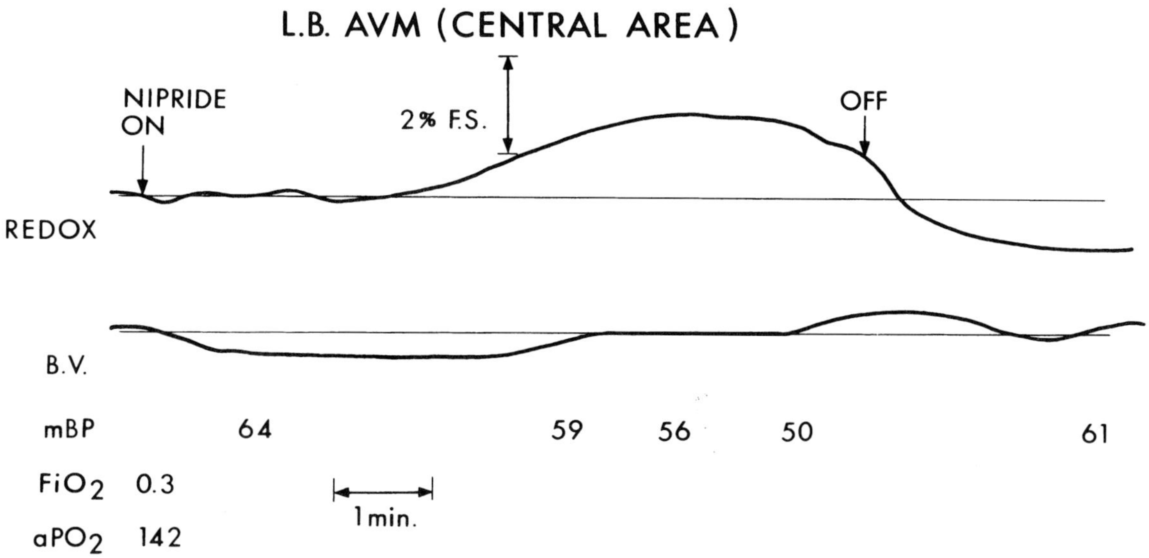

Figure 1. Redox changes in a patient during hypotension. The reduction level was lower than that reached during mild hypoxia (FiO_2 0.15), which is not shown here. See reoxidation starting during hypotension to MAP 50 mm Hg even before nitroprusside was discontinued. Simultaneous BV increase suggests one of the compensatory mechanisms of energy preservation during hypotension.

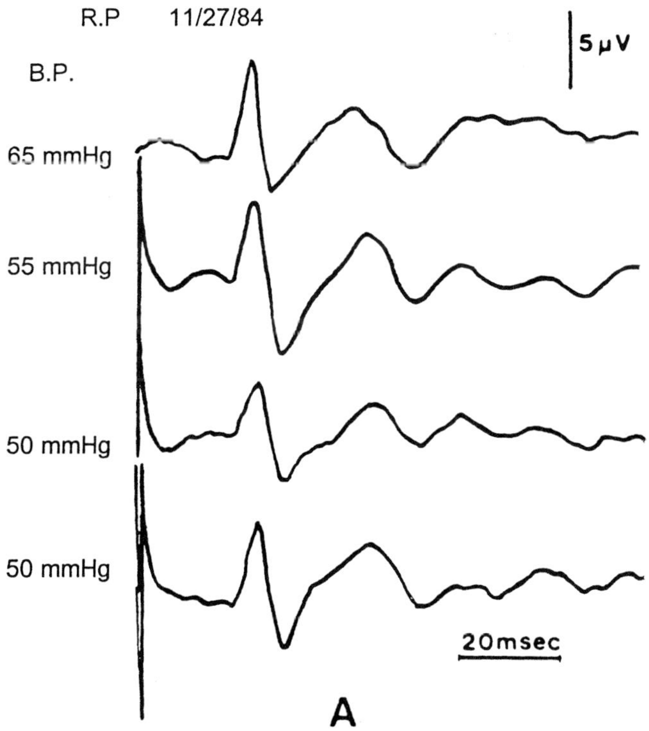

Figure 2A. SSEPs in humans. The wave pattern is unchanged during FiO_2 decrease to 0.15 and during hypotension down to 50 mm Hg. *Continued*

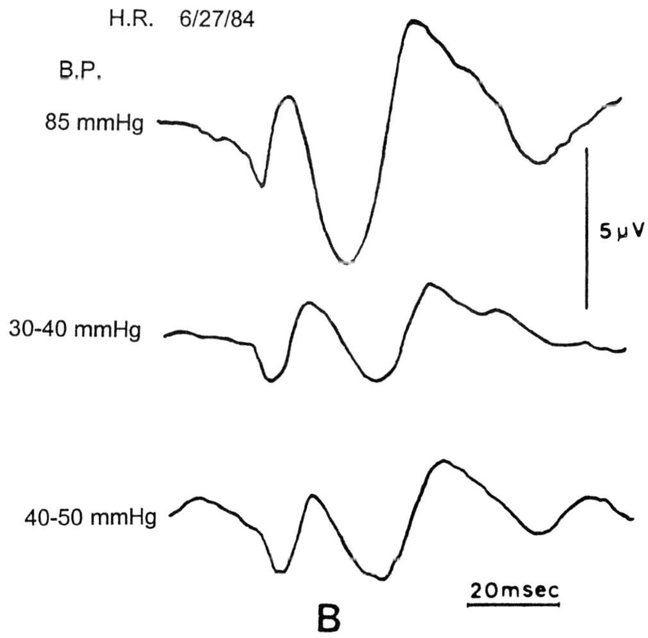

Figure 2B. SSEPs in humans. During hypotension with MAP below 40 mm Hg, latencies of the second and third waves are prolonged and their amplitudes are decreased. SSEPs recover when MAP returns above 40 mm Hg.

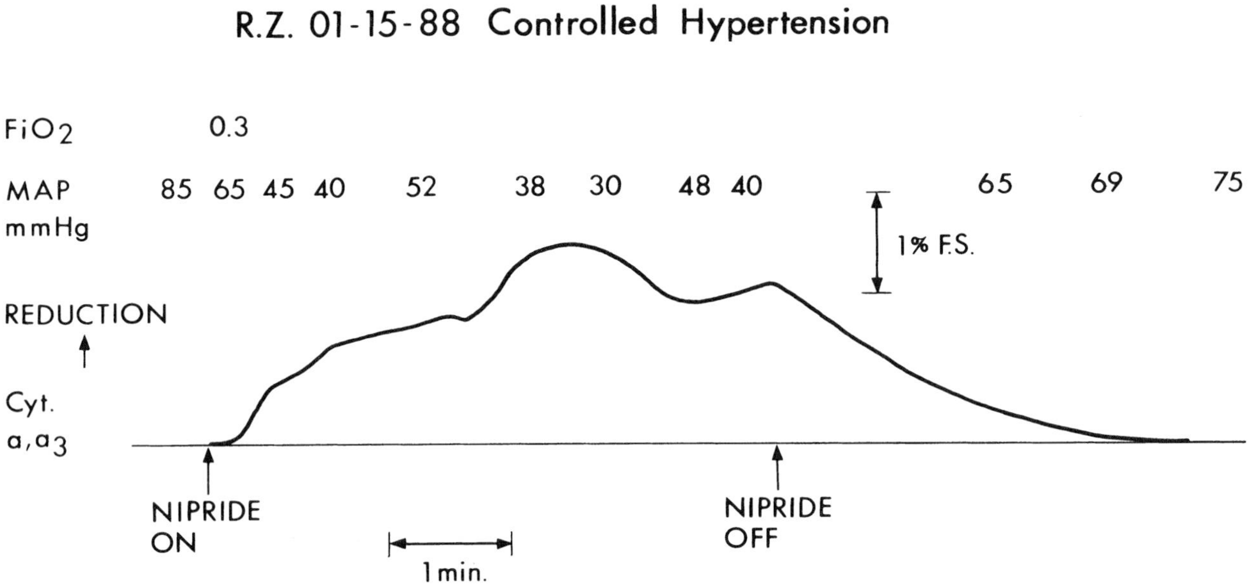

Figure 3. Slowly induced hypotension causes a stepwise increase in reduction level. See significant increase in reduction from 40–50 mm Hg to 30–40 mm Hg.

chrome became further reduced (Figure 3) and SSEPs were decreased in amplitude and delayed in latency (Figure 2B). Nevertheless, all four patients in whom the blood pressure fell between 25 and 40 mm Hg for approximately 45 minutes due to unexpected bleeding recovered without apparent physical or neurological sequelae.[36] SSEPs were better preserved when MAP fell to 35–40 mm Hg (Figure 2B) than when the fraction of inspired oxygen (FiO_2) decreased to 0.15 (which caused the PO_2 to fall to 70 mm Hg), indicating that energy preservation was still at an acceptable level (Figures 1 and 3).

Discussion

Spectrophotometry of cytochrome oxidase and the recording of SSEPs offer significant advantages for neurosurgical monitoring. These measurements can be recorded continuously throughout the procedures and appear to sensitively indicate metabolic trends. This is in contrast to other methods used for signaling the metabolic situation in the brain, which are either limited in temporal resolution (PET) or require a very expensive and cumbersome apparatus (MRS).

The authors' human and animal studies[36,37] show that hypoxemia of mild to moderate intensity will provoke shifts toward reduction of the mitochondrial electron transport carriers without changing SSEPs. This situation in the brain may be parallel to the "cushioning" in isolated mitochondria, wherein large changes in redox states can be provoked without corresponding changes in oxygen consumption.[6] Whether what is seen in an electrophysiologically intact brain results from decreased electron transport or from increased glycolytic activity that increases the supply of reducing equivalents (hydrogen ions and electrons) to the respiratory chain[6] remains unknown. What is apparent, however, is that shifts toward cytochrome reduction may warn of blood flow and oxygenation decline prior to the onset of conditions that threaten brain survival. The authors found, for example, that all patients recovered their neurological and physical status after 6 hours of hypotension.[34,35,37] However, when the MAP was lowered below 40 mm Hg, the further reduction of cytochrome a,a_3 with concomitant deterioration of SSEPs suggests that progressive metabolic insult is predromal to energy failure and pathological consequences. This suggested outcome was observed in cat experiments: a MAP below 40 mm Hg provoked large shifts toward reduction of cytochrome a,a_3, and rapid deterioration of SSEPs, which was followed by loss of responses to stimulation at 30 mm Hg and below.[36,37] This corresponds to data obtained by Lassen and Astrup (1987)[21] and Symon (1980).[32] Evidence is overwhelming that an insufficiency of adenosine triphosphate (ATP) and creatinine phosphate[23,26,31] initiates a cascade of events that block synaptic transmission, cause loss of ion homeostasis[1,4,23,30,35] with accumulation of calcium in the cytoplasm, and produce irreversible electrical failure, lipid peroxidation,[40] and histopathology.[13,30]

Energy production and consumption in chronically low blood flow, such as that seen in cerebrovascular occlusive diseases and blood flow diversion (steal) with large AVMs, are discussed elsewhere.[7,9,10,11,17,19,22,36,37,39]

In conclusion, the use of reflection spectrophotometry along with SSEPs has demonstrated that both methods parallel each other in signaling energy failure and brain damage during acute controlled hypotension. Inasmuch as the use of reflection spectrophotometry is difficult under ordinary clinical conditions, the use of SSEPs is recommended as a useful clinical monitor of controlled hypotension in cerebrovascular surgery.

Section 2

Magnetic Source Imaging for Arteriovenous Malformations in the Sensorimotor Area

Shokei Yamada, MD, PhD, Christopher Gallen, MD, PhD, and Russell R. Lonser, MD

AVMs located in sensorimotor functional areas can be safely removed despite the fact that the AVM core is directly in contact with functioning motor and sensory neurons.

Surgically, superselective microarteriovenous shunt obliteration is essential for preserving or improving neurological function. Application of this approach was facilitated by the recent technological development of a noninvasive magnetoencephalographic technology, magnetic source imaging (MSI), which allows for detailed, precise, presurgical mapping of functional sensorimotor cortices in relation to the AVM. The accuracy and reliability of MSI localization of sensorimotor cortices based on phase reversal of the motor or sensory potentials have been demonstrated. Functional mapping by MSI in cases in which the AVM is subjacent to the primary sensorimotor cortices allows informed decisions as to whether and how to apply superselective microarteriovenous shunt obliteration. This section focuses on the correlation of MSI mapping with intraoperative SSEPs, and the importance of the preoperative identification of motor and sensory areas.

Materials and Methods

The authors' series includes 20 patients who underwent surgical resection of AVMs and preoperative and/or postoperative sensorimotor mapping. The MSI studies were performed at Scripps Research Institute either before surgery (12 patients), postoperatively only (5 patients) or both preoperatively and postoperatively (3 patients). AVMs were localized in the sensorimotor area in 17 patients or partially in the sensory or motor area in 3 patients. The technical details for MSI recordings were described elsewhere.[3–6,8–10] The basic method includes: (1) stimulation of the lower lips (LL), 1st (D1) and 2nd (D2) digits, feet and toes bilaterally with a pulse of pressure exerted by a pneumatically driven tactile stimulator for sensory cortex mapping, and movement of the body specific for the recording of a segment; and (2) recording of electromagnetic fields generated by stimulation via the Magnes 37-channel biomagnetometer (Biomagnetic Technologies Inc., San Diego, CA).

Magnetic Source Imaging[4,5,8–10]

MSI refers to the integration of an anatomical image (e.g., from MRI or computed tomography [CT]) with the location of the sources of cerebral electromagnetic activity reflected in the extracranial neuromagnetic field. This activity is detected using a biomagnetometer that is sensitive to the electromagnetic field (50–100 femto Teslas [fT]) generated by the electrical current flow through the dendrites of the pyramidal cells. Detector coils within the biomagnetometer are connected to a superconducting quantum interference device (SQUID) sensor to determine the infinitesimal electromagnetic signals. Following amplification and processing of the signals, x, y, and z cartesian coordinates are developed and then can be translated into MRI or CT coordinates by nature of identification of the common fiducial markers and computation of the coordinate transformation. The functional areas are thus superimposed on the MRI or CT scan (Figure 4).

Surgical Techniques

The safe and effective resection of AVMs in functional areas can be accomplished using the microsurgical technique described in Chapter 1. The surgical techniques are slightly different, depending on the anatomical relationship between the AVM and sensorimotor area,[7] i.e.: (1) the AVM is surrounded by sensory and motor neurons; (2) the AVM extends beyond the sensory and motor cortices; and (3) a part of the AVM extends into the sensorimotor area. Intra-

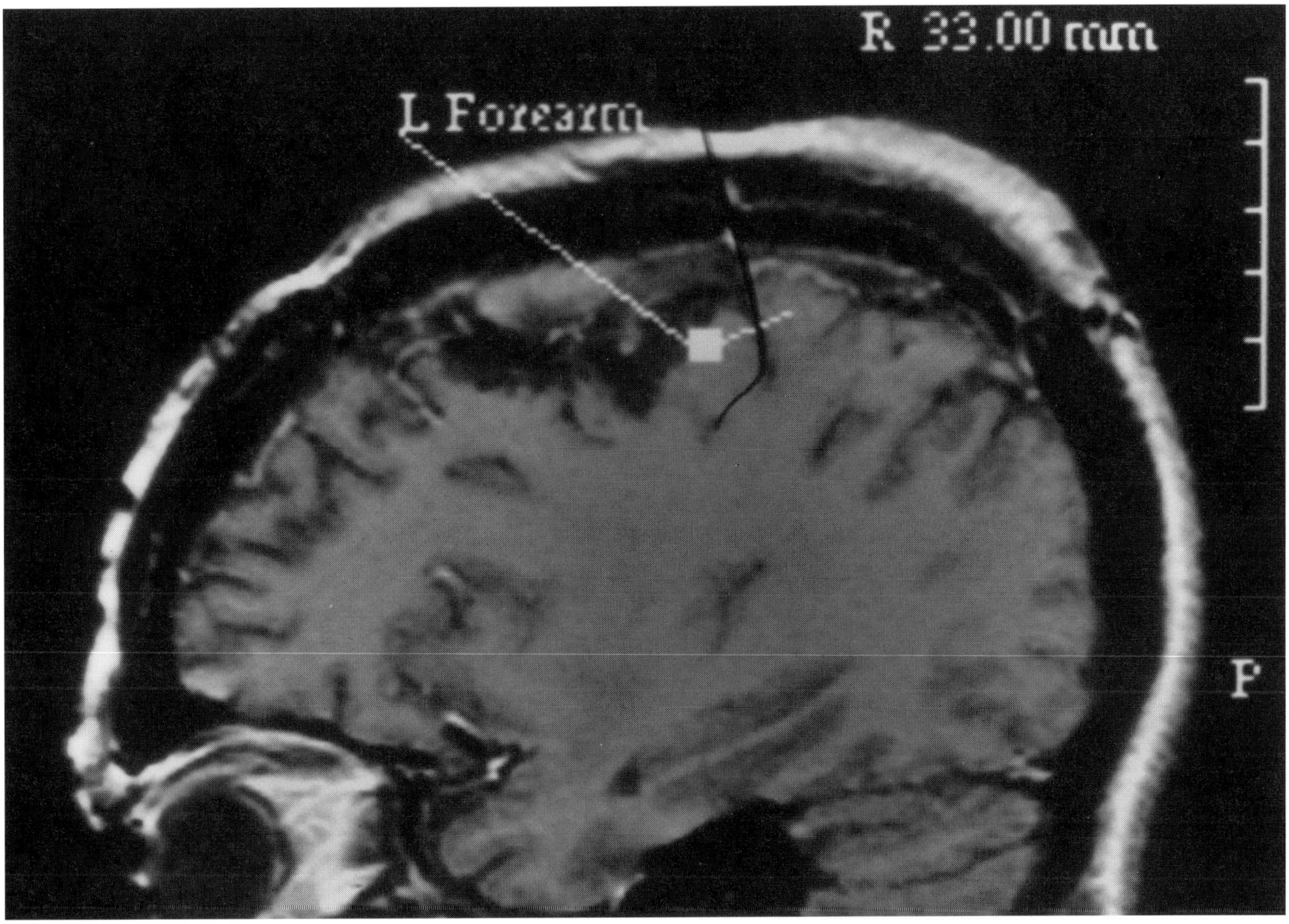

Figure 4. The sagittal view of the MRI shows the location of the left forearm in direct contact with the AVM.

operative mapping maybe done as described previously by some authors.[1,2,7]

Case Reports

Two cases of patients who underwent surgical resection of their AVMs after preoperative sensory and motor localization by MSI are presented.

Case 1

This 51-year-old woman suffered an adversive seizure. An MSI performed 1 month later showed a 5 cm (diameter) AVM, located in the premotor area and its posterior pole underneath the motor cortex. The patient underwent resection of the AVM, and within a few weeks was able to resume her normal household activities (Figure 5).

Case 2

This 42-year-old woman's case was presented in Chapter 1, illustrative case 3.

Comment

Compact AVMs can be removed by dissection without damaging the cortex overlying the AVM core. This is in contrast to the approach to gliomas in and adjacent to the sensorimotor area, in which the tumor is only excised outside of this area.

Discussion

The natural history of AVMs lends itself to a substantial level of morbidity and mortality, especially

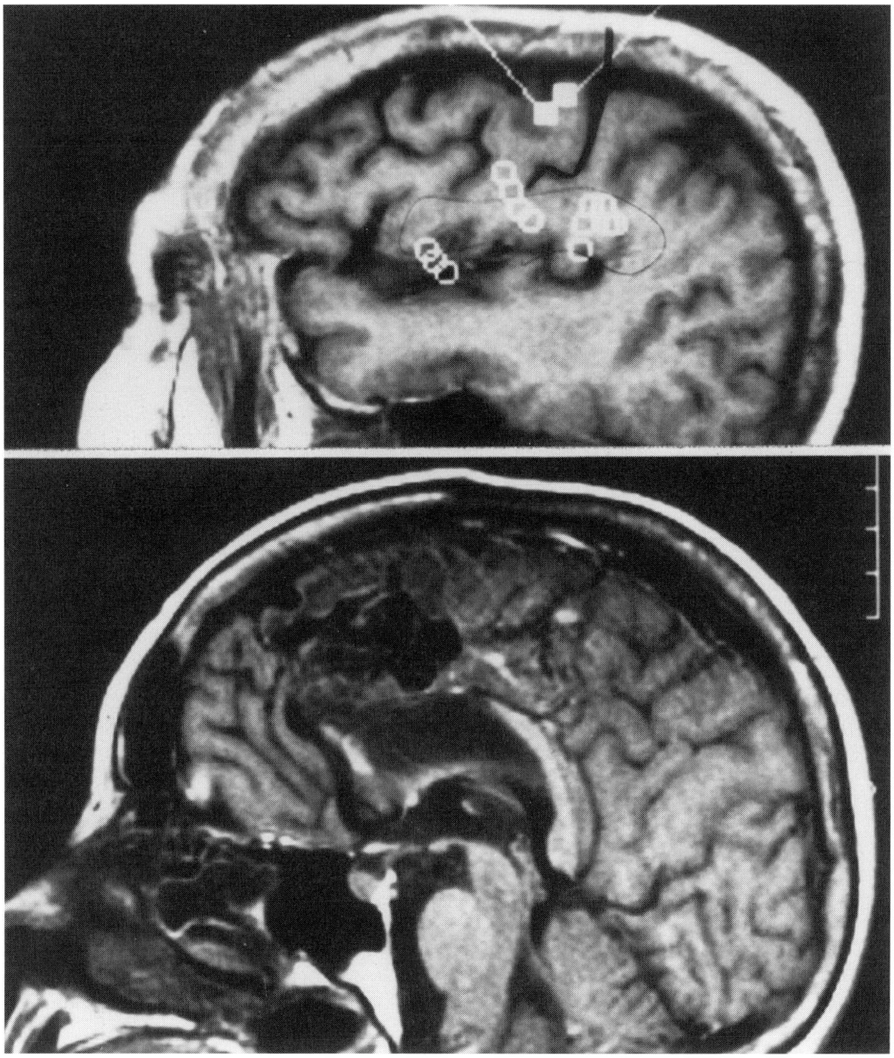

Figure 5. In this imaging study, the AVM is located in the premotor area. Intraoperative SSEPs confirmed that the AVM extended to the subcortical motor area. The sensory area (squares) is located anterior to the anatomically determined central sulcus.

those located in functional areas. Thus, surgical intervention utilizing the technique described is essential to prevent progressive neurological sequelae. Although diagnostic studies such as MRI, CT, and angiography can localize AVMs, the advent of MSI further enhances the presurgical mapping of the anatomical relationship between the AVM and the sensorimotor cortices. MSI will provide the neurosurgeon with additional insight into the surgical planning and safe resection of the sensorimotor AVM.

Section 3

Color Doppler Ultrasonography

Shokei Yamada, MD, PhD, and Glenn Rouse, MD

Resection of AVMs in functional areas requires special cautions in approaching and dissecting the AVM core. It is essential to distinguish shunting arterioles from angiographically demonstrated feeding arteries since the feeding arteries send branches to functional brain tissue as well as to the AVM. The authors use color Doppler ultrasonography[1–5] for identifying feeding arteries and draining veins in the area of the AVM core.[6] Sonography helps the surgeon avoid obliterating those arteries that have many branches to the AVM and to the surrounding brain. Similarly, the surgeon will avoid obliterating the major draining vein hidden between the AVM compartments.

Materials and Methods

Fifteen patients with AVMs in functional areas of the brain underwent color Doppler sonography during AVM surgery. Of these patients, four with a large or giant AVM underwent multistaged procedures. An appropriately sized craniotomy exposed the dura covering the subcortical AVMs.

A Diasonics VST masters series ultrasound (Diasonics, Santa Clara, CA) and a transducer covered with a sterile drape were used. The transducer, 20 mm in dimension, was either a linear or a sector array operating at 6–12 mHz. The AVM core was located, and the site and depth of the lesion were identified. Feeding arteries and draining veins were noted before surgical dissection was started.

Surgical Techniques Pertinent to Ultrasonography

Surgical procedures were performed based on technical principles gained from the use of ultrasonography. The technical details used specifically during the use of ultrasonography included the following:

1. The AVM is identified clearly and can be compared to the CT, MRI, and/or angiography findings.

2. The size, depth, and shape are more accurately measured than in other imaging studies, in relation to the craniotomy site and exposed cortices.

3. Feeding arteries and draining veins are demonstrated. Blue indicates vessels with their flow direction away from the transducer and red those with flow toward the transducer. From these images, the surgeon forms a three-dimensional (3-D) reconstruction of the AVM.

4. The portions of the AVM inside the sulcus and in the brain can be distinguished.

5. The silent area (no color demonstration) is considered to be glioma, cystic tumor, or hematoma.[4] Abnormal vasculature around the silent area after AVM resection is likely to indicate a residual AVM.

6. There is a correlation between the feeding artery (ultrasonographic) and surrounding shunting arterioles (microsurgical); that is, the surgeon finds crowded shunting arterioles around the feeding artery and focuses his/her attention on this area for interrupting arterioles.

7. The surgeon can confirm total elimination, either total resection or subtotal resection, and thrombosis of a small portion. Conversely, it is possible to find a residual AVM or satellite AVM.

8. An aneurysmal dilation of a venous loop of the core can be clearly identified. It is extremely important to recognize the size and flow of the aneurysmal dilatation that is a part of the draining vein. Cauterization and shrinking of the aneurysmal dilatation must still maintain the circulation of the draining vein.

9. 3-D imaging allows the ultrasonographer and surgeon to follow the course of the feeding arteries and draining veins and some large venous loops of the AVM core.

10. In addition to color Doppler imaging, ultrasonography assists in determining the flow velocity of the feeding arteries and draining veins, allowing the degree of obliteration of the AVM core (with one compartment) or special compartment.

11. Color ultrasonography may be the only means to diagnose some AVMs or vascular malformations. It also provides the accurate size of the AVM.

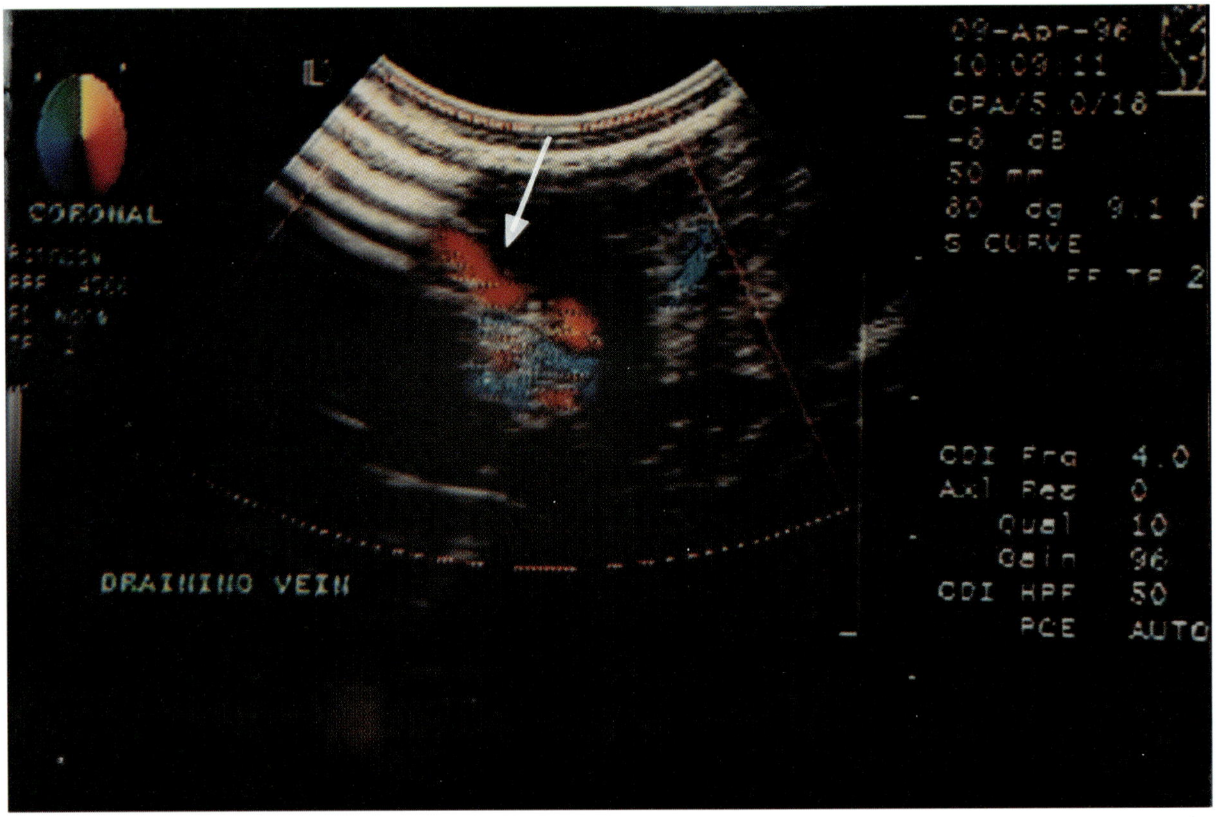

Figure 6. The arrow indicates the major draining vein which was connected to the AVM core underlying the Wernicke's area.

Case Report

This 37-year-old woman had a 2-month history of episodic severe throbbing headaches followed by speech difficulty. These symptoms were sometimes associated with motor seizures on the right side of her body. Neurologically, she was intact unless she was in the post-ictal state, at which time she showed receptive aphasia and visual agnosia. Angiography demonstrated a large AVM (60 cm^3) in the left posterior temporoparietal area.

At surgery, the major draining vein was followed into the sulcus, as correlated with color ultrasonographic images (Figure 6). The imaging study at the second operation showed that more than one-half of the AVM was thrombosed as a result of the isolation and coagulation. The feeding artery and its branches were identified as the AVM was approached anteriorly and isolated deep into the white matter. All shunting arterioles were interrupted, and this feeding artery and its larger branches maintained their normal circulation at the time of AVM removal.

Results

All of the patients who underwent color Doppler sonography during surgery did well, except for temporary mild weakness that lasted a few days to a few weeks in one-third of the cases. All patients had been out of work or on the verge of losing his/her job preoperatively, but all have returned to work postoperatively.

Discussion

Color Doppler sonography can be performed in the operating room during surgery. AVMs can be distinguished from vascular tumors, and the technical safety of the resection can be enhanced by properly interrupting the shunting arterioles and communicating venules and preserving the draining vein.[6] For these reasons, color Doppler ultrasonography is a great asset to the surgical refinement of AVM resection.

Section 4

Endoscopy for Arteriovenous Malformation Surgery

Shokei Yamada, MD, PhD, George Mandybur, MD, and Daniel Won, MD

The increased magnification and light intensity of the modern microscope enable surgeons to enhance their precision far beyond that achieved during the days of naked-eye surgery. Endoscopy provides even greater magnification and illumination, and has facilitated further advancement in surgical techniques.[1–5]

Endoscopy-assisted microsurgery provides specific precision in the following procedures: (1) superselective interruption of shunting arterioles and communicating venules; (2) dissection of AVMs extending into the ventricle from within the ventricle; and (3) identification and resection of occult AVMs hidden in the hematoma cavity underneath the functional area cortex.[6,8,9]

It is imperative to follow the surgical principles described in Chapter 1 and to use special techniques to reach AVMs that are located in the deep functional area (capsulostriatothalamic area or in the optic radiation) or underneath the functional area cortex, and to identify intraventricular AVMs or occult AVMs that have caused an intracerebral hematoma.

Materials and Methods

Materials were described in detail in a recent publication.[11] An endoscope manufactured by Medtronics-PS Medical-Clarus (Salinas, CA)[10] was used in the surgical procedures for the following AVMs (Figure 7).

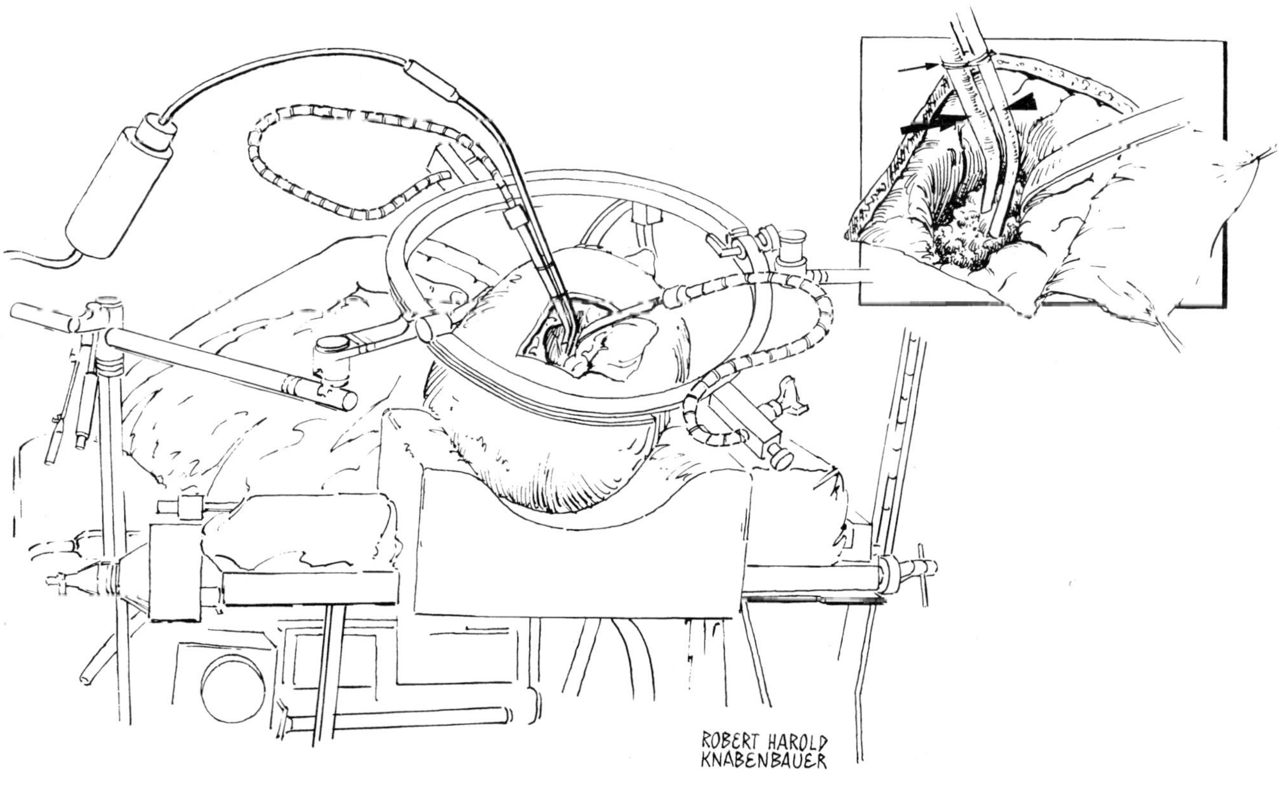

Figure 7. The drawing shows the endoscope (arrowhead) held to the 4 mm retractor by rubber bands (small arrow). The flexible retractor arm (large arrow) is adjusted to maintain the endoscope's stability, but some flexibility is permitted so that the operator can adjust the endoscope position with his/her fingertips.

AVMs in the Sensorimotor, Speech, Visual, and Dominant Posterior Parietal Areas

Endoscopy-assisted microsurgery is performed for specific purposes.

1. Isolation of draining veins.[6–8] After the external end of the draining vein is exposed, this vein must be isolated from the surrounding sulcal cortex. Endoscopy-assisted microsurgery enhances the techniques to identify and accurately coagulate and section communicating venules without damaging the sulcal cortex.

2. Interruption of arterioles and venules directly connected to the AVM core.[6–9] Endoscopy-assisted microsurgical dissection of the AVM core is performed with minimum bleeding and preserving surrounding brain tissue as shunting arterioles (50–250 μ) and communicating venules (50–200 μ) are cauterized and sectioned (Figures 8A-C). Endoscopy confirms adequate coagula formation in these tiny vessels. The endoscope inserted into the cleavage formed between the core and brain tissue facilitates interruption of arterioles and venules, particularly in the deep side of the AVM core (Figure 9). A curved endoscope (Clarus Murphy Scope, Model 2125–161, Medtronic, PS Medical-Clarus, Salinas, CA),[10] is helpful in visualization and identification of the hidden shunting arterioles and communicating venules in the dead angle, and minimizes retraction of core vessels or surrounding brain. An approach through the premotor area dissecting the multicompartment AVM underneath the sensorimotor cortex can be greatly enhanced with the endoscope passed underneath these cortices (Figure 10).

3. Localization of a bleeding point. When bleeding occurs from one of the core vessels during AVM dissection, usually due to disconnection of a shunting arteriole or communicating venule, the core vessel must be immediately grasped around the

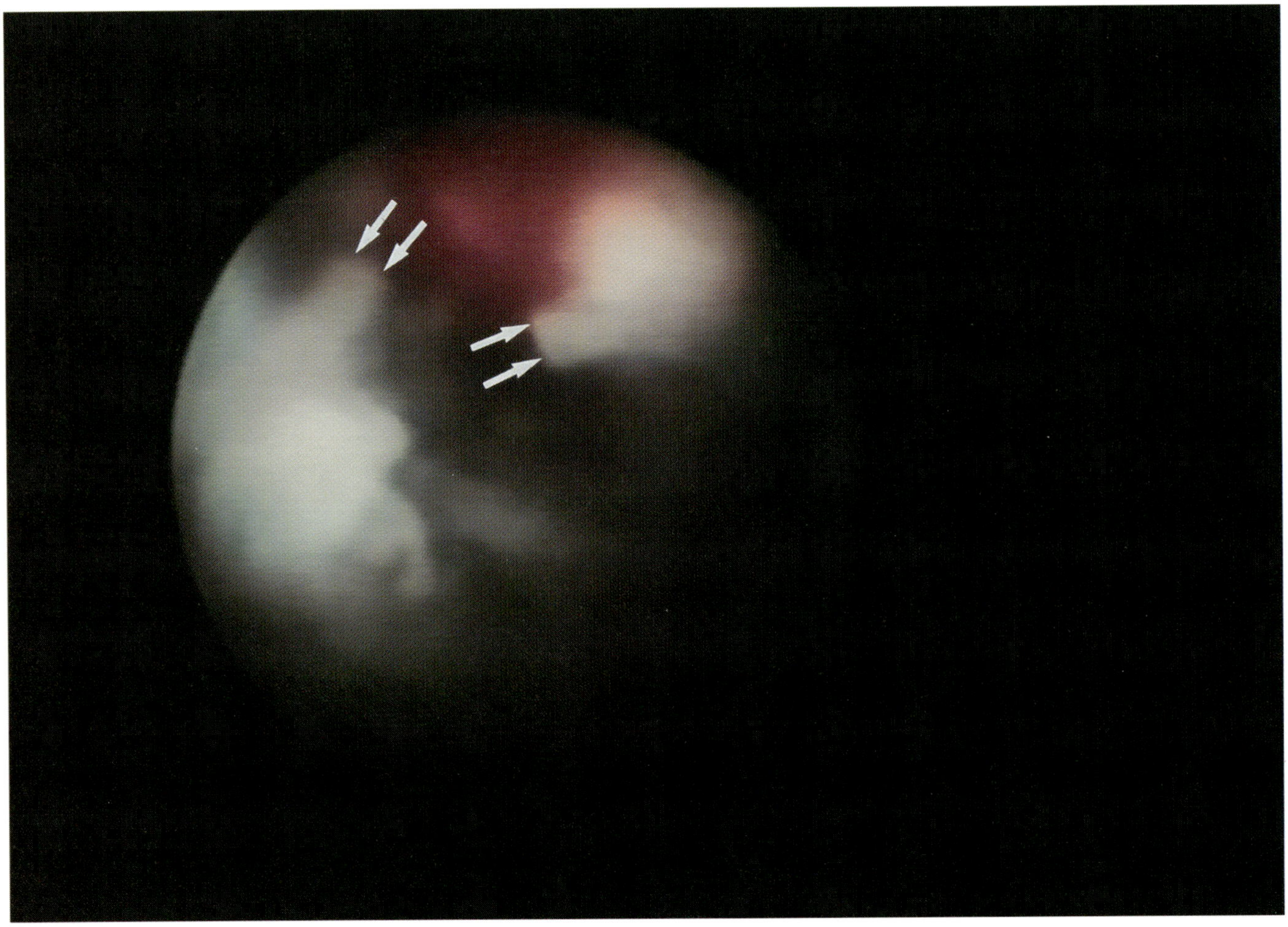

Figure 8A. A cauterized and sectioned shunting arteriole (200 μ) is shown in the video of the endoscope. The AVM vessels are located on the left. After an arteriole is sectioned, both ends (arrows) remain free in the cleavage formed between the AVM core and surrounding brain. Another deep shunting arteriole is seen faintly in the middle of the photograph. *Continued*

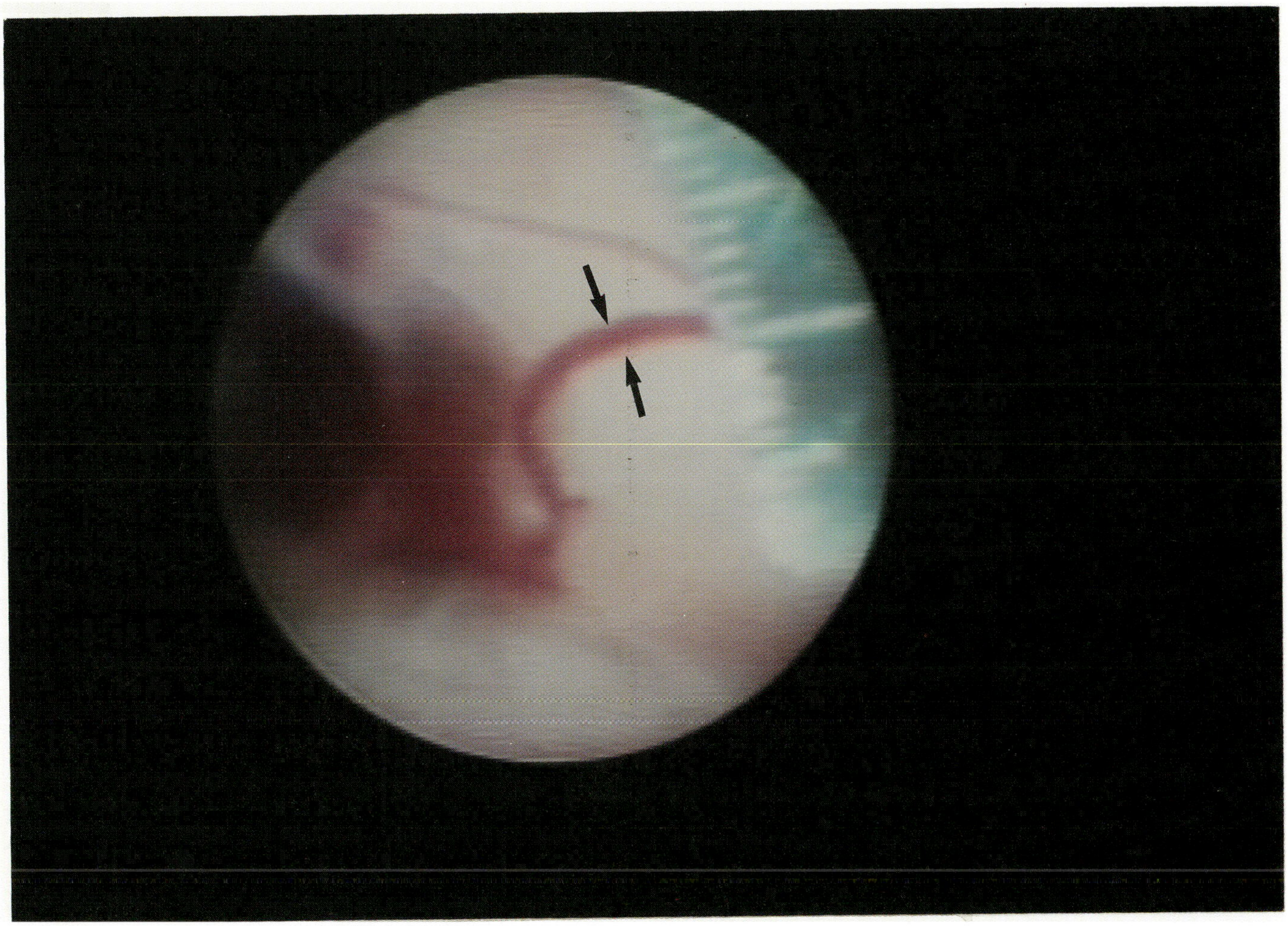

Figure 8B. This communicating venule (100 μ in diameter) (arrows) is shown to connect to an AVM core vessel at its lower end. One end of the sectioned venule contracts toward the core loop, and when using the surgical microscope, the other end contracts and seems to disappear into the brain; however, endoscopy allows the clear identification of both ends of the sectioned venule as seen in Figure 8A. *Continued*

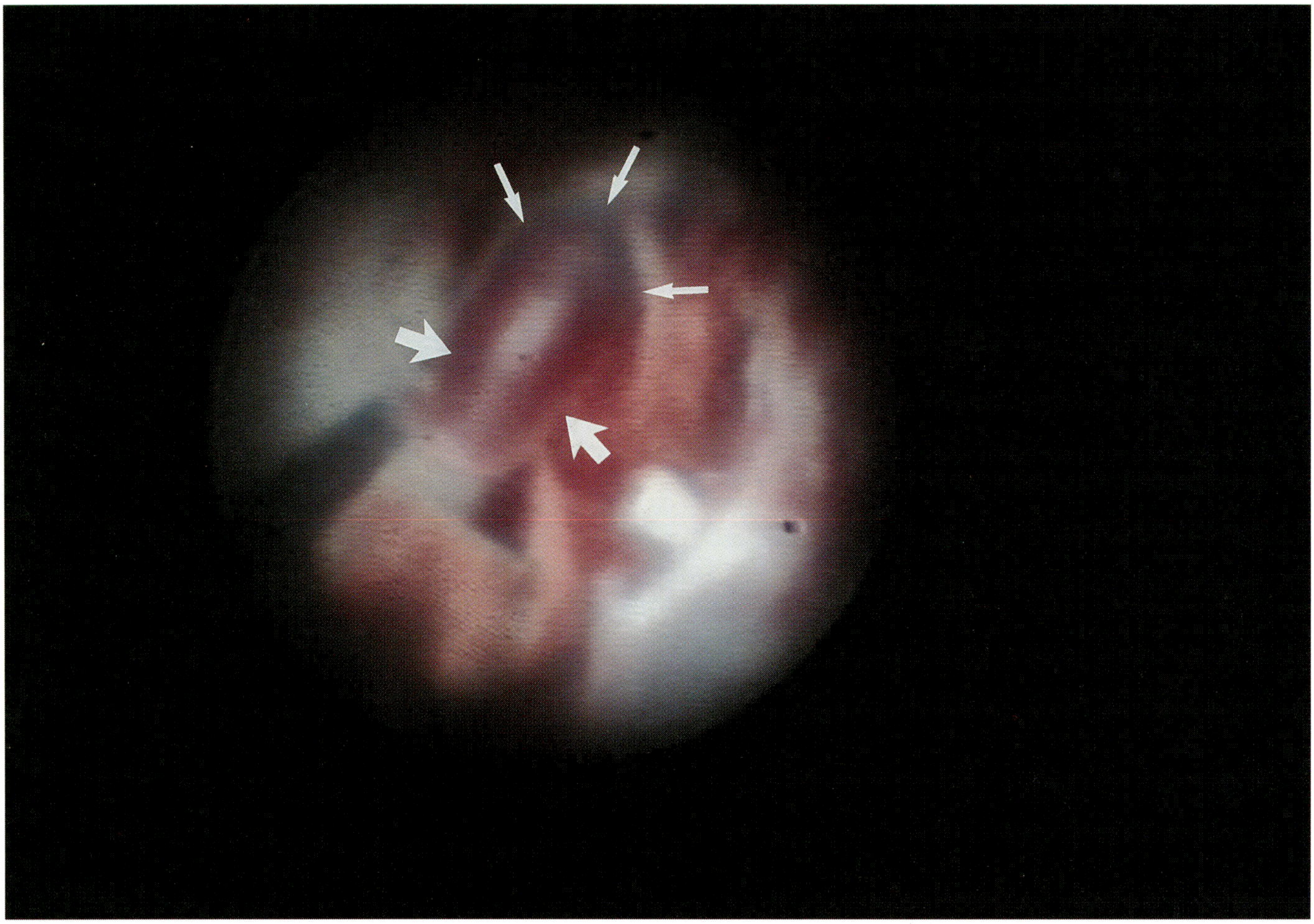

Figure 8C. A juxtanidal vein (large arrows) connects one part of the AVM core to another part of the AVM, or to cortical veins, and is seen to enter the white matter of the brain (small arrows). Juxtanidal veins are often spiral shaped and must be cauterized at their entrance to the brain, for pursuit of these veins into the brain results in uncontrollable hemorrhage and unwarranted removal of the brain tissue surrounding the veins.

bleeding hole by a fine bipolar coagulating forceps and cauterized until adequate coagula is formed locally. With endoscopy, this tiny hole can be easily identified, and subsequently, local coagulation can be accomplished. The entire loop should not be coagulated, because obstruction of this loop may result in increased pressure in the lumen and may rupture previously coagulated and sectioned junctions to arterioles and venules.

Intraventricular AVMs

Trigonal AVMs

Surgical resection of AVMs in the trigonal area extending into the ventricle carries a high risk for three reasons.

1. Approaches to a trigonal AVM must be transcortical, because no major draining vein is found from the hemispheric convexity that can be utilized for access to the AVM core.

2. Morbidity of AVM resection through the posterior temporal and parietal area is high, particularly in the dominant hemisphere.

3. Dissection of the AVM from the cortical side tends to cause spilling of blood into the ventricle. The surgeon may not realize that blood is pooling not only in the affected ventricle but also in the other ventricles. Unrecognized bleeding is partly due to a lack of visualization of the intraventricular portion of the AVM and inadequate tamponade or cauterization of bleeding vessels.

Surgical Procedure: Through a small (3 cm^2) occipitoparietal craniotomy, with its center located 7 cm

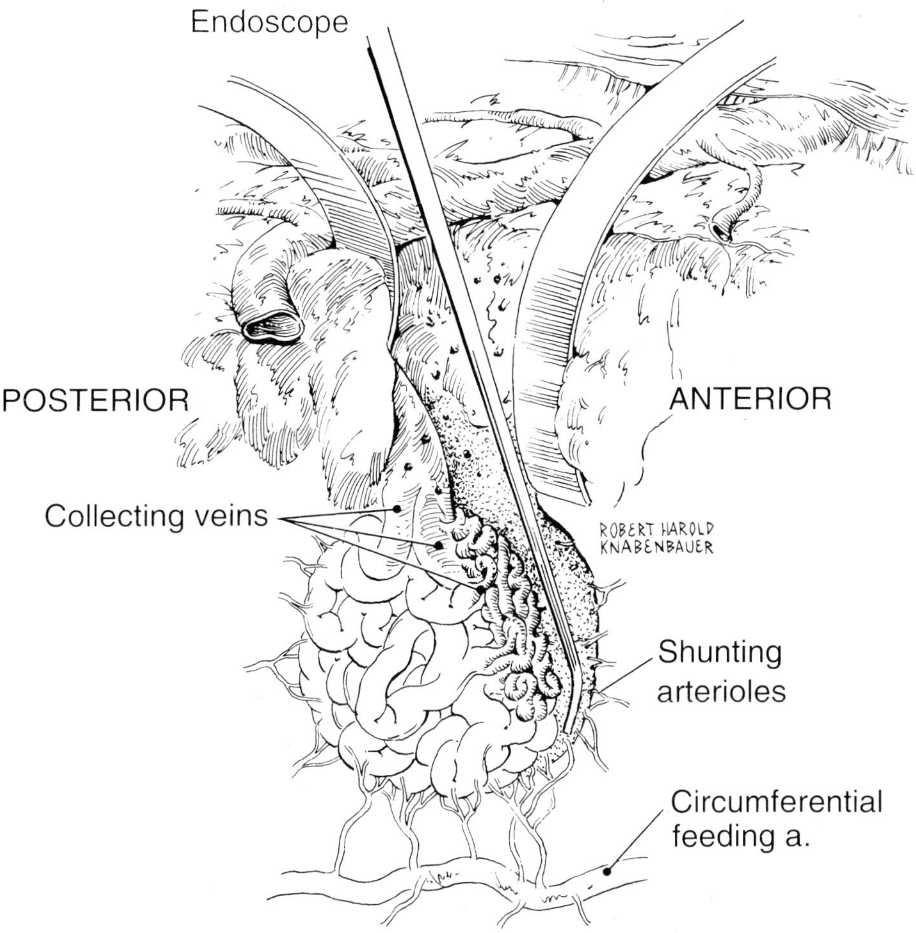

Figure 9. As soon as the AVM core is reached, shunting arterioles and communicating venules are interrupted first on the superficial side of the AVM core, and then on its deep side. The Murphy-Scope is useful in identifying and interrupting these small vessels in the dead angle behind the deep vessels of the AVM core.

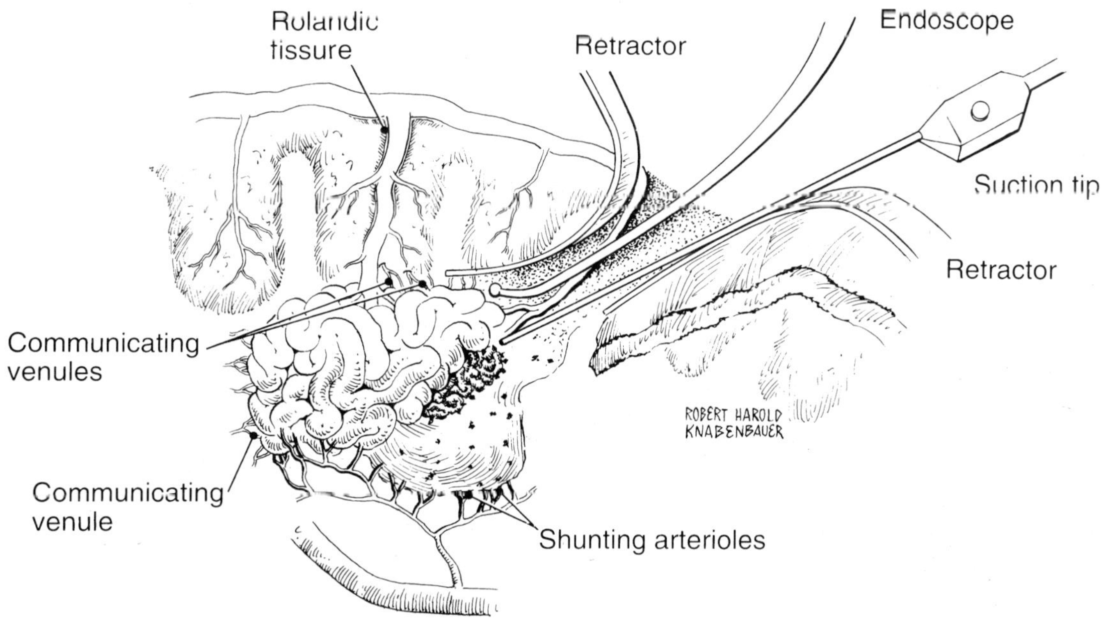

Figure 10. A large AVM is isolated from the sensorimotor cortices while these cortices are gently retracted outward away from the AVM. Endoscopy helps to identify communicating venules that are connected to the subcortical veins as well as to shunting arterioles. The cauterized shrunken core vessels (next to the suction tip) are shown medioanterior to the lateral compartment, which is still patent with arterial blood flow.

above the inion and 3 cm lateral to the midline, a ventricular needle or preferably a catheter is inserted into the trigone for the occipital ventriculostomy. A thin layer of brain tissue is resected around the ventricular catheter. After withdrawal of the catheter, two narrow retractors (3–5 mm wide) are placed through the cortical window and then the endoscope is inserted into the ventricular space (Figure 11). Using the curved endoscope, a direct view of a pulsatile AVM, passively dilated with arterial blood, is obtained on the lateral posterior wall of the ventricle (Figure 12). (If the microscope was used, the same approach to the intraventricular AVM would have provided only a tangential view of the ventricular wall, making it difficult to clearly identify the intraventricular portion of the AVM.) The intraventricular AVM is followed to the ventricular wall; there, the intracerebral portion of the AVM core is dissected by endoscopy- assisted microsurgery, interrupting shunting arterioles and communicating venules. Cauterization of small vessels is facilitated and confirmed by endoscopic observation.

Capsulostriatothalamic AVMs

AVMs in this location are frequently diffuse. It is impossible to totally remove large AVMs in this area without causing significant deficits, such as sensory, motor, speech, or visual field defects. For large AVMs, only the portion that has spread diffusely in the caudate nucleus, the putamen, and the dorsal part of the thalamus should be obliterated. The internal capsule, the nucleus ventralis posterior lateralis et medialis, and the lateral and medial geniculate bodies must be excluded from AVM cauterization.

With the currently available treatment, large AVMs that involve this area may be partly coagulated surgically until the size of the AVM decreases to the irradiation-effective range.

Surgical Procedure: A small craniotomy, 3 cm in diameter, is performed with its center 3 cm lateral to the midline, anterior to the coronal suture. A (usually) freehand stereotactic localization of the body of the lateral ventricle is performed by placing a ventricular catheter, similar to the technique used for a ven-

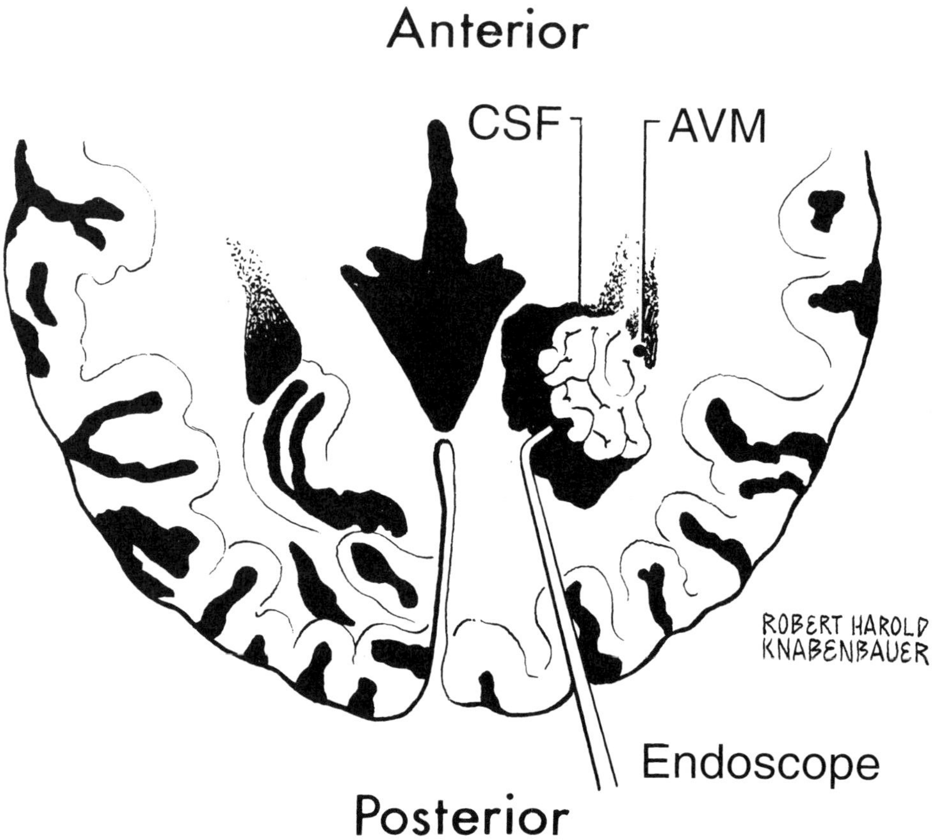

Figure 11. The endoscope insertion through the occipitoparietal cortical opening is schematically shown.

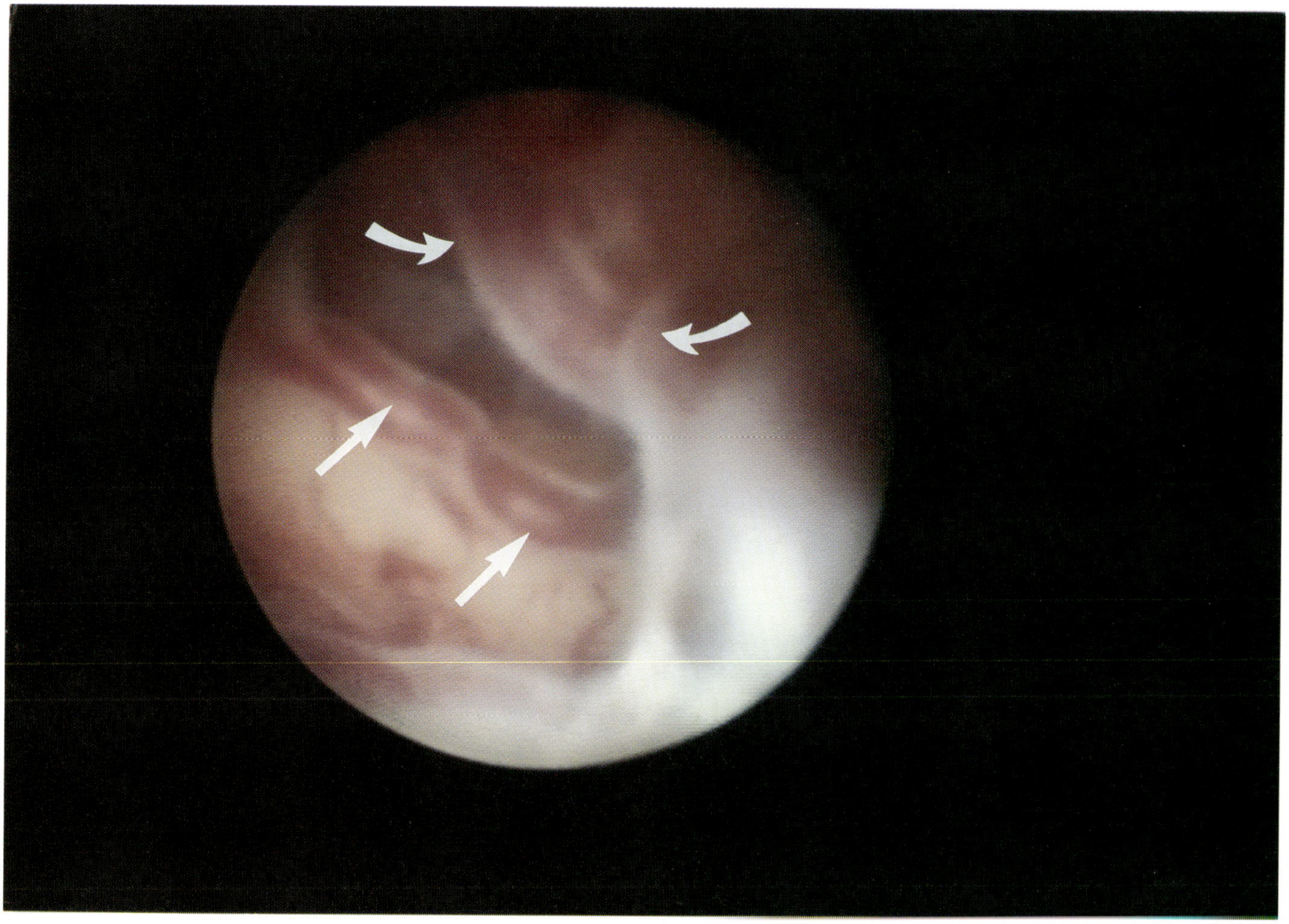

Figure 12. The endoscopic view of the intraventricular portion of the trigonal AVM clearly demonstrates the core in the lateral ventricular wall (curved arrows) and the medial wall, which has veins dilated passively with arterial blood (straight arrows). The white membrane in the right lower quadrant which covers the core vessels was formed as the result of hemorrhage from the AVM rupture.

triculostomy of the anterior horn. The direction of the catheter is toward the midpoint of the orbitomeatal line in the lateral view, 5° medially to the sagittal plane in the anteroposterior view. Color Doppler ultrasonography is a valuable adjunct to direct the insertion of the catheter. After draining a few milliliters of cerebrospinal fluid, a thin layer of brain tissue is removed from the region immediately around the ventricular needle, until the ventricular wall is reached. A straight endoscope is then inserted into the ventricle, allowing immediate identification of AVM vessels dispersed in the brain caudate nucleus anterior to the foramen of Monro. These vessels are cauterized segment by segment until each of the cauterized AVM vessels in the caudate nucleus and putamen is obliterated. Cauterization of blood vessels in the basal ganglia does not cause clinically significant motor dysfunction. However, cauterization of an AVM in the stria terminalis and thalamostriate veins should be avoided.

The posterior portion of the AVM, which is mainly in the thalamus, must be approached through the posterior route, as described for trigone AVM resection, except that the ventricular opening should be placed slightly more anteriorly. The major portion of the AVM in the dorsal thalamus is cauterized to minimize its size without functional impairment. (See illustrative case 9 in Chapter 1.)

Occult AVMs Within the Hematoma Cavity

Hematomas are often the result of rupture of occult subcortical AVMs or AVMs immediately outside of the capsulostriatothalamic structure. Evacuation of hematomas located underneath the functional cortex must be done by inserting a ventricular needle or catheter through the silent area. An extensive and meticulous search for an occult AVM must be done. The brain is retracted in various directions while the blood clot is removed by irrigation and suction, and by piecemeal removal with a large biopsy forceps along the hematoma wall. After the clot is totally removed and the hematoma cavity is collapsed, the retractor is inserted anteriorly, laterally, medially, and posteriorly until the inferior wall of the cavity is visualized. An AVM is usually found in the medioinferior wall of the cavity. Endoscopy minimizes retraction of the brain, and allows prompt detection of a tuft of blood vessels on the cavity wall. The AVM can be safely resected by endoscopy-assisted microsurgery, even if the AVM is located adjacent to the internal capsule.

Discussion and Summary

Improved visualization of deep structures provides a great advantage for endoscopy-assisted microsurgery, particularly in the ventricles, the subarachnoid spaces,[1–5] and the cleavage between the AVM core and surrounding brain tissue. It minimizes retraction of brain tissue and the AVM core, yet permits the surgeon to expose entire lesions. A curved endoscope allows for enlargement of the visual field when the tip of the endoscope is rotated in different directions. Surgical trauma is minimized, while surgical results are maximized.

Endoscopy-assisted microsurgery enables the surgeon to easily avoid the removal of brain tissue, to preserve microcirculation in the functional area, and to maintain circulation in the major draining veins until the core vessels are completely isolated. It assists in preserving cortical tissue overlying the AVM core and of all of the cortical veins that are passively dilated with arterial blood. Elucidation of 50–250 μ shunting arterioles by endoscopy is important in selecting these vessels from the AVM core in functional areas, particularly along its deep side.

Intraventricular endoscopy has several advantages: (1) direct visualization of the AVM through ventriculostomy; (2) dissection of AVMs from the ventricle side; (3) detection of large arteries or veins connected to the AVM deep in the brain; and (4) avoidance of blood pooling in the ventricles.

When the AVM is large, endoscopic surgery reduces the number and extent of various approaches. Several examples illustrate this: (1) A large AVM located under the sensorimotor cortex can be approached from the premotor area alone, rather than by two separate approaches from the premotor and from the posterior parietal areas (see illustrative case 3 in Chapter 1). (2) Intraventricular AVMs can be excised from the ventricular side alone, rather than combining the ventricular and cerebral cortical approaches. (3) AVM venous loops adherent to the arachnoid membrane and surrounding scar tissue, which is often found after subarachnoid hemorrhage, can be clearly identified and safely dissected without causing unexpected rupture of these venous loops, shunting arterioles, or communicating venules. In general, neurosurgical procedures are performed through a cylindrical or conical opening into the brain; endoscopy-assisted microscopic surgery can minimize the size of the opening. Finally, endoscopy provides a higher detection rate of occult AVMs in the hematoma cavity and a decreased operating time.

MRI, magnetic resonance angiography (MRA), CT, CT angiography magnetoencephalography (especially MSI), and intraoperative color Doppler ultrasonography all contribute to the successful removal of AVMs in the functional area. The authors emphasize that the additional powerful instrumentation is available as an intraoperative aid to microsurgery.

References

Section 1: Somatosensory Evoked Potential References

1. Astrup J, Symon L, Branston NM, et al. Cortical evoked potential and extracellular K^+ and H^+ at critical levels of brain ischemia. Stroke 8:51–57, 1977.
2. Austin G, Haugen G, LaManna J. Cortical oxidative metabolism following microanastomosis for brain ischemia. In Jobsis FF (ed): Oxygen and Physiological Function. Dallas: Professional Information Library, 1977, pp 531–544.
3. Awad I, Little JR, Furlan AJ, et al. Correlation of clinical and angiographic findings in brain ischemia and regional blood flow measured by the Xenon inhalation technique. Neurosurgery 11:1–5, 1982.
4. Branston NM, Hope DT, Symon L. Barbiturates in focal ischemia of primate cortex: effects of blood flow distribution, evoked potential and extracellular potassium. Stroke 10:647–653, 1979.
5. Carter LP, Raudens PA, Gaines C, et al. Somatosensory evoked potentials and cortical blood flow during craniotomy for vascular disease. Neurosurgery 15:22–28, 1984.
6. Chance B, Williams GR. The respiratory chain and oxidative phosphorylation. Adv Enzymol 12:65–134, 1956.
7. Diemer NH, Siemkovicz E. Increased 2-deoxy glucose-uptake in hippocampus, globus pallidus and substantia nigra after cerebral ischemia. Acta Neuron Scand 61:56–63, 1984.
8. Drake CG. Cerebral arteriovenous malformations: considerations for and experience with surgical treatment in 166 cases. Clin Neurosurg 26:145–208, 1979.
9. Duckrow RB, LaManna JS, Rosenthal M. Disparate recovery of resting and stimulated oxidative metabolism following transient ischemia. Stroke 12:677–686, 1981.
10. Evans RB, Austin GM. Psychological evaluation of patients undergoing microneurosurgical anastomosis for cerebral ischemia. In Austin GM (ed): Microsurgical Anastomosis for Cerebral Ischemia. Springfield: Charles C. Thomas, 1974, pp 320–326.
11. Fein JM, Olinger R. Cortical nicotinamide adenine dinucleotide (NADH) kinetics in patients undergoing extracranial-intracranial bypass. Neurosurgery 10: 428–439, 1982.
12. Ganz E. Positron emission tomography and nuclear magnetic resonance. Clin Neurosurg 31:441–455, 1984.
13. Garcia JH, Kalimo H, Kamijyo Y, et al. Cellular events during partial cerebral ischemia. I. Electron microscopy of feline cerebral cortex after middle cerebral-artery occlusion. Virchows Arch Zellpathol 25: 191–206, 1977.
14. Giannotta SL, Kindt G. Total morbidity and mortality rates of patients with surgically treated intracranial aneurysms. Neurosurgery 4:125–136, 1979.
15. Grubb RL Jr, Raichle ME, Phelps ME, et al. Effects of increased intracranial pressure on cerebral blood volume, blood flow and oxygen utilization in monkeys. J Neurosurg 43:385–398, 1975.
16. Heilbrun MP, Reichman OH, Anderson RE, et al. Regional cerebral blood flow studies following superficial temporal-middle cerebral artery anastomosis. J Neurosurg 43:706–716, 1975.
17. Hoffman WE, Charbel FT, Edelman G, et al. Brain tissue gases and pH during arteriovenous malformation resection. Neurosurgery 40:294–301, 1997.
18. Jobsis FF, Keizer JH, LaManna JC, et al. Reflectance spectrophotometry of cytochrome a,a_3 in vivo. J Neurophysiol 43:858–972, 1977.
19. Kogure K, Busto R, Schwartzman RJ, et al. The dissociation of cerebral blood flow, metabolism, and function in the early stages of developing cerebral infarction. Ann Neurol 8:278–290, 1980.
20. LaManna JC, Sick TJ, Pikarsky SM, et al. Detection of oxidizable fraction of cytochrome oxidase in intact rat brain. Am J Physiol 253:c477–483, 1987.
21. Lassen NA, Astrup J. Ischemic penumbra. In Wood JH (ed): Cerebral Blood Flow. New York: McGraw-Hill, 1987, pp 458–466.
22. LeBlanc R, Tyler JL, Mohr G, et al. Hemodynamic and metabolic effects of cerebral revascularization. J Neurosurg 66:529–535, 1987.
23. Michenfelder JD, Theyre RA. The effects of anesthesia and hypothermia on canine cerebral ATP and lactate during anoxia produced by decapitation. Anesthesiology 33:430–439, 1970.
24. Pilcher C. Angiomatous malformations of the brain. Ann Surg 123:766–784, 1946.
25. Powers WJ, Raichie ME. Positron emission tomography in cerebrovascular disease. Clin Neurosurg 31: 107–116, 1984.
26. Rosenthal M, LaManna JC. Oxidative metabolism and electrophysiological activity in intact central nervous system. In Jobsis FF (ed): Oxygen and Physiological Function. Dallas: Professional Information Library, 1977, pp 515–530.
27. Rosenthal M, Martel D, LaManna JC, et al. In situ studies of oxidative energy metabolism during transient cortical ischemia in cats. Exp Neurol 50:477–494, 1976.
28. Rosenthal M, Sick T. Brain oxygenation: monitoring techniques and insights into brain function and survival. In Bailliere (ed): Clinical Anaesthesiology Vol 3, No 3, 1989; pp 647–674.
29. Schmiedek P, Gratzl O, Spetzler R, et al. Selection of patients for extraintracranial arterial bypass surgery based on rCBF measurements. J Neurosurg 44: 303–312, 1976.
30. Siesjo BK. Cerebral circulation and metabolism. J Neurosurg 60:883–908, 1984.
31. Sundt TM Jr, Michenfelder JD. Focal transient cerebral ischemia in the squirrel monkey: effect on brain adenosine triphosphate and lactate levels with electrocorticographic and pathologic correlation. Circ Res 30: 703–712, 1972.
32. Symon L. The relationship between CBF, evoked potentials, and clinical features in cerebral ischemia. Acta Neurol Scand 62(Suppl 78):175–190, 1980.

33. Winn HR, Morii S, Berne RM. The role of adenosine in autoregulation of cerebral blood flow. Ann Biomed Eng 13:321–328, 1985.
34. Yamada S. Arteriovenous malformations in the functional area: surgical treatment and regional cerebral blood flow. Neurol Res 4:283–322, 1983.
35. Yamada S, Brauer FS, Knierim DS. Direct approach of arteriovenous malformations in functional areas of a cerebral hemisphere. J Neurosurg 72:418–425, 1990.
36. Yamada S, Brauer F, Knierim D, et al. Can somatosensory evoked potential monitoring predict energy dynamics during controlled hypotension. Neurol Res 14: 325–329, 1992.
37. Yamada S, Brauer F, Knierim D, et al. Safety limits of controlled hypotension in humans. Acta Neurochir (Suppl 42):14–17, 1988.
38. Yamada S, Brauer FS, Purtzer T, et al. MCA occlusion during STA-MCA anastomosis does not compromise cerebral metabolic or electrical activity. In Spetzler RF, Carter LP, Selman WR, et al (eds): Cerebral Revascularization for Stroke. New York: Theime-Stratton, 1985, pp 287–291.
39. Yamada S, Cojocaru T. Arteriovenous malformations. In Wood JH (ed): Cerebral Blood Flow. New York: McGraw-Hill, 1987, pp 580–590.
40. Yatsu JM, Moss SA. Brain lipid change following hypoxia. Stroke 2:587–593, 1971.
41. Yonekura M, Austin G, Poll N, et al. Evaluation of cerebral blood flow in patients with transient ischemic attacks and minor stroke. Surg Neurol 15:58–65, 1981.

Section 2: Magnetic Resonance Imaging References

1. Allison T, McCarthy G, Wood CC, et al. Human cortical potentials evoked by stimulation of the median nerve. I. Cytoarchitectonic areas generating short-latency activity. J Neurophysiol 62:694–710, 1989.
2. Berger MS, Cohen WA, Ojemann GA. Correlation of motor cortex brain mapping data with magnetic resonance imaging. J Neurosurg 72:383–387, 1990.
3. Gallen CC, Schwartz BJ, Bucholz RD, et al. Presurgical localization of functional cortex using magnetic source imaging. J Neurosurg 82:988–989,1001, 1995.
4. Gallen CC, Schwartz BJ, Pantev C, et al. Detection and localization of delta frequency activity in human stroke. In Hoke M (ed): Biomagnetism: Clinical Aspects. Amsterdam: Elsevier, 1992, pp 301–305.
5. Gallen CC, Schwartz B. Rieke K, et al. Intrasubject reliability and validity of somatosensory source localization using a large array biomagnetometer. Electroencephalogr Clin Neurophysiol 90:145–156, 1994.
6. Gallen CC, Sobel DF, Waltz T, et al. Noninvasive presurgical mapping of somatosensory cortex. Neurosurgery 33:260–268, 1993.
7. Martin N, Grafton S, Vinuela F, et al. Imaging techniques for cortical functional localization. Clin Neurosurg 38:132–165, 1992.
8. Pantev C, Gallen C, Hampson S, et al. Reproducibility and validity of neuromagnetic source localization using a large array biomagnetometer. Am J Electroencephalogr Technol 31:83–101, 1991.
9. Sobel DF, Gallen CC, Schwartz BJ, et al. Locating the central sulcus: comparison of MR anatomic and magnetoencephalographic functional methods. AJNR 14: 915–925, 1993.
10. Yamada S, Gallen CC. Biomagnetic technologies: magnetic source imaging (MSI): Magnes™ biomagnetometer. Neurosurgery 33:166–168, 1993.

Section 3: Color Doppler Ultrasonography References

1. Babcock DS, Barr LL, Crone KR. Intraoperative uses of ultrasound in the pediatric neurosurgical patient. Ped Neurosurg 18:84–91, 1992.
2. Black KL, Rubin JM, Chandler WF, et al. Intraoperative color-flow Doppler imaging of AVMs and aneurysms. J Neurosurg 68:635–639, 1988.
3. Goodkin R, McKhann GM 2nd, Haynor DR, et al. Persistent feeding arteries to angiographically completely embolized arteriovenous malformation demonstrated by intraoperative color-flow Doppler testing: report of two cases. Surg Neurol 44:326–332, 1995.
4. Kitazawa K, Nitta J, Okudera H, et al. Color Doppler ultrasound imaging in the emergency management of an intracerebral hematoma caused by cerebral arteriovenous malformations: technical case report [in Process Citation]. Neurosurgery 42:405–407, 1998.
5. Rubin JM, Hatfield MK, Chandler WF, et al. Intracerebral arteriovenous malformations: intraoperative color Doppler flow imaging. Radiology 170(1 Pt 1):219–222, 1989.
6. Yamada S, Rouse G, Iacono RP, et al. Color Doppler ultrasonography during arteriovenous malformation (AVM) surgery. Annual Meeting, Section on Cerebrovascular surgery of AANS and CNS, Poster # 51. Anaheim: February 4–6, 1997, p 96.

Section 4: Endoscopy for AVM Surgery References

1. Apuzzo MLJ, Heifitz MD, Weiss MH, et al. Neurosurgical endoscopy using the side- viewing telescope: technical notes. J Neurosurg 46:398–400, 1977.
2. Cohen AR, Perneczky A, Rodziewicz GS, et al. Endoscope-assisted craniotomy: approach to the rostral brain stem. J Neurosurg 36:1128–1130, 1995.
3. Fries G, Perneczky A. Endoscope-assisted microneurosurgery: three years experience in clinical application. Annual meeting of the American Association of Neurological Surgeons. San Diego: April 9–14, 1994, Poster # 1239.
4. Grateir L, Andre J. Endoscope-assisted craniotomy. Techniques in Neurosurgery 1:201–213, 1996.
5. Grotenhuis JA. Manual of Endoscopic Procedures in Neurosurgery. Nijmegen: Uitgevery Machaon, 1995.
6. Yamada S. Arteriovenous malformations in the functional area: surgical treatment and regional cerebral blood flow. Neurol Res 4:283–322, 1982.
7. Yamada S, Brauer F, Iacono RP. The surgical importance of venous channels in arteriovenous malformations. In Hakuba A (ed): Surgery of the Intracranial Venous Systems. Tokyo: Springer, 1996, pp 499–505.

8. Yamada S, Brauer FS, Knierim DS. Direct approach of arteriovenous malformations in functional areas of a cerebral hemisphere. J Neurosurg 72:418–425, 1990.
9. Yamada S, Brauer F, Knierim D. Feeding arteries to arteriovenous malformations. Neurosurg Forum. J Neurosurg 3:477–478, 1990.
10. Yamada S, Iacono RP, Mandybur GT, et al. Endoscopic procedures for AVMs in functional areas of the brain. Annual meeting of the American Association of Neurological Surgeons. Denver: April 12–17, 1997, p 72, Abstract #1102.
11. Yamada S, Iacono RP, Mandybur GT, et al. Endoscopic procedures for resection of arteriovenous malformations. Surg Neurol (in press).

Chapter 11

Vasculogenesis and Angiogenesis in Relation to Arteriovenous Malformations of the Brain

Nikolay I. Baev, MD, PhD, John H. Wong, MD, MSc, and Issam A. Awad, MD, MSc

Introduction

The morphogenesis of cranial arteries and veins in the human embryo has been well described.[11,35,36] The adult vascular system consists of large arteries that are internally lined by a monolayer of endothelial cells and are ensheathed by smooth muscle cells. They branch into progressively smaller vessels and terminate in precapillary arterioles and capillaries, the latter of which are composed almost entirely of endothelial cells that are only occasionally coated by pericytes. Capillaries then feed into postcapillary venules that connect further into progressively larger venous vessels.

Two processes form the vasculature: vasculogenesis and angiogenesis (Figure 1). The differentiation of angioblasts from mesoderm after gastrulation, and the formation of primitive blood vessels from angioblasts at or near their site of origin are the two distinct steps of vascularization in the embryo that define *vasculogenesis*. *Angiogenesis,* which occurs in both the embryo and the adult, is the process in which pre-existing vessels send out capillary sprouts to produce new vessels. Vasculogenesis and angiogenesis are interrelated, and vascular endothelial cells play a central role in both processes. Proliferating endothelial cells migrate and assemble into tubular structures with tight intercellular connections. Pericytes and smooth muscle cells are then recruited to encase these endothelial tubes and provide maintenance and modulatory functions to these vessels. The establishment and remodeling of blood vessels is controlled in part by paracrine signals, intercellular contacts and cell adhesion molecules, and the extracellular matrix.

Vasculogenesis

The earliest stages of vascular development, vasculogenesis, include the differentiation, expansion, and interconnection of endothelial cell precursors into the primary vascular network.[39] Of the three germ layers, mesoderm and endoderm are derived from the embryonic epiblast by the process of gastrulation. At the time blood islands form, the mesodermal layer is gradually split by the advancing extraembryonic coelom that is contiguous with the intraembryonic coelom. Members of the fibroblast growth factor (FGF) and transforming growth factor-β (TGF-β) families (see below) induce mesoderm formation. Vasculogenesis seems to be regulated negatively by the ectoderm and positively by the endoderm.

Blood vessel development is morphologically first evident outside the embryo on the yolk sac, where focal aggregations of mesenchymal cells form *blood islands.* The cells on their periphery, called *angioblasts,* transform later into endothelial cells and form vesicles that fuse with one another to form extraembryonic vascular channels. These primitive channels branch and elongate toward the embryo. The first intraembryonic angioblasts appear shortly after

From Yamada S (ed): *Arteriovenous Malformations in Functional Areas of the Brain.* © Futura Publishing Co, Inc, Armonk, NY, 1999.

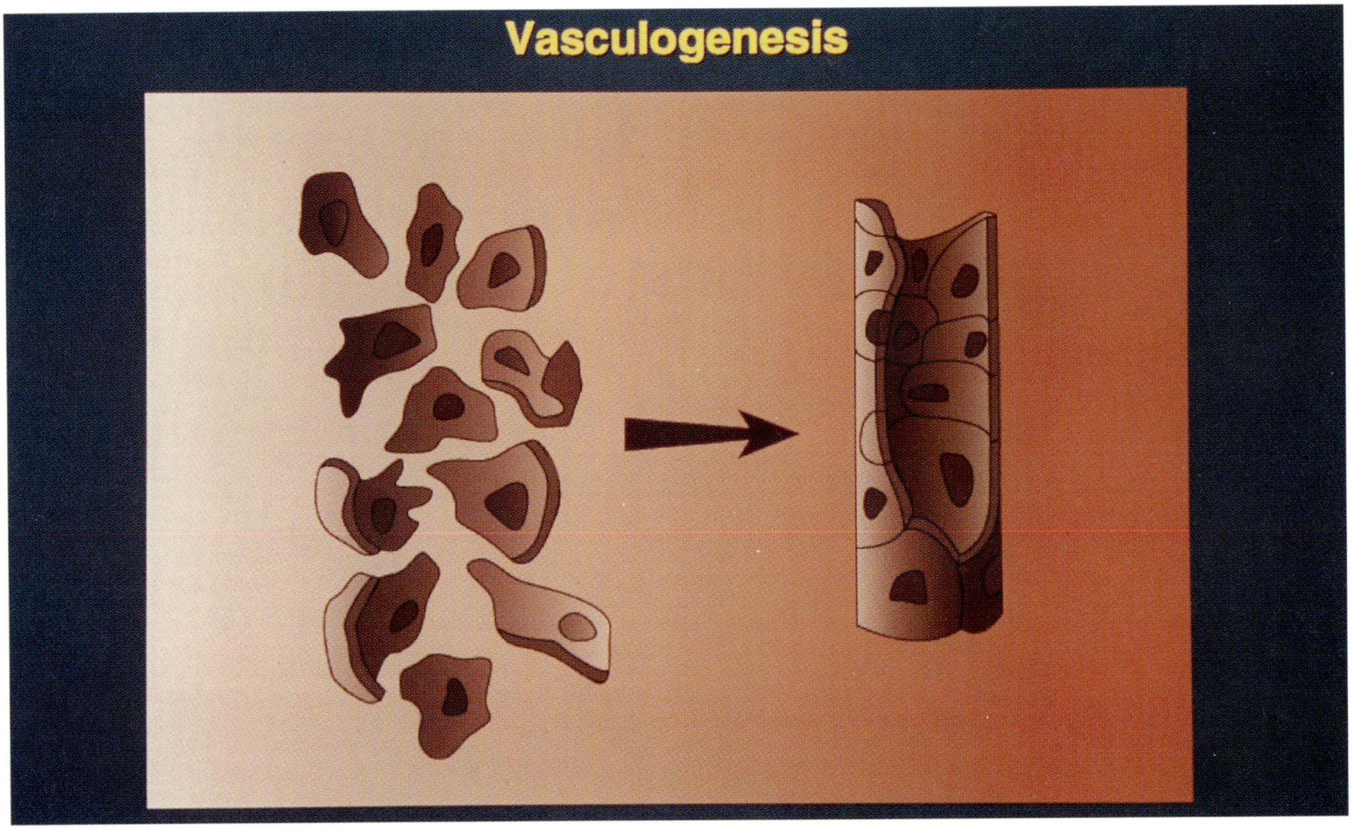

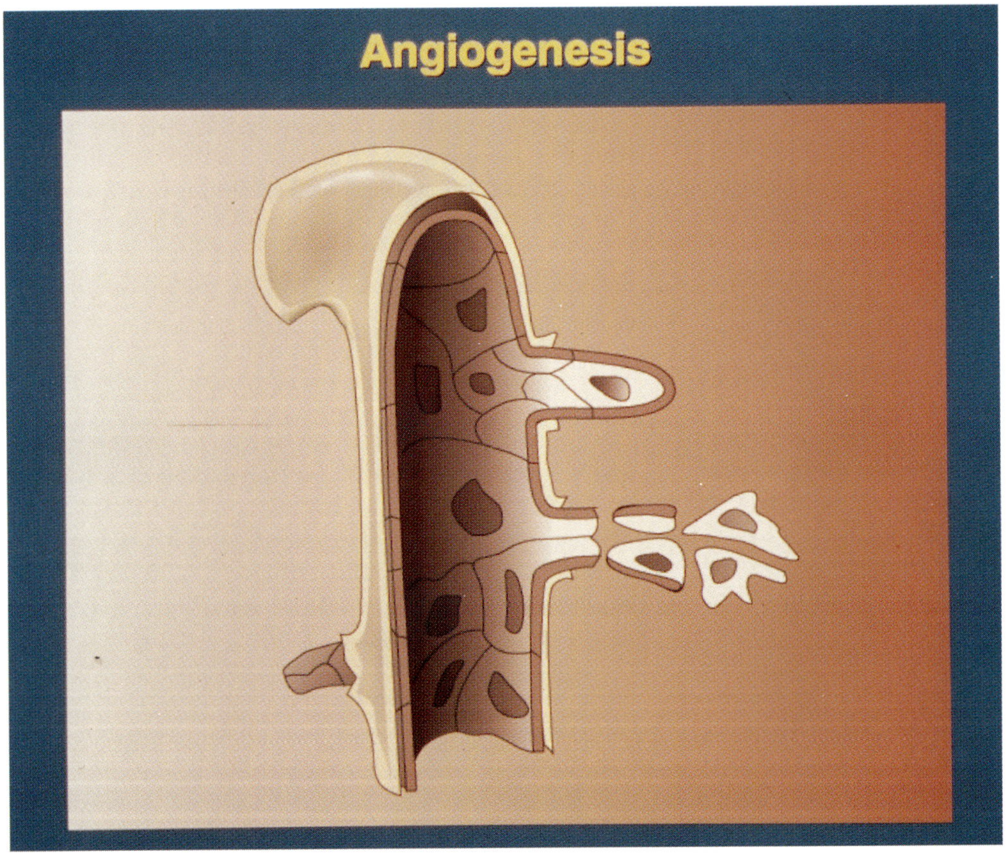

Figure 1. Illustrations of vasculogenesis and angiogenesis.

their extraembryonic counterparts, and are first seen in the single somite stage at the lateral edges of the anterior intestinal portal ventral to the somites and in close contact with the endoderm. Angioblast strands then develop along the lateral edges of the somites, which represent the primordia of the dorsal aorta. At the two-somite stage, the interconnection between extraembryonic and intraembryonic vascular primordia is already established. Cranial to the anterior intestinal portal, the endocardial primordia and the ventral aorta are formed at the midline.

The craniofacial mesenchyme is composed of the neural crest and three mesodermal populations: the prechordal plate, lateral mesoderm, and paraxial mesoderm. All paraxial and lateral mesodermal populations contain precursors of vascular endothelial cells. Some of these angioblasts differentiate in situ, contributing directly to pre-existing vessels or forming isolated nonpatent cords that subsequently vesiculate and fuse with nearby vessels. The angioblasts migrate in all directions, invading embryonic mesenchymal and epithelial tissues, and participate in new blood vessel formation at distant sites. The interactions leading to proper spatial formation of the craniofacial skeletal, muscular, vascular, and peripheral neural tissues are not fully understood. Current studies indicate that connective tissue precursors, regardless of their origin, contain spatial pattern information used by the developing muscular, vascular, and peripheral nervous system. The major events of embryonic vascular pattern formation, which are described extensively in the classic literature, and the details of head mesenchyme vascularization have been reviewed elsewhere.[34]

Several receptor protein kinases expressed on endothelial and smooth muscle cells, and their corresponding ligands, are involved in blood vessel formation.[13,17,56] Vascular endothelial growth factor (VEGF), a 40–45 kDa homodimeric protein, and its receptors play a central role in vasculogenesis.[23,51] Human VEGF monomers exist as five different isoforms of 121, 145, 165, 189, and 206 amino acids that are produced by alternate splicing from a single gene containing eight exons.[37,52] $VEGF_{121}$ and $VEGF_{165}$ are the most abundant of these isoforms and each differs somewhat in its biological properties.

VEGF binds to two receptor tyrosine kinases, VEGFR-1 (Flt-1)[8,45] and VEGFR-2 (KDR/Flk-1),[33,50] whose expression is restricted to endothelial cells and their embryonic precursors. Flk-1 marks the putative common embryonic endothelial and hematopoietic precursor, the hemangioblast, and is essential for yolk sac blood island formation in early vasculogenesis and hematopoiesis.[43,44] Disruption of the gene for the other receptor, Flt-1, interferes with a later stage of vasculogenesis, resulting in thin-walled vessels of larger than normal diameter.[14,15]

Recently, a third VEGF receptor, $VEGF_{165}R$, has been identified and found identical to human neurophilin-1.[46] In the developing embryo, neurophilin-1 is a receptor for the collapsin/semaphorin family that mediates neuronal cell guidance. Neurophilin-1, which is expressed widely in human adult tissues outside the brain, modulates $VEGF_{165}$ binding to Flk-1 and subsequent bioactivity and may therefore regulate VEGF-induced vasculogenesis and angiogenesis. Since both neurons and blood vessels display branching and directional migration, neurophilin-1 may play an essential role also in blood vessel guidance.

Members of the FGF family are potent inducers of ventral mesoderm, which in the amphibious *Xenopus laevis* embryo includes muscular and hematologic cells.[21,24] Despite reports that one member, basic FGF (bFGF), is a potent stimulator of angiogenesis in vitro and in vivo,[12] there is no convincing evidence that it plays a major role in the actual development of the vasculature.

The fully developed vertebrate circulatory system is composed of arteries and veins (with an interposing capillary bed), which were traditionally defined only by the direction of blood flow and by anatomical and functional differences. Until recently, all models of angiogenesis have considered the developing endothelial network of arteries and veins as a homogeneous population. It is clear now, however, that arterial and venous endothelial cells are molecularly distinct from the earliest stages of blood vessel formation. Ephrin-B2, an Eph family transmembrane ligand, has been found to mark arterial but not venous endothelial cells from the onset of angiogenesis.[25] In contrast, Eph-B4, a receptor for ephrin-B2, marks veins but not arteries. Ephrin-B2 knockout mice display defects in angiogenesis in both arteries and veins in the capillary networks of the head and yolk sac as well as in myocardial trabeculation. The differences between arteries and veins seem to be in part genetically determined, and reciprocal signaling between these two types of vessels appears to be crucial for the morphogenesis of the capillary bed.

Angiogenesis

The primary capillary plexus, which is formed entirely of endothelial cells during the initial stages of vasculogenesis, is remodeled by a process referred to as angiogenesis.[40] A newly discovered group of cytokines, angiopoietins[6,31] and their protein-tyrosine kinase receptors, Tie-1 and Tie-2/Tek, play an important role in angiogenesis and remodeling.[42] Unlike VEGF, angiopoietin-1 (Ang-1), the first identified ligand for Tie-2, is neither a mitogen for endothelial cells nor does it induce endothelial tube formation. Instead, Ang-1 seems to regulate the recruitment of pericytes and smooth muscle cell precursors to the cell wall.[49] Angiopoietin-2 (Ang-2), an Ang-1 relative, is the naturally occurring antagonist for Ang-1 and Tie-2.[31]

In humans, the most common errors of vascular morphogenesis are the venous malformations. They are composed of dilated, serpiginous channels, whose walls are variably thickened with smooth muscle while some mural regions lack smooth muscle altogether. A missense mutation in the kinase domain of Tie-2 was found to increase the activity of Tie-2 and segregated with dominantly inherited venous malformations in two unrelated families.[31] Upregulation of Tie-2 in the vasculature of arteriovenous malformations (AVMs) has also been demonstrated.[19] Thus an apparent defect in vascular remodeling can result either from an activating mutation of the receptor, from the absence of the ligand, or from a deficiency of the Tie-2 receptor itself.

Platelet-derived growth factor (PDGF) plays an important role in peri-endothelial cell signaling and in the development of specific subsets of smooth muscle cells.[28] The PDGF family consists of homodimers, PDGF-AA or PDGF-BB, or heterodimers, PDGF-AB, that are made from the pairwise assembly of two related PDGF chains, A and B. The three PDGF isoforms differ in their effect on a given cell type, primarily due to the repertoire of PDGF receptors expressed by that particular cell. In a similar manner, the receptors consist of dimers of the α and β subtypes of the PDGF tyrosine kinase receptor, PDGF-Rα and PDGF-Rβ. PDGF-Rα can bind both PDGF chains, whereas the β receptor is selective for the PDGF-B chain. Therefore, αα receptor dimers can bind all three PDGF isoforms, αβ heterodimers can bind AB or BB, and the ββ receptor dimer binds only PDGF-BB. PDGF-B promotes the proliferation and migration of mesenchymal cells in vitro.[20]

PDGF is involved in the paracrine recruitment of mural cell precursors to the vessel wall, based on the observations that PDGFR-β and PDGF-B ligand-null mice die from hemorrhage in the perinatal period and have no pericytes in their renal vasculature.[30,47] In separate experiments, PDGF-B-deficient mice lacked microvascular pericytes and developed brain capillary microaneurysms that ruptured at late gestation.[29] The endothelial cells of the sprouting capillaries in these mutant mice appeared to be unable to attract PDGF-Rβ-positive pericyte progenitor cells that may normally contribute to the mechanical stability of the capillary wall.

A number of serine-threonine kinase receptors have been identified. Most of these are type I or type II receptors for proteins in the TGF-β superfamily. The type I or type II receptors form heteromeric receptor complexes after ligand binding and transduce intracellular signals.[38] TGF-β RI requires TGF-β RII for ligand binding, and TGF-β RII needs TGF-β RI for signaling. TGF-β binds directly to receptor II, which is a constitutively active kinase. Bound TGF-β is recognized by TGF-β RI and is then recruited into the complex becoming phosphorylated by TGF-β RII. Phosphorylation allows TGF-β RI to propagate the signal to downstream substrates. TGF-β causes mesenchymal cells to differentiate into pericytes and smooth muscle cells and inhibits endothelial cell proliferation. Under experimental conditions, 50% of TGF-β null mice die from a defect resulting from improper interaction between epithelial and mesenchymal cells during vasculogenesis.[9]

In humans, endoglin (CD105), a TGF-β binding protein of endothelial cells and component of the TGF-β receptor complex,[57] was identified as the gene responsible for hereditary hemorrhage telangiectasia (HHT) type 1, a disease of inherited AVMs affecting multiple organs including skin, lung, and brain.[32] Mutations in the activin receptor-like kinase 1 (ALK-1) gene, the prototypic TGF-β RI, are the cause of HHT type 2, another form of the disease.[16,22]

Tissue factor, a high-affinity receptor and cofactor for plasma factor VII/VIIa and the primary cellular initiator of blood coagulation, may also play a role in blood vessel development. Inactivation of the tissue factor gene in a mouse knockout model resulted in abnormal circulation from yolk sac to embryo beyond embryonic day 8.5, leading to embryo wasting and death.[5] Vitelline vessels from null mice were found deficient in smooth muscle α-actin-expressing mesenchymal cells, which normally participate in the organization of the vessel wall.

The formation of new microvessels requires a number of interactions that must be coordinated in a spatially and temporally specified manner. These events are likely mediated by adhesion molecules and extracellular matrix molecules that provide endothelial cells with instructions as they migrate into the perivascular space and assemble into new vessels with surrounding supportive cells.[2] Members of four families of cell adhesion molecules—integrins, immunoglobulin superfamily members, cadherins, and selectins—have been described in blood vessels undergoing vascular remodeling. The αvβ3 integrin can bind a wide range of different ligands such as vitronectin, fibronectin, von Willebrand factor, fibrinogen, PECAM-1 (CD31), and matrix metalloproteinase-2. It is expressed in growing but not quiescent blood vessels and clearly participates in both angiogenesis[3,4] and vasculogenesis.[10] VE-cadherin was found to play a role during angiogenesis by specifying endothelial cell organization and differentiation into mature vessels.[7] PECAM-1 (CD31) may also be involved in angiogenesis based on its expression and localization in sprouting blood vessels.[1] E-selectin is associated with essential components of angiogenesis, endothelial cell proliferation, migration, capillary formation, and neovascularization.[25,26] However, the mechanisms by which E-selectin contributes to angiogenesis is likely to be subtle since E-selectin knockout mice are viable and reproduce normally.[27] With the exception of the αv integrins, relatively little is known, however, about the mechanisms by which cell adhesion molecules function in angiogenesis.

Possible Roles in AVM Development

Although the molecular mechanisms of vascular differentiation remain to be fully elucidated and understood, advances in molecular biology allow speculation into the genesis, progression, and recurrence of cerebral AVMs (Figure 2). The genesis of vascular malformations is potentially related to local abnormal embryonic development and differentiation of the circulation. Since cerebral AVMs lack the normal interposing capillary bed, studies on capillary morphogenesis may shed light on the pathogenesis of AVMs. Wang et al. have described differential expression of ephrin-B2 on arterial endothelial cells and Eph-B4 on endothelial cells destined to line the venous circulation.[54] This work suggests that the endothelium of the vasculature may not be a homogeneous population as previously thought and that the ephrin and Eph receptor family may not only direct axonal growth and maintain neuronal boundaries, but may also differentiate the arterial and venous circulations on a cellular level.

The inherited propensity of persons with HHT or Osler-Weber-Rendu disease to develop AVMs of the brain, viscera, and skin suggest that the development of AVMs may be genetically determined. It also illustrates that AVMs can develop later in life (and not just during vasculogenesis) and may mature and grow over time. Studies have revealed a significant

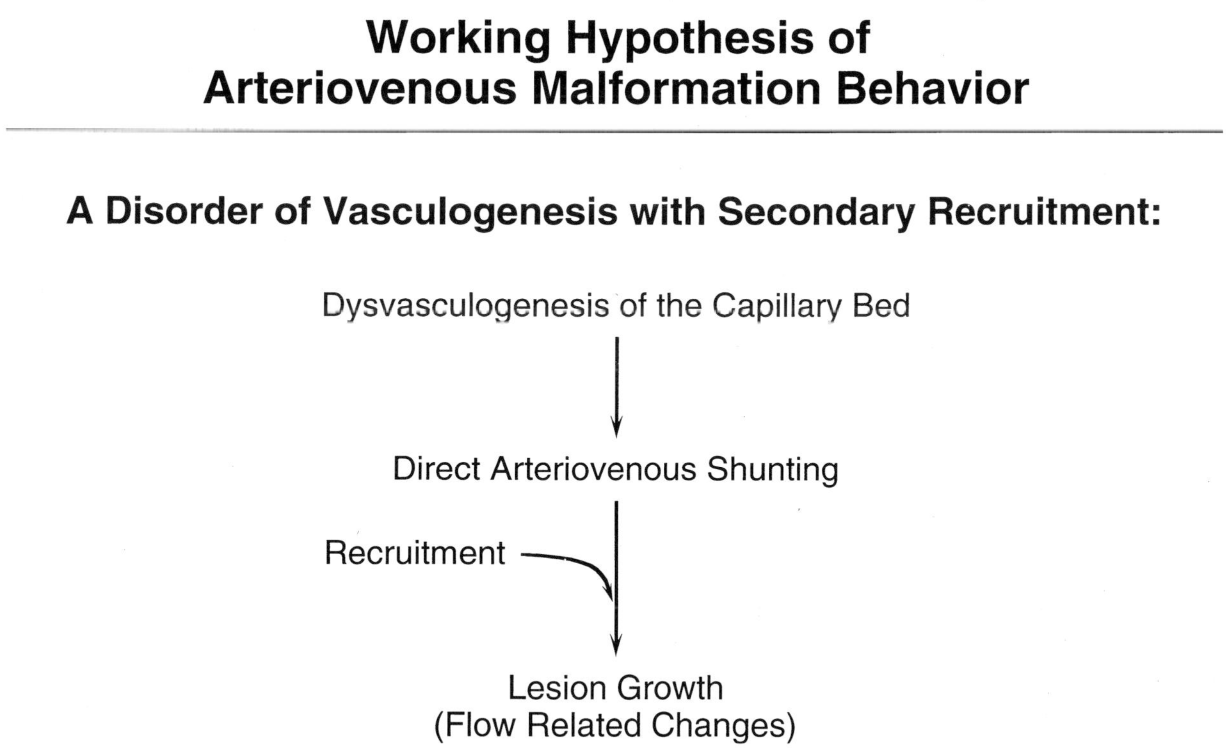

Figure 2. Hypothesis of potential roles of abnormal vasculogenesis and angiogenesis in the genesis and development of cerebral AVMs. Dysvasculogenesis of the capillaries, occurring in the embryonic or mature vascular bed, may lead to direct arteriovenous shunting. Subsequent local cellular signaling mechanisms may result in recruitment of feeding vessels from adjacent vascular territories and growth of the lesion.

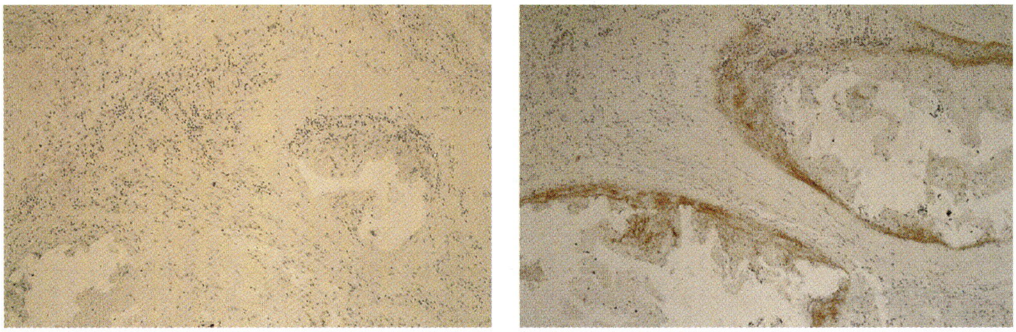

Figure 3. Expression of VEGF shown by immunohistochemistry, in comparison to negative control **(left)**, in the vessels of a cerebral AVM **(right)**. Used with permission from Rothbart et al.[54]

role of endoglin in lesion development as it was identified on chromosome 9 as the gene responsible for HHT type 1,[32] and mutations in the ALK-1 gene are the cause of HHT type 2.[16,22] Endoglin (CD105) has been recognized as a TGF-β binding protein of endothelial cells and a component of the TGF-β receptor complex,[57] but its exact influence on AVM development is unknown. As previously discussed, a missense mutation in the kinase domain of Tie-2, the receptor for Ang-1, increased the activity of Tie-2 and was found to be associated with inherited venous malformations.[53]

Other avenues of investigation have further suggested a central role of angiogenesis in AVM development. Using immunohistochemical methods, Rothbart and co-workers demonstrated angiogenic activity in both cerebral AVMs and cavernous malformations surgically resected from human patients, by finding increased expression of VEGF and bFGF in the vasculature of these lesions (Figure 3).[41] Other investigators using immunohistochemistry and in situ hybridization techniques have demonstrated the upregulation of Tie-2, a receptor tyrosine kinase specific to endothelial cells, and VEGF mRNA and protein in human AVMs and surrounding brain parenchyma.[18] Although these studies suggest a role of angiogenesis in the development of brain AVMs, these results should be tempered by the fact that angiogenic activity may be influenced not only by the biological activity of the AVM but also by local phenomena related to flow or ischemia. Further study is required to dissect out the exact role of angiogenesis related to the AVM itself versus such secondary factors.

Ongoing angiogenesis may also influence the growth or recurrence of AVMs. Sonstein and co-workers described several pediatric patients who developed recurrent AVMs despite normal postoperative angiography after surgical resection.[48] Based on elevated levels of VEGF found on immunocytochemistry staining in these recurrent AVMs as compared to nonrecurrent AVM specimens, they hypothesized that raised production of VEGF by perilesional astrocytes may lead to AVM formation or recurrence, possibly as a result of immature cerebral vascularization or dysregulated angiogenesis. The recognized recurrence of AVMs after partial embolization and propensity of AVMs for recruitment of feeding vessels from distant vascular beds are additional clinical scenarios pointing to the possibility of angiogenic paracrine signaling pathways that remain to be delineated. Rhoten and co-workers found that endothelin-1, a peptide with vasoconstrictory properties that normally regulates gene expression and vascular remodeling, is repressed in human AVMs, both in histological specimens and in endothelial cells cultured from pathological tissue.[38] These investigators hypothesize that lack of endothelin-1 secretion by AVM endothelium may explain the dysautoregulation and resultant high-flow hemodynamic state associated with AVMs that predispose these lesions to local ischemia and hemorrhage.

The molecular dissection of cerebral vascular malformations will likely shed light on mechanisms of AVM development and holds the even greater promise of producing novel diagnostic and therapeutic avenues for these lesions. Further understanding of AVMs on a cellular level may eventually allow genotyping of AVMs to identify vascular malformation subtypes, isolation of somatic mutations in sporadic AVMs, genetic modification to promote regression, inhibit recurrence or recruitment of abnormal vasculature, and predict or prevent lesion genesis in predisposed hosts. Although much work clearly remains to be accomplished, integrating advances in molecular biology into the clinical realm may offer new insights into the genesis and behavior of cerebral AVMs.

References

1. Berger R, Albelda SM, Berd D, et al. Expression of platelet-endothelial cell adhesion molecule-1 (PECAM-1) during melanoma-induced angiogenesis in vivo. J Cutan Pathol 20:399–406, 1993.
2. Bischoff J. Cell adhesion and angiogenesis. J Clin Invest 100:S37–39, 1997.
3. Brooks PC, Clark RA, Cheresh DA. Requirement of vascular integrin alpha v beta 3 for angiogenesis. Science 264:569–571, 1994.
4. Brooks PC, Montgomery AM, Rosenfeld M, et al. Integrin alpha v beta 3 antagonists promote tumor regression by inducing apoptosis of angiogenic blood vessels. Cell 79:1157–1164, 1994.
5. Carmeliet P, Mackman N, Moons L, et al. Role of tissue factor in embryonic blood vessel development. Nature 383:73–75, 1996.
6. Davis S, Aldrich TH, Jones PF, et al. Isolation of angiopoietin-1, a ligand for the TIE2 receptor, by secretion-trap expression cloning. Cell 87:1161–1169, 1996.
7. Dejana E. Endothelial adherens junctions: implications in the control of vascular permeability and angiogenesis. J Clin Invest 98:1949–1953, 1996.
8. de Vries C, Escobedo JA, Ueno H, et al. The fms-like tyrosine kinase, a receptor for vascular endothelial growth factor. Science 255:989–991, 1992.
9. Dickson MC, Martin JS, Cousins FM, et al. Defective haematopoiesis and vasculogenesis in transforming growth factor-beta 1 knockout mice. Development 121: 1845–1854, 1995.
10. Drake CJ, Cheresh DA, Little CD. An antagonist of integrin alpha v beta 3 prevents maturation of blood vessels during embryonic neovascularization. J Cell Sci 108: 2655– 2661, 1995.
11. Evans HM. On the development of the aortae, cardinal and umbilical veins, and the other blood vessels of vertebrate embryos from capillaries. Anat Rec 3: 498–518, 1909.
12. Fernig DG, Gallagher JT. Fibroblast growth factors and their receptors: an information network controlling tissue growth, morphogenesis and repair. Progr Growth Factor Res 5:353–377, 1994.
13. Folkman J, D'Amore PA. Blood vessel formation: what is its molecular basis? Cell 87:1153–1155, 1996.
14. Fong GH, Klingensmith J, Wood CR, et al. Regulation of flt-1 expression during mouse embryogenesis suggests a role in the establishment of vascular endothelium. Dev Dyn 207:1–10, 1996.
15. Fong GH, Rossant J, Gertsenstein M, et al. Role of the Flt-1 receptor tyrosine kinase in regulating the assembly of vascular endothelium. Nature 376:66–70, 1995.
16. Guttmacher AE, Marchuk DA, White RI, Jr. Hereditary hemorrhagic telangiectasia. N Engl J Med 333: 918–924, 1995.
17. Hanahan D. Signaling vascular morphogenesis and maintenance. Science 277:48–50, 1997.
18. Hatva E, Kaipainen A, Mentula P, et al. Expression of endothelial cell-specific receptor tyrosine kinases and growth factors in human brain tumors. Am J Pathol 146:368–378, 1995.
19. Hatva E, Jaaskelainen J, Hirvonen H, et al. Tie endothelial cell-specific receptor tyrosine kinase is upregulated in the vasculature of arteriovenous malformations. J Neuropathol Exp Neurol 55:1124–1133, 1996.
20. Heldin CH. Structural and functional studies on platelet-derived growth factor. EMBO J 11:4251–4259, 1992.
21. Isaacs HV. New perspectives on the role of the fibroblast growth factor family in amphibian development. Cell Mol Life Sci 53:350–361, 1997.
22. Johnson DW, Berg JN, Baldwin MA, et al. Mutations in the activin receptor-like kinase 1 gene in hereditary haemorrhagic telangiectasia type 2. Nat Genet 13: 189–195, 1996.
23. Keck PJ, Hauser SD, Krivi G, et al. Vascular permeability factor, an endothelial cell mitogen related to PDGF. Science 246:1309–1312, 1989.
24. Knochel W, Grunz H, Loppnow-Blinde B, et al. Mesoderm induction and blood island formation by angiogenic growth factors and embryonic inducing factors. Blut 59:207– 213, 1989.
25. Koch AE, Halloran MM, Haskell CJ, et al. Angiogenesis mediated by soluble forms of E-selectin and vascular cell adhesion molecule-1. Nature 376:517–519, 1995.
26. Kraling BM, Razon MJ, Boon LM, et al. E-selectin is present in proliferating endothelial cells in human hemangiomas. Am J Pathol 148:1181–1191, 1996.
27. Labow MA, Norton CR, Rumberger JM, et al. Characterization of E-selectin-deficient mice: demonstration of overlapping function of the endothelial selectins. Immunity 1:709–720, 1994.
28. Lindahl P, Betsholtz C. Not all myofibroblasts are alike: revisiting the role of PDGF-A and PDGF-B using PDGF-targeted mice. Curr Opin Nephrol Hyperten 7:21–26, 1998.
29. Lindahl P, Johansson BR, Leveen P, et al. Pericyte loss and microaneurysm formation in PDGF-B-deficient mice. Science 277:242–245, 1997.
30. Leveen P, Pekny M, Gebre-Medhin S, et al. Mice deficient for PDGF B show renal, cardiovascular, and hematological abnormalities. Genes Dev 8:1875–1887, 1994.
31. Maisonpierre PC, Suri C, Jones PF, et al. Angiopoietin-2, a natural antagonist for Tie2 that disrupts in vivo angiogenesis. Science 277:55–60, 1997.
32. McAllister KA, Grogg KM, Johnson DW, et al. Endoglin, a TGF-beta binding protein of endothelial cells, is the gene for hereditary haemorrhagic telangiectasia type 1. Nat Genet 8:345–351, 1994.
33. Millauer B, Wizigmann-Voos S, Schnurch H, et al. High affinity VEGF binding and developmental expression suggest Flk-1 as a major regulator of vasculogenesis and angiogenesis. Cell 72:835–846, 1993.
34. Noden DM. Development of craniofacial blood vessels. In Feinberg RN, Sherer GK, Auerbach R (eds): The Development of the Vascular System. Basel: Karger, 1991, pp 1– 24.
35. Padget DH. The development of the cranial arteries in the human embryo. Carnegie Contrib Embryol 32: 206–261, 1948.
36. Padget DH. The development of the cranial venous sys-

tem in man, from the viewpoint of comparative anatomy. Carnegie Contrib Embryol 36:80–140, 1957.
37. Poltorak Z, Cohen T, Sivan R, et al. VEGF145, a secreted vascular endothelial growth factor isoform that binds to extracellular matrix. J Biol Chem 272: 7151–7158, 1997.
38. Rhoten RL, Comair YG, Shedid D, et al. Specific repression of the preproendothelin-1 gene in intracranial arteriovenous malformations. J Neurosurg 86:101–108, 1997.
39. Risau W, Flamme I. Vasculogenesis. Ann Rev Cell Dev Biol 11:73–91, 1995.
40. Risau W. Mechanisms of angiogenesis. Nature 386: 671–674, 1997.
41. Rothbart D, Awad IA, Lee J, et al. Expression of angiogenic factors and structural proteins in central nervous system vascular malformations. Neurosurgery 38: 915–924, 1996.
42. Sato TN, Tozawa Y, Deutsch U, et al. Distinct roles of the receptor tyrosine kinases Tie-1 and Tie-2 in blood vessel formation. Nature 376:70–74, 1995.
43. Shalaby F, Rossant J, Yamaguchi TP, et al. Failure of blood-island formation and vasculogenesis in Flk-1-deficient mice. Nature 376:62–66, 1995.
44. Shalaby F, Ho J, Stanford WL, et al. A requirement for Flk1 in primitive and definitive hematopoiesis and vasculogenesis. Cell 89:981–990, 1997.
45. Shibuya M, Yamaguchi S, Yamane A, et al. Nucleotide sequence and expression of a novel human receptor-type tyrosine kinase gene (flt) closely related to the fms family. Oncogene 5:519–524, 1990.
46. Soker S, Takashima S, Miao HQ, et al. Neuropilin-1 is expressed by endothelial and tumor cells as an isoform-specific receptor for vascular endothelial growth factor. Cell 92:735–745, 1998.
47. Soriano P. Abnormal kidney development and hematological disorders in PDGF beta-receptor mutant mice. Genes Dev 8:1888–1896, 1994.
48. Sonstein WJ, Kader A, Michelsen WJ, et al. Expression of vascular endothelial growth factor in pediatric and adult cerebral arteriovenous malformations: an immunocytochemical study. J Neurosurg 85:838–845, 1996.
49. Suri C, Jones PF, Patan S, et al. Requisite role of angiopoietin-1, a ligand for the TIE2 receptor, during embryonic angiogenesis. Cell 87:1171–1180, 1996.
50. Terman BI, Dougher-Vermazen M, Carrion ME, et al. Identification of the KDR tyrosine kinase as a receptor for vascular endothelial cell growth factor. Biochem Biophys Res Commun 187:1579–1586, 1992.
51. Tischer E, Gospodarowicz D, Mitchell R, et al. Vascular endothelial growth factor: a new member of the platelet-derived growth factor gene family. Biochem Biophys Res Commun 165:1198–1206, 1989.
52. Tischer E, Mitchell R, Hartman T, et al. The human gene for vascular endothelial growth factor: Multiple protein forms are encoded through alternative exon splicing. J Biol Chem 266:11947–11954, 1991.
53. Vikkula M, Boon LM, Carraway KL, 3rd, et al. Vascular dysmorphogenesis caused by an activating mutation in the receptor tyrosine kinase TIE2. Cell 87:1181–1190, 1996.
54. Wang HU, Chen ZF, Anderson DJ. Molecular distinction and angiogenic interaction between embryonic arteries and veins revealed by ephrin-B2 and its receptor Eph-B4. Cell 93:741–753, 1998.
55. Wrana JL, Attisano L, Wieser R, et al. Mechanism of activation of the TGF-beta receptor. Nature 370: 341–347, 1994.
56. Yancopoulos GD, Klagsbrun M, Folkman J. Vasculogenesis, angiogenesis, and growth factors: ephrins enter the fray at the border. Cell 93:661–664, 1998.
57. Zhang H, Shaw AR, Mak A, et al. Endoglin is a component of the transforming growth factor (TGF)-beta receptor complex of human pre-B leukemic cells. J Immunol 156:564– 573, 1996.

Chapter 12

Future of Treatment for Arteriovenous Malformations in Functional Areas

Shokei Yamada, MD, PhD, FACS

Arteriovenous malformations (AVMs) in functional areas of the brain had been considered unapproachable. It is through the efforts of a limited number of neurosurgeons that these AVMs have become operable without serious complications. Intravascular procedures and radiosurgery have joined microneurosurgery in an effort to perfect the elimination of difficult AVMs.

This book covers each mode of AVM treatment separately or in combination with one or two other modes. Basic understanding of the hemodynamic anatomy of AVMs has made treatment safer and more effective. It must be realized that it is critical to avoid damage to the brain tissue surrounding the AVM and to preserve the smallest arterial branches supplying functional brain tissue. This surgical principle must also be maintained when using embolization and radiosurgery.

The author and his associates have described the surgical treatment of AVMs in functional areas of the brain to the maximum degree that neurosurgeons can achieve with microsurgery. Others have made valuable contributions in conquering the problems that were considered insurmountable until recently. Beyond the technical achievements described in other chapters, microsurgical treatment of functional area AVMs faces three main barriers: (1) diffuse AVMs that are located mainly in the basal ganglia and brain stem; (2) extremely large AVMs (greater than half the hemisphere) tend to develop thrombosis of important cortical veins (e.g., veins of Trolard, Labbé, Rosenthal); and (3) deep-seated brain stem AVMs that are surrounded by critically functional nuclei and long tracts. These are the areas where other modes of treatment are needed to achieve effective results. In contrast, cavernous hemangiomas are only treated surgically at this time. It has been proved that cavernous hemangiomas are mixed with venous malformations. AVMs often consist of typical arteriovenous structures interspersed by nonfunctioning brain tissue, venous malformations, and cavernous hemangiomas (Liwinicz B, Yamada S, unpublished paper). Venous malformations and cavernous hemangiomas that tend to bleed will become the focus of microsurgical treatment.

Embolization has been considered to be an adjunct to microsurgery, and is used as such at present for the treatment of functional area AVMs. Small AVMs can be eliminated by embolization only if the AVM nidus or core is embolized (Moret J, personal communication, 1990). The author speculates that either: (1) embolization must obliterate all shunting arterioles (50–200 μ) and type 2 (200–300 μ) and type 1 (0.5–2 mm) final feeding arteries to completely interrupt the arterial blood supply, or (2) obliterate the entire core or nidus with or without embolizing the above-mentioned terminal arteries or their branches. Other factors must be considered. If emboli are small enough to pass through these small terminal branches, draining veins could be obstructed before the entire core is obliterated. Naturally, expansion and rupture of the AVM or congestion of the surrounding cerebral veins can occur. The early obstruction of the draining vein may occur more easily with isobutyl cyanoacrylate embolization than with other methods. Controlled hypotension may be used dur-

From Yamada S (ed): *Arteriovenous Malformations in Functional Areas of the Brain.* © Futura Publishing Co, Inc, Armonk, NY, 1999.

ing the embolization procedure to prevent emboli from quickly reaching the draining veins (Debrun G, personal communication, 1982). Embolization of proximal arteries of diffuse, particularly large AVMs in the capsulocaudatothalamic area may be complicated with higher morbidity. From the author's surgical experience with cauterizing peripheral arterial branches first (see Chapter 1, case 10), it is advisable to embolize the peripheral branches of these arteries first, and gradually extend embolization toward the proximal portion of the artery as the patient is closely observed for subtle neurological changes.

Radiosurgery or irradiation of AVMs of the brain in general was reported with a high rate of success by Steiner:[7] 95% with total obliteration within 2 years, if the size of the AVM was limited to 2.5 cm or less. A similar success rate was reported by Fabrikant,[2] who treated AVMs with high-energy particle (helium) irradiation, by Kjellberg using proton beam,[4] by Lunsford with the gamma knife,[5,6] and later by Colombo and Friedman, who used a linear accelerator.[1,3] However, some shortcomings have been noted with irradiation: (1) the success rate decreased to 65%[8] for AVM patients with angiographic follow-up; (2) incidence of hemorrhages is significant while waiting for obliteration; and (3) no statistics are available for irradiation of functional area AVMs. In this respect, Chapter 8 of this book is extremely valuable.

Imaging studies are helpful, particularly for localization, estimating shapes, and calculating the volume by contrast-enhanced computed tomography (CT). Understanding blood flow to AVMs and the dynamic mechanisms of AVM obliteration will further advance irradiation therapy. No matter which mode of treatment is chosen, the future goal of treatment for functional area AVMs is to limit necrosis of surrounding brain to microns instead of millimeters in thickness.

The concept of multiple compartments in large AVMs is well recognized, and compartmental dissection of these AVMs in functional areas is mandatory. The concept was originally proposed by radiologists, based on the extent of the partial obliteration during embolization. Further detailed definitions of the compartmental structure of AVMs by intravascular interventionists is needed. Fractionated irradiation of large AVMs has been advocated by some radiosurgeons (Heifetz M, personal communication, 1997). The author believes that radiosurgery of these AVMs also requires compartmental obliteration; perhaps irradiation of each compartment less than 2.5–3 cm would be more effective than irradiating the entire mass at the same time.

Ancillary studies such as magnetic resonance imaging (MRI), angiography, CT angiography, color Doppler studies, magnetic source imaging or functional MRI, holography, and somatosensory evoked potentials must be fully utilized for surgical planning and precision work.

In the near future, the understanding of AVM angiogenesis will lead to the further advancement of treatment, as well as preventing the growth of this complex disorder.

The Western pioneer's song echoes neurosurgeons' ambition to achieve the goal: "I want to go somewhere nobody has ever been, I want to see something nobody has ever seen, and I want to do something nobody has ever done."

References

1. Colombo F, Pozza F, Chierego G, et al. Linear accelerator radiosurgery of cerebral arteriovenous malformations: an update. Neurosurgery 34:14–21, 1994.
2. Fabrikant JI, Levy RP, Steinberg GK, et al. Charged-particle radiosurgery for intracranial vascular malformations. Neurosurg Clinic North Am 3:99–103, 1992.
3. Friedman WA, Bova FJ. LINAC radiosurgery for arteriovenous malformations. In Alexander E, Loeffler JS, Lunsford LD (eds): Stereotactic Radiosurgery. New York: McGraw-Hill, 1993, pp 147–155.
4. Kjellberg R, Hanamura T, Davis K, et al. Bragg-peak proton beam therapy for arteriovenous malformations of the brain. N Engl J Med 309:269–274, 1983.
5. Kondziolka D, Lunsford LD, Flickinger JC. Gamma knife stereotactic radiosurgery for cerebral vascular malformations. In Alexander E, Loeffler JS, Lunsford LD (eds): Stereotactic Radiosurgery. New York: McGraw-Hill, 1993, pp 136–146.
6. Lunsford L, Kondziolka D, Flickinger J, et al. Stereotactic radiosurgery for arteriovenous malformations of the brain. J Neurosurg 75:512–524, 1991.
7. Steiner L. Radiosurgery in cerebral arteriovenous malformations. In Fein JM, Flamm ES (eds): Cerebrovascular Surgery, Vol 4. New York: Springer Verlag, 1985, pp 1161–1215.
8. Yamamoto M, Kobayashi T, Jokura H, et al. Gamma knife radiosurgery for cerebral arteriovenous malformations: a multi-institutional study in Japan. Annual Meeting of American Association of Neurological Surgeons, Philadelphia, April 25–30, 1988.

Index